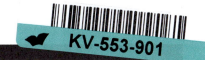

New Ischemic Syndromes

Beyond Angina
and Infarction

Sponsored by the Council on
of the International Society

Molecular and Cellular Cardiology
and Federation of Cardiology

New Ischemic Syndromes

Beyond Angina and Infarction

Editors

Derek M. Yellon, Ph.D., D.Sc., Hon. M.R.C.P., F.E.S.C., F.A.C.C.
Director of Institute and Head of Division of Cardiology
The Hatter Institute and Center for Cardiology
University College Hospital and Medical School
Grafton Way
London, United Kingdom

Shahbudin H. Rahimtoola, M.B., F.R.C.P., M.A.C.P.
Distinguished Professor
George C. Griffith Professor of Cardiology
Professor of Medicine
Chairman, Griffith Center
University of Southern California
Los Angeles, California

Lionel H. Opie, M.D., D.Phil., F.R.C.P.
Professor of Medicine and
Director, Medical Research Council
Ischemic Heart Disease Unit
University of Cape Town
Cape Town, South Africa
and
Visiting Professor
Division of Cardiovascular Medicine
Stanford University Medical Center
Stanford, California

With contributions by:
Carl S. Apstein, G. F. Baxter, William E. Boden, Roberto Bolli, C. Richard Conti, Franz R. Eberli, Roberto Ferrari, Gerd Heusch, David P. Jenkins, Robert B. Jennings, Robert A. Kloner, R. Schultz, Marcus F. Stoddard, and Niraj Varma.

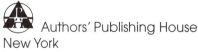 Authors' Publishing House
New York

Lippincott–Raven Publishers
Philadelphia   New York
1997

Every effort has been made to check generic and trade names, and to verify drug doses as correct according to the standards accepted at the time of publication. The ultimate responsibility lies with prescribing physicians based on their professional experience and knowledge of the patient to determine dosages and the best course of treatment for the patient. The reader is advised to check the product information currently provided by the manufacturer of each drug to be administered to ascertain any change in drug dosage, method of administration, or contraindications. In no case can the institutions with which the authors are affiliated or the publisher be held responsible for the view expressed in the book, which reflects the combined opinions of several authors. Please call any errors to the attention of the authors.

ISBN: 1-881063-06-2

Printed in the United States of America

CONTENTS

Carl S. Apstein, M.D.
Professor of Medicine and Physiology
Director, Cardiac Muscle Research Laboratory
Boston University Medical Center
80 East Concord Street, W611
Boston, Massachusetts 02118-2394

Gary F. Baxter, Ph.D.
Honorary Lecturer and Research Fellow
The Hatter Institute and Center for Cardiology
University College London Hospitals and Medical School
Grafton Way
London WC1E 6DB
United Kingdom

William E. Boden, M.D.
Department of Veterans Affairs
800 Irving Avenue
Syracuse, New York 13210

Roberto Bolli, M.D.
Chief, Division of Cardiology
Distinguished University Scholar
Department of Medicine
University of Louisville
550 South Jackson Street
Louisville, Kentucky 40292

C. Richard Conti, M.D.
Professor of Medicine
Chief, Division of Cardiology
University of Florida
1600 Archer Road
P.O. Box 100277
Gainesville, Florida 32610-0277

Franz R. Eberli, M.D.
Assistant Professor of Medicine
Cardiac Muscle Research Laboratory
Boston University Medical Center
80 East Concord Street, W611
Boston, Massachusetts 02118-2394

Roberto Ferrari, M.D., Ph.D.
Professor of Cardiology
Fondazione Salvatore Maugeri
Clinica del Lavoro e della Riabilitazone
Centro di Fisiopatologia Cardiovasculare
Via Pinidolo, 23
25064 Gussago (Brescia)
Italy

Gerd Heusch, M.D., Ph.D., F.E.S.C.
Professor and Director of the Department of Pathophysiology
Center for Internal Medicine
University Clinic
University of Essen
Hufelandstr 55
45122 Essen
Germany

David P. Jenkins, B.Sc., M.B., B.S., F.R.C.S.
Research Fellow
The Hatter Institute and Center for Cardiology
University College London Hospitals and Medical School
Grafton Way
London WC1E 6DB
United Kingdom

Robert B. Jennings, M.D.
James B. Duke Professor of Pathology
Department of Pathology
Duke University Medical Center
P.O. Box 3712
Durham, North Carolina   27710

Robert A. Kloner, M.D., Ph.D.
Director of Research Heart Institute
Hospital of the Good Samaritan
Professor of Medicine
University of Southern California
Los Angeles, California <zipcode>

Lionel H. Opie, M.D., D.Phil., F.R.C.P.
Professor of Medicine
Director, Medical Research Council Unit for Research
in Ischemic Heart Disease
University of Cape Town
Director, Hypertension Clinic
Groote Schuur Hospital
Cape Town
South Africa
and
Visiting Professor
Division of Cardiovascular Medicine
Stanford University Medical Center
Stanford, California

Shahbudin H. Rahimtoola, M.D., F.R.C.P., M.A.C.P.
Distinguished Professor
George C. Griffith Professor of Cardiology
Professor of Medicine
Chairman, Griffith Center
University of Southern California
2025 Zonal Avenue
Los Angeles, California 90033

Rainer Schulz, M.D.
Department of Pathophysiology
Center for Internatal Medicine
University Clinic
University of Essen
Hufelandstr 55
45122 Essen
Germany

Marcus F. Stoddard, M.D.
Associate Professor of Medicine
Director, Non-Invasive Laboratory
Department of Medicine
Division of Cardiology
University of Louisville
550 South Jackson Street
Louisville, Kentucky 40292

Niraj Varma, M.D., M.R.C.P.
Assistant Professor of Medicine
Cardiac Muscle Research Laboratory
Boston University Medical Center
80 East Concord Street, W611
Boston, Massachusetts 02118-2394

Derek M. Yellon, Ph.D., D.Sc., Hon. M.R.C.P., F.E.S.C., F.A.C.C.
Director of Institute and Head of Division of Cardiology
The Hatter Institute and Center for Cardiology
University College London Hospitals and Medical School, Grafton Way
London WC1E 6DB
United Kingdom

Ischemia of the myocardium is the most important identifiable cause of cardiovascular and total mortality and morbidity in the United States and other Western societies. Yet ischemia is difficult to define and to fully understand. In brief, ischemia means too little blood to the myocardium, and clinically includes the well-understood anginal syndromes that are classically identified by typical chest pain. Today, however, it is known that ischemia can manifest itself in clinically unexpected ways, termed the new ischemic syndromes. As each of these has clinical importance, cardiologists and physicians must be updated on recent developments in an informed yet practical manner. This is the aim of this book.

The first chapter by Lionel H. Opie explains what the new ischemic syndromes are and outlines how each can contribute to left ventricular dysfunction and heart failure. He emphasizes that there are no less than four ischemic syndromes: (1) silent ischemia, (2) preconditioning, (3) stunning, and (4) hibernation. Of these, silent ischemia is described by C. Richard Conti, lead investigator on a large ongoing trial that attempts to assess the best treatment for this condition (whether medical or surgical).

The section on preconditioning is edited by Derek M. Yellon, who points out that deprivation of the blood supply to the heart, although commonly thought to have adverse effects, is in fact protective. That is, episodes of ischemia protect against subsequent ischemia, and this is the phenomenon of preconditioning. Derek M. Yellon and co-workers describe the basic biology, and the likely metabolic signal pathways that are involved. Pharmacologic manipulation of the latter is likely to lead to the development of new cardioprotective drugs. Other clinical implications of preconditioning are examined by Robert A. Kloner, one of the pioneers in describing the new ischemic syndromes.

Stunning is a phenomenon of increasing importance. Every time there is myocardial ischemia, whether silent ischemia or angina, or whenever the heart is reperfused by thrombolytic therapy during myocardial infarction, it is now thought that there is stunning. Various stages and degrees of stunning explain the very complex picture of postinfarction left ventricular dysfunction, and stunning may also contribute to postinfarct heart failure. These complexities are discussed by Lionel H. Opie, and Carl S. Apstein emphasizes how stunning and diastolic heart failure are interrelated. Roberto Bolli, a pioneer in the area of stunning, writes about the many clinical manifestations of stunning, a condition so common and important to clinicians that it must be considered in the full assessment of any patient with angina or past myocardial infarction, or whenever thrombolytic therapy is applied in an acute heart attack. In a truly important chapter, Roberto Bolli writes specifically for clinicians on the implications of recognizing this important condition.

Hibernation is the state whereby the heart muscle can go to "sleep," only to wake up with operative intervention. This crucially important phenomenon has great implications for health care, because identification of the hibernating myocardium by sophisticated modern techniques can mandate whether or not an expensive bypass operation is needed. Gerd Heusch describes animal models of hibernation, Roberto Ferrari the clinical identification of hibernation, and Shahbudin H. Rahimtoola the clinical management of the hibernating myocardium.

By combining laboratory and clinical approaches to these problems, the authors have produced a book that should demystify the new ischemic syndromes for clinical cardiologists while providing sufficient background material to be of interest to research workers and others in the field.

Derek M. Yellon
Lionel H. Opie
Shahbudin H. Rahimtoola

New Ischemic Syndromes

Beyond Angina and Infarction

CHAPTER 1

Ischemia and the New Ischemic Syndromes

Lionel H. Opie

Although there still is some argumentation about the definition of myocardial ischemia (Hearse, 1994), in the end the concept is simple: Ischemia means that the blood supply to the myocardium is inadequate. The Greek *ischo* means "to hold back" and *haima* means "blood." The fundamental concept of supply/demand imbalance came from an exercising limb:

> In health when we excite the muscle action to more energetic action than usual, we increase the circulation in every part. If, however, we call into vigorous action a limb around which we with a moderate degree of tightness applied a ligature, we find then that the member can only support its action for a very short time; for now its supply of energy and its expenditure do not balance each other. (Burns, 1809)

The early phase of ischemia is recognized when it is sufficiently severe to cause characteristic metabolic, mechanical, and electrocardiographic (ECG) changes that are reversible when the ischemia ceases. Ischemia therefore, by definition, starts off as a reversible deficiency of the myocardial blood supply. As ischemia progresses, it becomes irreversible and ultimately a state of infarction develops. Infarction (literally, *stuffed in*) is the pathological term indicating that the cell is so damaged that myocyte death can be recognized by light microscopy. Necrosis is a closely related term (*necro*, meaning death).

The relatively clear conceptual distinctions between the reversible and irreversible stages of ischemia have now become blurred as a result of the keen clinical interest in achieving reperfusion by thrombolysis as early as possible after the onset of symptoms of the condition that will develop into acute myocardial infarction, while there is in fact reversible ischemia rather than irreversible infarction. Thrombolysis can be expected to benefit cells reversibly damaged by ischemia, but not those cells irreversibly damaged and necrotic. Thus, in clinical terminology, the term *acute myocardial infarction* has come to encompass the whole spectrum of events starting with the initial chest pain, which is thought to indicate the time of the coronary occlusion, and hence to herald the onset of ischemia of those cells that are threatened with cell death if the ischemia persists.

The emphasis on reperfusion has led to fresh knowledge that there is a whole group of new conditions, some arising in the wake of reperfusion, called the *new ischemic syndromes*.

BIOCHEMICAL MARKERS OF ISCHEMIA

There are a host of biochemical markers of ischemia, including lactate output, increased glycolysis with inhibition of pyruvate entry into the citrate cycle, formation of inorganic phosphate and adenosine, as well as accumulation of the reduced cofactor, lactate, and protons in the ischemic tissue. Each and every one of these can be explained by the simple concept of Jennings (1970), which states that there is a change from aerobic to anaerobic metabolism. The defect of the clinical use of such markers is that they require coronary sinus catheterization to measure arteriovenous differences, and even then local metabolic changes may not be evident in the coronary sinus blood that is inevitably diluted by blood drained from the nonischemic myocardium.

Fortunately the clinician can turn to a simple noninvasive test—the ECG. ST-segment deviations indirectly reflect a simple biochemical marker of ischemia, namely potassium loss. Potassium loss from ischemic zones is fundamental in explaining the early ECG features of ischemia. Very soon after the onset of coronary artery ligation in the dog, there is ST-segment elevation and a prominent, peaked T-wave in the epicardial ECG (Kondo et al., 1996). About 60% of these changes are attenuated by glibenclamide, the blocker of the adenosine triphosphate (ATP)-dependent potassium channel, showing the importance of potassium loss in these ECG changes (Fig 1-1). Metabolically there is coincidence of the loss of potassium with that of inorganic phosphate, derived ultimately from high-energy phosphates (Opie et al., 1973), which could explain opening the ATP-dependent potassium channel. The opening of this channel in ischemia is a complex event (Coetzee, 1992) and may be simplified as follows. Normally this channel is inhibited by the high intracellular level of ATP (Fig 1-2). During ischemia, breakdown products of ATP, such as adenosine diphosphate (ADP) and adenosine, help to open the channel even when ATP levels are still relatively high. The loss of potassium during ischemia is nonetheless complex (Wilde & Aksnes, 1995). The loss of only 1% of cellular potassium, raising the intracellular potassium from 4.0 to 9.6 mM, can markedly decrease the resting membrane potential and the action potential duration (Holland & Brooks, 1977). In addition, an increased cytosolic calcium very probably also contributes to early depolarization, especially when the heart rate is very rapid (Clusin, 1987).

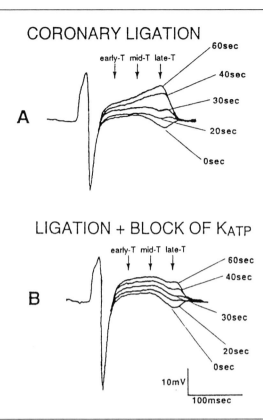

Figure 1-1. *Note rapid ST-elevation and T-wave peaking within 60 seconds of coronary artery ligation in the dog. The role of potassium loss via the ATP-dependent potassium channel (K_{ATP}) is shown in the lower panel (ligation plus channel block by glibenclamide). (Data from Kondo and colleagues [1996] by permission of authors and publisher.)*

FUNCTIONAL MARKERS OF ISCHEMIA

The basic concept was laid in the mid-1930s. Tennant and Wiggers (1935) showed that coronary artery ligation in the dog was rapidly followed by cessation of contractile function. Such mechanical failure is now known to be biochemical in origin (Table 1-1). Blood flow and function go together, says Rahimtoola (1994). How best to measure contractile dysfunction is a clinical challenge. Echocardiography is a technique that is widely available and is clinically useful to evaluate abnormalities of contraction due to ischemia induced by exercise, dobutamine, or high-dose dipyridamole. Some clinical indices of ischemia-induced contractile dysfunction include

1. Echocardiographic wall-motion abnormalities induced by exercise or by high-dose dipyridamole (Coletta et al., 1995), dobutamine (Diagianti et al., 1995; Senior & Lahiri, 1995), or arbutamine (Cohen et al., 1995)
2. Dyspnea or fatigue on effort stress test

Recently, another sympathomimetic, arbutamine, has been successfully used (Cohen et al., 1995).

TABLE 1-1. CAUSES OF IMPAIRED CONTRACTILITY IN ISCHEMIA

Proposed mechanism
Accumulation of metabolites
Intracellular acidosis with displacement of Ca^{2+} from intracellular binding sites(1980);
Accumulation of inorganic phosphate, which interacts with calcium
Accumulation of neutral lactate
Changes in ATP level or availability
Decreased turnover of ATP
Decreased level of ATP in a "contractile" subcompartment
Decreased free energy change of ATP hydrolysis
Mechanical effects of decreased coronary flow
Reversed "garden hose" or "erectile" effect

Ca^{2+} = calcium; ATP = adenosine triphosphate.

IMPAIRED CORONARY BLOOD FLOW

Central to the concept of ischemia is a decrease in coronary blood flow (Fig 1-3). Hence the "gold standard" for detection of coronary ischemia would be the absolute measurement of coronary blood flow (e.g., by nitrogen-13 at rest and during exercise) and then deciding whether or not the blood flow is defective. Unfortunately the range of normal coronary flow is so large and the response to exercise so variable, that this is not a viable diagnostic test on its own. Therefore, a number of indices of impaired myocardial perfusion, used as indirect markers of ischemia, give a more definite answer. For example, impaired myocardial uptake of thallium or of technetium-99m is used. Some clinical indices of impaired myocardial perfusion (other than coronary angiography) include

1. Thallium-201 with single-photon emission cardiac-computed tomography (SPECT) (Marie et al., 1995)
2. Technetium-99m-sestamibi with SPECT (Sandler et al., 1995; Berman et al., 1995)
3. Nitrogen-13 with positron emission tomography (Dilsizian & Bonow, 1993) (measures coronary flow)
4. Coronary angiography (still the "gold standard")

Ideally these should be further combined with an index of impaired metabolism, such as enhanced glucose extraction (Sandler et al., 1995). This dual isotope procedure gives excellent sensitivity, a good specificity, and a positive predictive value (Sandler et al., 1995). In practice, though, such complex techniques may not be available and myocardial ischemia is more often diagnosed by (1) a clinical history and (2) effort stress testing using an electrocardiographic, echocardiographic, or radionuclide technique. The presence of coronary disease shown on angiography does not demonstrate ischemia but does suggest that the correct clinical setting for ischemia is present.

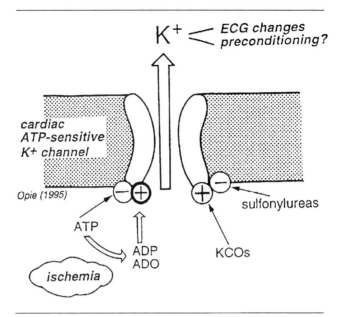

Figure 1-2. *Proposed role of ATP-sensitive potassium channel in causing the early ECG changes of ischemia, acting via potassium ion egress and accumulation on the outer surface of the ischemic myocytes. Ischemia breaks down ATP to adenosine diphosphate (ADP) and adenosine (ADO)—a change that opens this channel. The results include shortening of the action potential duration, diastolic depolarization and ST-segment and T-wave changes (see Fig 1-1). Hypothetically, opening of this channel as a result of prior ischemia may mediate preconditioning. The potassium channel-opening (KCO) drugs may mediate protection against ischemia by a local cardioplegic effect of the increased external potassium ion concentration, whereas the sulfonylureas such as glibenclamide act on a site not integral to the pore to inhibit opening (i.e., to close the channel). (Figure copyright 1995, L. H. Opie.)*

ANGINAL CHEST PAIN

Myocardial ischemia is often clinically suspected by the presence of chest pain, typically on exertion. Anginal chest pain, as typically taught to medical students, remains a valuable indicator of ischemia, yet the existence of painless ischemia cannot be doubted. Even myocardial infarction can be painless. Silent ischemia by definition is painless and is an important condition (see Chapter 3). The pain threshold varies substantially from patient to patient. One explanation may be that those with silent ischemia more readily release beta-endorphins that mask the pain (Sheps et al., 1995). When typical ischemic pain does occur, the two main biochemical hypotheses for the pain are (1) formation of adenosine (Sylven, 1993) and (2) release of ATP from the cytoplasm of ischemic cells (Kennedy & Leff, 1995).

In general, anginalike pain indicates ischemia. Anginal pain can occur without coronary disease, when the prognosis is good (Lichtlen et al., 1995). The mechanism for such pain is not at all understood. When anginalike pain is detected in patients with early-phase acute myocardial infarction, there is a reasonable chance that at least some of the ischemic tissue is still salvable. Typically, a current indication for the use of thrombolytic agents is the combination of prolonged anginalike pain, but within 4 to 12 hours of the onset, and ST-segment elevation in at least two of the precordial leads.

New Ischemic Syndromes

Not only is conventional ischemia difficult to define and to understand fully, but the recent addition of the new ischemic syndromes has added to the potential confusion. The first of these new syndromes to be widely recognized by clinicians was *silent ischemia,* initially described in 1974 (Stern & Tzivoni, 1974) and well accepted by 1978 (Maseri, 1978). After acute myocardial infarction, silent ischemia increases the risk of death, nonfatal myocardial infarction, or unstable angina two- to threefold (Gill et al., 1996). Nonetheless, exactly how to manage silent ischemia remains a matter of contention (see Chapter 3).

At about the same time, Heyndrickx and colleagues (1975) described their innovative work, which led to the recognition of *stunning* by Braunwald and Kloner (1982). This is the delayed mechanical recovery despite full reperfusion after ischemia. "Brief periods of coronary occlusion result in prolonged impairment of regional myocardial function which could not have been predicted from the rapid return of the electrogram and coronary flow" (Heyndrickx, 1975). More recently, stunning has been divided into an acute condition, in which mechanical function recovers within minutes and hours, and a chronic condition, in which recovery is measured in weeks or months. When the recovery is incomplete, the condition is called the *maimed myocardium* (Boden et al., 1995) (see Chapter 9).

In 1984, Rahimtoola proposed the concept of *hibernating* myocardium to describe "a state of persistently impaired

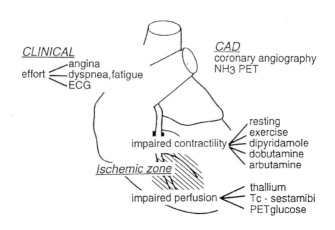

Figure 1-3. Proposed measures to detect myocardial ischemia in humans. CAD = coronary artery disease; Tc = technetium; PET = positron emission tomography.

myocardial and left ventricular function at rest due to reduced coronary blood flow that can be partially or completely restored to normal if the myocardial oxygen supply/demand relationship is favorably altered, either by improving blood flow and/or by reducing demand" (Rahimtoola, 1985). Recently the essential role of reduced coronary flow at rest has been questioned, so that in my view the current sine qua non concepts would be threefold: (1) impaired contractile activity; (2) the presence of significant, severe coronary artery disease; and (3) recovery of mechanical function after revascularization or similar procedures.

Preconditioning, described in 1986 by Murry and associates, has perhaps been the most seminal of all the discoveries, making the postulate that transient ischemia could protect from subsequent ischemia, as follows:

> Given these salutary effects of intermittent ischemia and reperfusion with respect to sustained ischemia, we postulated that multiple brief ischemic episodes might actually protect the myocardium during a subsequent sustained ischemic insult so that, in effect, we could exploit ischemia to protect the heart from ischemic injury. (Murry et al., 1986)

In each case, whether it is silent ischemia, stunning, hibernation, or preconditioning, ischemia or ischemia followed by reperfusion seems to express a new manifestation of coronary artery disease. The result is that clinicians must now think beyond the traditional concepts of angina and infarction, and consider that every patient with significant coronary disease may also have one or more of the new ischemic syndromes.

REFERENCES

Berman DS, Hachamovitch R, Kiat H, et al. Incremental value of prognostic testing in patients with known or suspected ischemic heart disease: A basis for optimal utilization of exercise technetium-99m sestamibi myocardial perfusion single-photon emission computed tomography. *J Am Coll Cardiol* 1995; 26: 639.

Boden WE, Brooks WW, Conrad CH, et al. Incomplete, delayed functional recovery late after reperfusion following acute myocardial infarction: "maimed myocardium." *Am Heart J* 1995; 130: 922–932.

Braunwald E, Kloner RA. The stunned myocardium: prolonged, postischemic ventricular dysfunction. *Circulation* 1982; 66: 1146–1149.

Burns A. *Observations on some of the most frequent and important diseases of the heart*. Edinburgh: Bryce, 1809.

Clusin WT. What is the solution to sudden cardiac death: calcium modulation or arrhythmia clinics? *Cardiovasc Drugs Ther* 1987; 1: 335–342.

Coletta C, Galati A, Greco G, et al. Prognostic value of high dose dipyridamole echocardiography in patients with chronic coronary artery disease and preserved left ventricular function. *JACC* 1995; 26: 887–894.

Coetzee WA. ATP-sensitive potassium channels and myocardial ischemia: why do they open? *Cardiovasc Drugs Ther* 1992; 6: 201–208.

Cohen JL, Chan KL, Jaarsma W, et al. Arbutamine echocardiography: efficacy and safety of a new pharmacologic stress agent to induce myocardial ischemic heart disease and detect coronary artery disease. *J Am Coll Cardiol* 1995; 26: 1168–1175.

Coletta, et al. *J Am Coll Cardiol* 1995; 26: 887.

Diagianti A, Penco M, Agati L, et al. Stress echocardiography: Comparison of exercise, dipyridamole and dobutamine in detecting and predicting the extent of coronary artery disease. *J Am Coll Cardiol* 1995; 26: 18.

Dilsizian V, Bonow R. Current diagnostic techniques of assessing myocardial viability in patients with hibernating and stunned myocardium. *Circulation* 1993; 87: 1–20.

Gill JB, Cairns JA, Roberts RS, et al. Prognostic importance of myocardial ischemia detected by ambulatory monitoring early after acute myocardial infarction. *N Engl J Med* 1996; 334: 65–70.

Hearse DJ. Myocardial ischaemia: can we agree on a definition for the 21st century? *Cardiovasc Res* 1994; 28: 1737–1744.

Heyndrickx GR, Millard RW, McRitchie RJ, et al. Regional myocardial function and electrophysiological alterations after brief coronary occlusion in conscious dogs. *J Clin Invest* 1975; 56: 978–985.

Holland RP, Brooks H. TQ-ST segment mapping: critical review and analysis of current concepts. *Am J Cardiol* 1977; 40: 110–129.

Jennings RB. Myocardial ischemia—observations, definitions and speculations. *J Mol Cell Cardiol* 1970; 1: 345–349.

Kennedy C, Leff P. Painful connection for ATP. *Nature* 1995; 377: 385–386.

Kondo XX, Kuboa I, Tachibana H, et al. Glibenclamide attenuates peaked T-wave in early phase of myocardial ischemia. *Cardiovasc Res* 1996; 31: 683–687.

Lichtlen PR, Bargheer K, Wenzlaff P. Long-term prognosis of patients with angina-like chest pain and normal coronary angiographic findings. *J Am Coll Cardiol* 1995; 25: 1013–1018.

Marie P-Y, Danchin N, Durand J, et al. Long-term prediction of major ischemic events by exercise. Thallium-201 single-photon emission computed tomography. Incremental prognostic value compared with clinical, exercise testing, catheterization and radionuclide angiographic data. *J Am Coll Cardiol* 1995; 26: 879–886.

Maseri A, Severi S, De Nes M, et al. "Variant" angina: One aspect of continuous spectrum of vasospastic myocardial ischemia. Pathogenetic mechanisms, estimated incidence and clinical and coronary arteriographic findings in 138 patients. *Am J Cardiol* 1978; 42: 1019–1035.

Murry CE, Jennings RB, Reimer KA. Preconditioning with ischemia: a delay of lethal cell injury in ischemic myocardium. *Circulation* 1986; 740: 1124–1136.

Opie LH, Muller CA, Lubbe WF. Cyclic AMP and arrhythmias revisited. *Lancet* 1978; ii: 921–923.

Opie LH, Owen P, Thomas M, Samson R. Coronary sinus lactate measurements in the assessment of myocardial ischemia. Comparison with changes in the ratios lactate/pyruvate and beta-hydroxybutyrate/acetoacetate and with release of hydrogen, phosphate and potassium ions from the heart. *Am J Cardiol* 1973; 32: 295–305.

Patel TB, Olson MS. Regulation of pyruvate dehydrogenase complex in ischemic rat heart. *Am J Physiol* 1984; 246: H858–H864.

Rahimtoola SH. A perspective on three large multicenter randomized clinical trials of coronary bypass surgery for chronic stable angina. *Circulation* 1985; 72(Suppl V): 123–125.

Rahimtoola SH. The definition of ischemia. *Cardiovasc Res* 1994; 28: 1745–1746.

Sandler MP, Videlefsky S, Delbeke D, et al. Evaluation of myocardial ischemia using a rest metabolism/stress perfusion protocol with fluorine-18 deoxyglucose/technetium-99m MIBI and dual-isotope simultaneous-acquisition single-photon emission computed tomography. *J Am Coll Cardiol* 1995; 26: 870–878.

Senior R, Lahiri A. Enhanced detection of myocardial ischemia by stress dobutamine echocardiography utilizing the "biphasic" response of wall thickening during low and high dose dobutamine infusion. *J Am Coll Cardiol* 1995; 26: 26–32.

Sheps DS, Ballenger MN, De Gent GE, et al. Psychophysical responses to a speech stressor: correlation of plasma beta-endorphin levels at rest and after psychological stress with thermally measured pain threshold in patients with coronary artery disease. *J Am Coll Cardiol* 1995; 25: 1499–1503.

Stern S, Tzivoni D. Early detection of silent ischemic heart disease by 24-hour electrocardiographic monitoring of active subjects. *Br Heart J* 1974; 36: 481–486.

Sylven C. Mechanisms of pain in angina pectoris—a critical review of the adenosine hypothesis. *Cardiovasc Drugs Ther* 1993; 7: 745–759.

Tennant R, Wiggers CJ. The effect of coronary occlusion on myocardial contraction. *Am J Physiol* 1935; 112: 351–361.

Wilde AAM, Aksnes G. Myocardial potassium loss and cell depolarisation in ischaemia and hypoxia. *Cardiovasc Res* 1995; 29: 1–15.

CHAPTER 2

Ischemic Injury and Myocardial Protection: Evolving Concepts

Robert B. Jennings

This chapter is a highly selective review of the last 60 years of research on ischemia with the particular aim of showing the development of the idea that myocardium can be protected from the deleterious effects of ischemia. Also included is a brief description of the newer ischemic syndromes and their relationship to ischemia and reperfusion in general, and to myocardial protection in particular.

The idea that myocardium might be protected from ischemia originated from studies of two large groups of investigators. The first was composed primarily of surgeons, whose aim was (1) to arrest the heart transiently with total ischemia in order to repair valvular or other defects and (2) to restore the heart to full contractile function when the surgery was completed. The second group was basic scientists interested in understanding how the healthy heart worked in terms of contraction, electricity, viability, and so on, plus how these processes were altered by the onset of acute myocardial ischemia. The latter group eventually applied its skills to the study of ways of delaying the death of myocytes in evolving acute myocardial infarcts. Both groups wanted to keep ischemic myocytes alive and developed a common base of knowledge about myocardial ischemic injury, the major facets of which will be summarized in this chapter.

NEW ISCHEMIC SYNDROMES

The past 25 years have seen a massive research effort in the field of ischemia. As a consequence of this effort, our knowledge of the basic biology of myocardial ischemia has increased enormously and a variety of exciting new phenomena not dreamed of by earlier workers have appeared on the scene. In general, these new phenomena developed as investigators began to study the effects of reperfusion of ischemic myocardium in the experimental animal, particularly the effects of reperfusion on *living, reversibly injured* myocytes (i.e., the type of myocyte salvaged in humans by reperfusion after thrombolysis).

The most productive period in terms of new ischemic syndromes was the 8 years from 1978 to 1986, because during this time three new concepts were described. The first involved the appearance of persistent contractile defects in myocardium reperfused after an episode of reversible ischemic injury in the canine heart. This contractile defect first was noted in 1978 by Heyndrickx and colleagues. However, it did not become popular until 1982 when Braunwald and Kloner termed it *stunning*. When severe, this contractile failure persists during 24 to 48 hours of reperfusion. It undoubtedly is important in the management of patients with coronary artery disease.

The second phenomenon, *hibernation*, was described in humans in 1985 by Braunwald and associates. Hibernation (Rahimtoola, 1989) is the absence of contraction in viable areas of tissue receiving low arterial flow. A kind of down-regulation is hypothesized to occur that allows myocytes receiving inadequate flow to survive in an acontractile state. The basic concept is "little blood, little work" (Rahimtoola, 1989). Reperfusion of such regions is followed by resumption of function. This phenomenon occurs in living myocytes that are either resting (hibernating) or are unable to shorten against the in vivo pressure head. The hallmark of ischemia, anaerobic glycolysis, is absent in these areas. Unfortunately, hibernation has been difficult to reproduce in experimental animal hearts and, as usual in pathobiology, the absence of a good animal model has slowed the development of full understanding of the phenomenon. Moreover, increasingly precise studies of flow in areas identified as hibernating in humans have provided data indicating that flow sometimes may be normal in such areas. In this case the explanation for the contractile failure may be a kind of repetitive stunning (Conversano et al., 1996). In any event, hibernation appears to be important in terms of the total capacity of the myocardium to maintain the cardiac output in patients with coronary artery disease.

The third phenomenon, *preconditioning myocardium with ischemia*, was described by Murry and coworkers in 1986, who showed that myocardium exposed to a brief episode or episodes of ischemia tolerated a prolonged episode of ischemia much better than virgin myocardium. This preconditioning episode of ischemia delayed but did not prevent cell death; thus, it increased the time available to salvage myocytes during an evolving myocardial infarct. In addition, preconditioning proved to be effective against arrhythmias and stunning. The exploitation of these potential benefits in humans awaits the discovery of the mechanism or mechanisms involved in its development.

The concepts of stunning, hibernation, and preconditioning are objective signs of alterations induced by ischemia in living, reversibly injured myocytes. Stunning and preconditioning both have been used as measures of ischemic damage in pharmacological studies of myocardial protection. Here, the aim is to eliminate or accentuate these monuments of antecedent ischemia. Studies of preconditioning have revealed some distinctive features of the signaling processes occurring during a reversible episode of ischemia (Downey et al., 1994). A thumbnail sketch of the development of the concept of protection of the ischemic myocardium is presented in the next section in order to give the reader perspective on this topic.

CONCEPT OF PROTECTION

The idea of protecting myocardium from ischemic injury developed in the middle of the twentieth century from the work of two essentially unrelated groups. Most of the principal investigators in the first group were thoracic surgeons. Their aim was highly focused. They wanted to be able to arrest a heart long enough to allow the repair of a congenital cardiac defect or to bypass a diseased coronary artery. This required a significant amount of biomedical engineering in that they had to be able to perfuse the organism with oxygenated blood while maintaining the heart in an arrested, quiescent state. In addition, they had to protect the heart from any damage developing during the period of arrest. The success of a protective intervention was easy to measure in this mixture of engineering and science by observing whether or not reperfusion of the heart with arterial blood resulted in enough coordinated contractile function to keep the patient alive and well.

A second group were basic scientists who became involved in studies of myocardial protection. This group generally was interested in delaying or preventing myocyte death in evolving acute myocardial infarcts. Since arrested hearts are totally ischemic and areas undergoing infarction are receiving little and sometimes no arterial flow, both groups were studying ischemia, but from different points of view. Furthermore, interaction between these groups, with few exceptions, was uncommon. In fact, to the best of my knowledge, the two groups did not meet together until 1979. In June of that year, they met in New York City to discuss the general features of myocardial ischemia at a Cardioplegia Workshop. The meeting was held under the auspices of the Division of Cardiothoracic Surgery of Mt. Sinai Hospital Medical School and Baxter Laboratories.

The second group of scientists was heterogeneous. It was composed of cardiologists, cell biologists, electrophysiologists, pathologists, pharmacologists, physiologists, and others. Their goal was to understand the general biology of cardiac function and the biology of myocardial infarction. Only a few investigators were involved when studies on this subject began in the 1930s (Herrmann & Decherd, 1935; Himwich et al., 1934; Tennant & Wiggers, 1935; Tennant et al., 1936). However, more interest in this topic developed in the 1940s and 1950s, and this group of investigators gradually increased in number. These early investigators had wide-ranging interests and pursued subjects as diverse as intermediary metabolism of normal, anoxic, and ischemic myocardium; contractile mechanisms; ion currents; arrhythmic mechanisms; the mechanism of action of pharmacological agents against arrhythmias during ischemia; and so on. In the late 1960s, the interests of many members of the second group were focused on protection of ischemic myocardium because of availability of funding to support such investigations. Interest in protection originated from a study published in 1960 showing the duration of ischemic periods required to injure myocytes reversibly and irreversibly (Jennings et al., 1960) followed by the first direct attempts to salvage ischemic myocardium (Ginks et al., 1972; Maroko et al., 1971). There had been earlier attempts to affect infarct size with drug therapy, but the idea did not catch on because there was insufficient knowledge of myocardial biology. It is of interest that these primitive attempts to reduce myocardial infarct size with adrenocorticotrophic hormone (ACTH) or cortisone (Johnson et al., 1953; Wartman et al., 1955) were associated with disagreements with respect to whether or not therapy was beneficial, similar to some of the controversies seen in modern studies of protection some 30 to 40 years later.

The idea of protecting the ischemic myocardium was given further impetus in the 1960s by the Myocardial Infarction Research Units and Ischemia SCORs of the National Heart Institute of the National Institutes of Health. These units both performed and stimulated an enormous amount of research on basic mechanisms of myocardial ischemia. Also, in 1979 Rentrop and colleagues showed that one could eliminate the thrombus causing acute myocardial ischemia with streptokinase and thereby reperfuse the infarcting tissue with arterial blood. This eliminated the cause of the injury and, when done early in ischemia, salvaged myocytes in humans just as it did in the animal heart. In this scenario, one was not attempting to protect the myocytes, but rather to prevent their death by eliminating the cause of the injury. Moreover, the advent of reperfusion therapy in humans reinforced the need for an intervention that would delay myocyte death as long as possible and thereby increase the time available to salvage myocytes in an evolving infarct by reperfusion.

The widespread study of reperfusion, both in evolving infarcts and in cardioplegia, led some authors to postulate that myocytes were damaged by reoxygenation occurring during reperfusion. Since irreversibly injured myocytes accumulated Ca^{2+} (Shen & Jennings, 1972) and developed contraction band necrosis when they were reoxygenated by reperfusion in vivo (Herdson et al., 1965) and since a similar lesion, the calcium paradox, could be induced in the isolated perfused rat heart by eliminating Ca^{2+} transiently from the aerobic perfusate (Ganote & Nayler, 1985; Zimmerman et al., 1967; Zimmerman & Hulsmann, 1966), dramatic and potentially deleterious changes in myocytes clearly were mediated by calcium. Rosenkranz and Buckberg (1983) developed the concept that reperfusion might be injurious in detailed studies of cardiac functional capacity following the total ischemia of cardioplegia. They defined reperfusion injury as "those metabolic, functional, and structural consequences of restoring arterial flow . . . that can be avoided or reversed by a modification of the conditions of reperfusion" (Rosenkranz & Buckberg, 1983). Their goal was to maintain function after a period of prolonged ischemic arrest. They used interventions generally designed to maintain viability of reversibly injured myocytes and measured their efficacy against maintenance of the cardiac output.

In the mid-1980s, Bolli and associates (1988) showed that much of the stunning effect was related to reperfusion injury by showing that stunning could be prevented by preventing the action of the excess oxygen-derived (O_2-derived) free radicals that were generated in reperfused tissue. The most likely explanation for the stunning effect is altered Ca^2 control or availability, as discussed by Opie (see Chapter 7). Presumably, the O_2-derived free radicals impact on the membrane or on one or more intracellular or membrane proteins involved in the control of intracellular Ca^{2+}. Also proposed was the idea of lethal reperfusion injury (Jennings & Yellon, 1992). Here the hypothesis was that myocytes alive at the time of reperfusion were killed by some aspect of the reperfusion process. The concepts of stunning and lethal reperfusion injury led investigators to concentrate on protecting myocardium from the effects of reperfusion as well as to protecting it from ischemia itself.

Delaying death of ischemic myocytes in an evolving myocardial infarct with pharmacological agents was studied in great detail by the second group. However, since much basic knowledge was required to pursue this goal successfully, an enormous amount of general knowledge of molecular mechanisms involved in cardiac function was gained during the course of these studies. Since the zone of myocardial ischemia in an acute myocardial infarct is not contracting and the patient or experimental animal is still alive, the surgical goal of acute restoration of contractile function was less important to the second group. Their aim was to prevent the death of as many ischemic myocytes as possible.

Throughout the 1970s and 1980s, the idea that one could delay the death of myocytes in a zone of acute myocardial ischemia induced by acute occlusion of a coronary artery in the experimental animal with a pharmacological agent was studied intensively (Hearse & Yellon, 1984). Although more than 100 agents were reported to be cardioprotective, relatively few beneficial effects were confirmed experimentally in vivo and none of these therapies have proved to be efficacious in patients.

The models used in studies of the basic biology of ischemia have been reviewed in many articles and in several books (Hearse & de Leiris, 1979; Hearse & Yellon, 1984; Reimer & Jennings, 1992) and include isolated perfused hearts subjected to low-flow or total ischemia (Hearse & Chain, 1972; Hearse et al., 1976; Neely & Morgan, 1974; Opie and Mansford, 1971; Steenbergen et al., 1978; Williamson, 1966; Williamson et al., 1976), isolated rabbit septum perfusion studies (Harding & Poole-Wilson, 1980), total ischemia in vitro (Jennings et al., 1981; Reimer et al., 1981), nuclear magnetic resonance (NMR) studies of isolated perfused hearts (Malloy et al., 1986; Steenbergen et al., 1987), acute myocardial ischemia in vivo (Bolli et al., 1988; Braasch et al., 1968; Downey et al., 1994; Ginks et al., 1972; Maroko et al., 1971; Murry et al., 1986; Reimer & Jennings, 1979; Reimer et al., 1985), and the effects of anoxia (Ganote & Vander Heide, 1988) or ischemia (Vander Heide et al., 1990) on isolated myocytes. These studies revealed the general features of ischemic injury. Some of the important aspects of the biology of acute myocardial ischemia are summarized in the next section.

GENERAL FEATURES OF ANOXIA AND ISCHEMIA

The general features of the pathobiology of acute ischemia have been established by work in numerous laboratories around the world. Various facets of the subject have been reviewed elsewhere. A few representative references to papers or books are referred to in this chapter (Bing, 1965; Hearse & de Leiris, 1979; Hearse & Yellon, 1984; Jennings et al., 1990; Jennings et al., 1986; Neely & Morgan, 1974; Opie, 1968; Opie, 1976; Reimer & Jennings, 1992; Rosenkranz & Buckberg, 1983). The following sections summarize some of the major features of ischemia that are particularly relevant to the subject of myocardial protection.

Energy metabolism in aerobic heart

Myocardium is dependent virtually totally on aerobic metabolism to make enough energy to support the continuous contractile activity and the processes of growth and turnover associated with health. Aerobic metabolism takes place in the mitochondria, the importance of which is reflected in the fact that they occupy roughly one third of the volume of a myocyte. With an efficiency of roughly 50%, they metabolize fatty acids, amino acids, ketone bodies, and glucose to carbon dioxide (CO_2) and water (H_2O)with the liberation of much high-energy phosphate (~P). For example, 38 µmol of ~P are released from glucose converted to CO_2 and H_2O. The remaining energy is released as heat.

The ~P is utilized in an enormous number of reactions within the myocyte. Most of it is utilized to support the contractile effort, but some is required for phosphorylation reactions, protein synthesis, formation of cyclic-AMP, or the activity of enzymes like the Na/K_{ATP}ase and protein kinase C (PKC) or channels like the K_{ATP} channel. Because of its involvement in various processes that are important to maintaining cellular integrity, it is clear that ~P plays a very critical role in the metabolism of all cells; however, it is particularly important in the heart because contractile function cannot occur without ~P and absence of contractile function soon results in the death of the entire organism.

Ischemia

The simplest definition of ischemia is the absence of arterial flow (Jennings, 1970). When no flow is present, this is categorized as *total* or *global ischemia;* total ischemia results in an interrelated series of changes that begin within a few seconds of onset. The cause of the changes is the absence of arterial flow, which deprives the tissue of oxygen and substrate, and allows the accumulation of products of ischemic metabolism (Jennings et al., 1986). Within a few seconds of the cessation of flow, the O_2 trapped in the area is utilized together with the reserve ~P. Simultaneously, energy metabolism converts to the anaerobic form. As a consequence of the shift in metabolism, contractile function ceases, membrane potential decreases, and electrocardiographic changes appear. Moreover, because metabolism is continuing in the ischemic

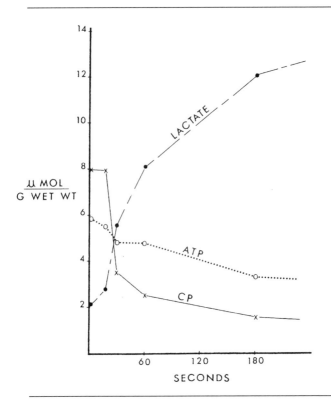

Figure 2-1. *The data of Braasch and colleagues (1968) is plotted in this figure in order to demonstrate the speed with which changes develop in ~P at 37°C in acutely ischemic canine myocardium. These investigators instantly froze biopsies of the center of an epicardial zone of acute ischemia. The biopsies were obtained 15, 30, 60, and 180 seconds after the onset. Note the speed with which creatinine phosphate (CP) declines and lactate rises. Changes in ATP occur more slowly. Contrast these changes to those seen in Figure 2-3, where the tissue was obtained from the subendocardial layer of the canine heart after longer intervals of ischemia. Because of the transmural gradient of ischemia observed following coronary occlusion (Reimer & Jennings, 1979), the subendocardial layer usually develops severe metabolic changes earlier and dies more quickly than the subepicardial layer studied by Braasch and colleagues (1968). (Reproduced with permission from Hearse & de Leiris [1979].)*

myocytes, they accumulate the products of ischemic metabolism such as lactate, hydrogen ion (H^+), inorganic phosphate, and so on—the so-called *osmotic load* (Jennings et al., 1986). Oxygen deficiency is the proximate cause of most of the metabolic changes in ischemia, but these reactions are influenced by the osmotic load and especially the acidosis that develops as a consequence of the absence of flow. Oxygen deficiency with continued flow in the isolated perfused heart, so-called *high-flow anoxia*, is a good model of anoxia and bad model of ischemia, because no osmotic load accumulates in the presence of flow (Jennings et al., 1986).

Energy metabolism in ischemia

Energy is required to maintain both myocardial viability and function. Thus, a brief summary of the changes in en-

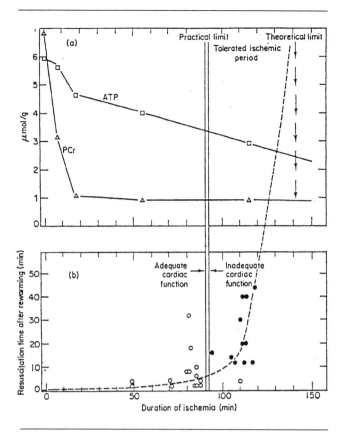

Figure 2-2. *This figure shows the effect of hypothermia on changes in ~P in the canine heart. The animals were anesthetized with pentobarbital and the heart was cooled to 15°C. At 15°C, CP disappears in minutes rather than in seconds (see Fig 3-1). Note that after 90 minutes of ischemia, ATP only has declined to 50% of control, whereas at 37°C in vivo, it is virtually 0 after only 40 minutes of severe ischemia (see Fig 2–3). The vertical double line shows that all hearts recovered good contractile function when warmed to 37°C when the ATP was 3.5 μmol/g wet or greater. On the other hand, lower tissue ATP levels were associated with insufficient function to maintain the circulation. (Reproduced with permission from Kubler & Spieckermann [1970].)*

ergy metabolism found in untreated ischemia is appropriate in terms of assessment of protection. The reader should note that there are species differences in energy requirements and in the enzymes involved in the destruction of the adenine nucleotide pool in severe ischemia; thus, results in various experimental models may differ in both a qualitative and a temporal fashion. However, the general result in terms of ~P is identical. Sooner or later, persistent severe ischemia results in depletion of ~P and in destruction of the adenine nucleotide pool.

The speed with which ~P is depleted is illustrated in Figure 2-1 using the data of Braasch and colleagues (1968). Note that the total reserve supply of ~P is small in mammalian hearts and consists primarily of CP and adenine nucleotides. After the onset of ischemia, only a few contractions are required to exhaust supplies of CP. This CP is used primarily to preserve the ~P of ATP via the action of creatine

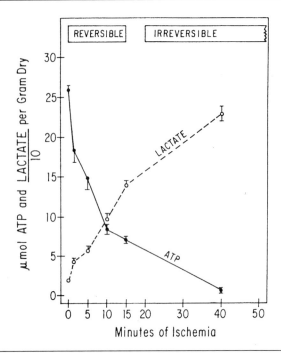

Figure 2-3. The effect of severe ischemia in vivo in the canine heart on adenosine triphosphate (ATP) depletion (-) and lactate production (- -) is shown in this graph. Results were obtained from the subendocardial region of four to six hearts of anesthetized, open-chest dogs subjected to occlusion of the circumflex branch of the left coronary artery. The tissue was frozen, dried, and analyzed after estimating collateral flow with microspheres. In no case was the collateral arterial flow >0.07 ml/min/g. Brackets indicate standard error of mean. The injury is considered to be reversible during the first 15 minutes and irreversible after 20 or more minutes of ischemia. (Reprinted with permission from Jennings and colleagues [1989].)

kinase (CK). However, as soon as CP is exhausted, ATP declines and ADP accumulates in the ischemic tissue.

The changes in ~P were studied in detail by investigators interested in cardioplegia. This group showed a clear relationship between preservation of ATP, prevention of acidosis, and the capacity of the myocardium to function when reperfused (Bretschneider, 1964; Bretschneider et al., 1975; Hearse et al., 1975; Kübler & Spieckermann, 1970; Lazar et al., 1980; Rosenkranz & Buckberg, 1983). A representative study is shown in Figure 2-2. As long as the ATP remained above 3.5 μmol/g wet weight during ischemic arrest in the canine heart, function returned to control levels when arterial flow was restored. Potassium arrest to eliminate contractile activity and hypothermia was shown to be extraordinarily efficient in preserving ATP and in slowing the development of acidosis (i.e., accumulation of lactate) (Bretschneider et al., 1975; Kübler & Spieckermann, 1970; Nayler & Williams, 1978). At 15°C (see Fig 2-2), ischemic metabolism proceeded at about one third the rate seen at 37° C, with the result that ~P was conserved at levels that made it possible to restore good function when the heart was reperfused.

In general, the studies of the surgical group were directed at preserving function while the studies of the basic science group were directed at understanding fundamental mechanisms of ischemia, especially those that might directly or indirectly cause the death of ischemic myocytes. The general underlying belief then and now was that full understanding of the mechanisms of ischemic injury would lead to the development of pharmacological interventions designed to slow or prevent the transition to cell death. The chief problem in ischemia was recognized by both groups as being the fact that the demand of ischemic tissue for ~P exceeded the supply (Bretschneider et al., 1975; Hearse et al., 1975; Jennings et al., 1990; Neely & Morgan, 1974; Williamson, 1966). The importance of ATP depletion, lactate, and H^+ ion accumulation with respect to cell death were noted somewhat later. However, it was known by the late 1970s that dead myocytes had virtually no ~P and a very large osmotic load due to continuing metabolism and the absence of flow (Jennings et al., 1990).

An explosion of information about the role of Ca^{2+} and other ions, the effect of catecholamines on glycolysis and contractile mechanisms, the cytoskeleton, sarcolemmal function, sodium-hydrogen, and sodium-calcium exchange, and so forth, became available to scientists interested in altering the progress of ischemia in infarction. Lack of space precludes review of the role of these phenomena in ischemic injury and in protection against ischemic injury except to state that slowing the rate of change in these variables, at a rate of one to two variables at a time, did not produce dramatic protective effects.

Effects of reperfusion

Most scientists now agree that reperfusion with arterial blood is the only means available to prevent cell death and that drug therapy induces only modest degrees of protection. Many therapies were used with the aim of delaying cell death during ischemia prior to reperfusion. Widely studied therapies include the effect of (1) beta-blockers, (2) Ca^{2+} channel blockers, (3) free radical scavengers, (4) agents inhibiting ion exchange, (5) phenothiazines, (6) hypertonic mannitol, and so on. Each of these interventions affected a theoretical mechanism that could lead to cell death. However, with few exceptions, none of these therapies had enough of an effect to be clinically useful. Some were added to cardioplegia solutions where they were reported to be beneficial (Rosenkranz & Buckberg, 1983). However, most of these drugs were not adapted widely by either surgeons or cardiologists.

Preconditioning myocardium with a brief episode of ischemia provides the strongest protective effect against infarction seen up to the present time (Murry et al., 1986). Moreover, it has been shown that endogenous mediators such as adenosine, bradykinin, α-1 agonists, and so on, will pharmacologically precondition an otherwise normal heart (Downey et al., 1994). Study of this distinctive new phenomenon has already revealed changes in intracellular signaling in ischemia that were previously unknown. Since alterations of these signaling sequences clearly are protective, understanding of the mechanism of preconditioning should contribute much to our understanding of cardiac protection. Also, Yellon and associates (1992a, 1992b) have shown that the protective effect of preconditioning returns in a somewhat weaker form after 24 hours of reflow and persists for several days. This so-called second window of protection is an attractive new area remaining to be explored in detail.

SUMMARY

Two general questions have led to much investigation in the field of ischemic injury: What are the molecular mechanisms involved in contraction and how is this process controlled? What are the mechanisms involved in maintaining the viability of myocytes and how does alteration of these processes lead to cell death? Variants of these questions are still being asked because they have never been fully answered; it is certain that much remains to be learned. Nevertheless, our understanding of the cell biology of the myocardium and our knowledge of ischemic injury have increased markedly. Moreover, much of this increased understanding has resulted from studies directed at protecting the myocardium from ischemic damage.

The recognition that myocytes died of ischemia as a function of the severity and duration of the ischemia, and that elimination of ischemia by reperfusion with arterial blood was the only means available to prevent the death of ischemic myocytes was an important advance that has contributed much to understanding the effects of ischemia on the myocyte. Use of reperfusion to prevent myocyte death also led to striking improvement in the treatment of acute ischemia resulting from coronary occlusion in man. However, reperfusion also induced deleterious effects such as stunning and perhaps hibernation. Stunning in particular, is a kind of reperfusion injury from which the myocyte needs protection.

Finally, it is clear that preservation of both cell function and viability is associated closely with preservation of high energy phosphates. Interventions that slow the inevitable depletion of $\sim$P in severely or totally ischemic myocardium are protective and can be induced by a variety of techniques including cooling, drugs, and a reduction in hemodynamic load. Slowing of energy metabolism is associated with slowing of the accumulation of the ischemic metabolites that comprise the osmotic load such as H^+, inorganic phosphate, and glycolytic intermediates. However, the relationship, if any, between changes in the osmotic load and protection has not been established.

ACKNOWLEDGMENT

The work described in this chapter was supported in part by NIH grants HL 27416 and HL 23138.

REFERENCES

Bing RJ. Cardiac metabolism. *Physiol Rev* 1965; 45: 171–213.

Bolli R, Patel BS, Jeroudi MO, et al. Demonstration of free radical generation in "stunned" myocardium of intact dogs with the use of the spin trap alpha-phenyl N-teriary butyl nitrone. *J Clin Invest* 1988; 82: 476–485.

Braasch W, Gudbjarnason S, Puri PS, et al. Early changes in energy metabolism in the myocardium following acute coronary artery occlusion in anesthetized dogs. *Circ Res* 1968; 23: 429–438.

Braunwald E, Hollingsworth C, Passamani E. Surgery in the treatment of coronary artery disease. Presented at the NHLBI Workshop. September 6 & 7, 1984. Bethesda, MD. Also in *Circulation* 1985; 72(Suppl V): V-1–V-2.

Braunwald E, Kloner RA. The stunned myocardium: prolonged, postischemic ventricular dysfunction. *Circulation* 1982; 66: 1146–1149.

Bretschneider HJ. Uberlebenszeit und Wiederbelebungszeit des Herzens bei Normo- und Hypothermie. *Verh Dtsch Ges Kreislaufforsch* 1964; 30: 11–34.

Bretschneider HJ, Hubner G, Knoll D, et al. Myocardial resistance and tolerance to ischemia: physiological and biochemical basis. *J Cardiovasc Surg* 1975; 16: 241–260.

Conversano A, Walsh JF, Geltman EM, et al. Delineation of myocardial stunning and hibernation by positron emission tomography in advanced coronary artery disease. *Am Heart J* 1996; 131: 440–450.

Downey JM, Cohen MV, Ytrehus K, Liu Y. Cellular mechanisms in ischemic preconditioning: the role of adenosine and protein kinase C. *Ann NY Acad Sci* 1994; 723: 82–98.

Ganote CE, Nayler WG. Contracture and the calcium paradox [editorial review]. *J Mol Cell Cardiol* 1985; 17: 733–745.

Ganote CE, Vander Heide RS. Irreversible injury of isolated adult rat myocytes. Osmotic fragility during metabolic inhibition. *Am J Pathol* 1988; 132: 212–222.

Ginks WR, Sybers HD, Maroko PR, et al. Coronary artery reperfusion. II. Reduction of myocardial infarct size at 1 week after the coronary occlusion. *J Clin Invest* 1972; 51: 2717–2723.

Harding DP, Poole-Wilson, PA. Calcium exchange in rabbit myocardium during and after hypoxia: effect of temperature and substrate. *Cardiovasc Res* 1980; XIV: 435–445.

Hearse DJ, Chain EB. The role of glucose in the survival and "recovery" of the anoxic isolated perfused rat heart. *Biochem J* 1972; 128: 1125–1133.

Hearse DJ, de Leiris J. *Enzymes in cardiology. Diagnosis and research.* New York: John Wiley & Sons, 1979: 1–586.

Hearse DJ, Stewart DA, Braimbridge MV. Hypothermic arrest and potassium arrest: metabolic and myocardial protection during elective cardiac arrest. *Circ Res* 1975; 36: 481–489.

Hearse DJ, Stewart DA, Braimbridge MV. Cellular protection during myocardial ischemia: the development and characterization of a procedure for the induction of reversible ischemia. *Circulation* 1976; 54: 193–202.

Hearse DJ, Yellon DM. *Therapeutic approaches to myocardial infarct size limitation.* New York: Raven Press, 1984: 1–255.

Herdson PB, Sommers HM, Jennings RB. A comparative study of the fine structure of normal and ischemic dog myocardium with special reference to early changes following temporary occlusion of a coronary artery. *Am J Pathol* 1965; 46: 367–386.

Herrmann G, Decherd G. Creatine and glycogen content of normal and infarcted héart muscle of the dog. *Proc Soc Exper Biol Med* 1935; 32: 1304–1305.

Heyndrickx GR, Baig H, Nellens P, et al. Depression of regional blood flow and wall thickening after brief coronary occlusions. *Am J Physiol* 1978; 234: H653–H659.

Himwich HE, Goldfarb W, Nahum LH. Changes of the carbohydrate metabolism of the heart following coronary occlusion. *Am J Physiol* 1934; 109: 403–408.

Jennings RB. Myocardial ischemia—observations, definitions and speculations [editorial]. *J Mol Cell Cardiol* 1970; 1: 345–349.

Jennings RB, Murry CE, Steenbergen Jr C, Reimer KA. The acute phase of regional ischemia. In: Cox RH, ed. *Acute myocardial infarction: emerging concepts of pathogenesis and treatment.* New York: Praeger Scientific, 1989: 67–84.

Jennings RB, Murry CE, Steenbergen Jr C, Reimer KA. Development of cell injury in sustained acute ischemia. *Circulation* 1990; 82(Suppl): II-2–II-12.

Jennings RB, Reimer KA, Hill ML, Mayer SE. Total ischemia, in dog hearts, in vitro. I. Comparison of high energy phosphate production, utilization and depletion and of adenine nucleotide catabolism in total ischemia in vitro vs severe ischemia in vivo. *Circ Res* 1981; 49: 892–900.

Jennings RB, Reimer KA, Steenbergen Jr C. Myocardial ischemia revisited. The osmolar load, membrane damage, and reperfusion [editorial]. *J Mol Cell Cardiol* 1986; 18: 769–780.

Jennings RB, Sommers H, Smyth GA, et al. Myocardial necrosis induced by temporary occlusion of a coronary artery in the dog. *Arch Pathol Lab Med* 1960; 70: 68–78.

Jennings RB, Yellon DM. Reperfusion injury: definitions and historical background. In: Yellon D, Jennings RB, eds. *Myocardial protection: the pathophysiology of reperfusion and reperfusion injury.* New York: Raven Press, 1992: 1–11.

Johnson AS, Schemberg SR, Gerisch RA, Saltzstein HC. Effect of cortisone on the size of experimentally produced myocardial infarcts. *Circulation* 1953; 7: 224–228.

Kübler W, Spieckermann PG. Regulation of glycolysis in the ischemic and anoxic myocardium. *J Mol Cell Cardiol* 1970; 1: 351–377.

Lazar HL, Buckberg GD, Manganaro AM, Becker H. Myocardial energy replenishment and reversal of ischemic damage by substrate enhancement of secondary blood cardioplegia with amino acids during reperfusion. *J Thorac Cardiovasc Surg* 1980; 80: 350–359.

Malloy CR, Matthews PM, Smith MB, Radda GK. Influence of propranolol on acidosis and high energy phosphates in ischemic myocardium of the rabbit. *Cardiovasc Res* 1986; 20: 710–720.

Maroko PR, Kjekshus JK, Sobel BE, et al. Factors influencing infarct size following experimental coronary artery occlusions. *Circulation* 1971; 43: 67–82.

Murry CE, Jennings RB, Reimer KA. Preconditioning with ischemia: a delay of lethal cell injury in ischemic myocardium. *Circulation* 1986; 74: 1124–1136.

Nayler WG, Williams A. Relaxation in heart muscle: some morphological and biochemical considerations. *Eur J Cardiol* 1978; 7 (Suppl): 35–50.

Neely JR, Morgan HE. Relationship between carbohydrate and lipid metabolism and the energy balance of heart muscle. *Ann Rev Physiol* 1974; 36: 413–459.

Opie LH. Metabolism of the heart in health and disease. Part I. *Am Heart J* 1968; 76: 685–698.

Opie LH. II. Metabolic regulation in ischemia and hypoxia. Effects of regional ischemia on metabolism of glucose and fatty acids. Relative rates of aerobic and anaerobic energy production during myocardial infarction and comparison with effects of anoxia. *Circ Res* 1976; 38(Suppl 1): I-52–I-68.

Opie LH, Mansford KRL. The value of lactate and pyruvate measurements in the assessment of the redox state of free nicotinamide-adenine dinucleotide in the cytoplasm of perfused rat heart. *Eur J Clin Invest* 1971; 1: 295–306.

Rahimtoola SH. The hibernating myocardium. *Am Heart J* 1989; 117: 211–221.

Reimer KA, Jennings RB. The "wavefront phenomenon" of myocardial ischemic cell death. II. Transmural progression of necrosis within the framework of ischemic bed size (myocardium at risk) and collateral flow. *Lab Invest* 1979; 40: 633–644.

Reimer KA, Jennings RB. Myocardial ischemia, hypoxia, and infarction. In*: The heart and cardiovascular system.* Fozzard HA, Jennings RB, Haber E, et al., eds. New York: Raven Press, 1992: 1875–1973.

Reimer, KA, Jennings RB, Cobb FR, et al. Animal models for protecting ischemic myocardium: results of the NHLBI cooperative study comparison of unconscious and conscious dog models. *Circ Res* 1985; 56: 651–665.

Reimer KA, Jennings RB, Hill ML. Total ischemia in dog hearts, in vitro. 2. High energy phosphate depletion and associated defects in energy metabolism, cell volume regulation, and sarcolemmal integrity. *Circ Res* 1981; 49: 901–911.

Rentrop KP, Blanke H, Kostering K, Karsch KR. Acute myocardial infarction: intracoronary application of nitroglycerin and streptokinase in combination with transluminal recanalization. *Clin Cardiol* 1979; 5: 354–360.

Rosenkranz ER, Buckberg GD. Myocardial protection during surgical coronary reperfusion. *J Am Coll Cardiol* 1983; 1: 1235–1246.

Shen AC, Jennings RB. Kinetics of calcium accumulation in acute myocardial ischemic injury. *Am J Pathol* 1972; 67: 441–452.

Steenbergen Jr C, Deleeuw G, Williamson JR. Analysis of control of glycolysis in ischemic hearts having heterogeneous zones of anoxia. *J Mol Cell Cardiol* 1978; 10: 617–639.

Steenbergen Jr C, Murphy E, Levy L, London RE. Elevation in cytosolic free calcium concentration early in myocardial ischemia in perfused rat heart. *Circ Res* 1987; 60: 700–707.

Tennant R, Grayzel DM, Sutherland FA, Stringer SW. Studies on experimental coronary occlusion. Chemical and anatomical changes in the myocardium after coronary ligation. *Am Heart J* 1936; 12: 168–173.

Tennant R, Wiggers CJ. The effect of coronary occlusion on myocardial contraction. *Am J Physiol* 1935; 112: 351–361.

Vander Heide RS, Rim D, Hohl M, Ganote CE. An in vitro model of myocardial ischemia utilizing isolated adult rat myocytes. *J Mol Cell Cardiol* 1990; 22: 165–181.

Wartman WB, Campbell LA, Craig RL. The effect of ACTH on experimental myocardial infarcts. *Circ Res* 1955; 3: 496–500.

Williamson JR. Glycolytic control mechanisms. II. Kinetics of intermediate changes during the aerobic-anoxic transition in perfused rat heart. *J Biol Chem* 1966; 241: 5026–5036.

Williamson JR, Safer B, Rich T, et al. Effects of acidosis on myocardial contractility and metabolism. *Acta Med Scand* 1976; 587: 95–111.

Yellon DM, Latchman DS. Stress proteins and myocardial protection during ischemia and reperfusion. In: Yellon DM, Jennings RB, eds. *Myocardial protection: the pathophysiology of reperfusion and reperfusion injury.* New York: Raven Press, 1992a: 185–195.

Yellon DM, Pasini E, Cargnoni A, et al. The protective role of heat stress in the ischemic and reperfused rabbit myocardium. *J Mol Cell Cardiol* 1992b; 24: 895–907.

Zimmerman ANE, Daems W, Hulsmann WC, et al. Morphological changes of heart muscle caused by successive perfusion with calcium-free and calcium-containing solutions (calcium paradox). *Cardiovasc Res* 1967; 1: 201–209.

Zimmerman ANE, Hulsmann WC. Paradoxical influence of calcium ions on the permeability of the cell membranes of the isolated rat heart. *Nature* 1966; 211: 646–647.

CHAPTER 3

Silent Ischemia

C. Richard Conti

WHAT IS SILENT ISCHEMIA?

In order to define asymptomatic or silent myocardial is-chemia, one has to define *myocardial ischemia*. Unfortunately there still remains considerable confusion about the clinical definition of myocardial ischemia (see Chapter 1).

In humans, silent myocardial ischemia can be demon-strated during balloon coronary angioplasty. Balloon occlu-sion of a coronary artery obviously decreases coronary blood flow and alters the regional flow/demand ratio. A decrease in coronary sinus regional PO_2 can be demon-strated followed by abnormalities of regional ventricular re-laxation and contraction, rise in LVEDP, ECG changes, and finally chest pain (Sigwart et al., 1984) (Fig 3-1).

Electrocardiography

In patients with chest pain, transient electrocardiographic abnormalities such as ST-segment elevation or depression and T-wave peaking or inversion seen on the 12-lead ECG during rest or exercise generally indicates myocardial is-chemia. Ambulatory ECGs [AECGs] are also used to iden-tify myocardial ischemia during daily life activities. The question can be asked: Are transient ST changes on a 2-lead AECG sufficient and accurate enough to represent myocar-dial ischemia? If the AECG changes are transient and asso-ciated with chest discomfort, the diagnosis of myocardial ischemia is highly suspect. The problem with silent myocar-dial ischemia is that the patient has no chest discomfort as-sociated with transient ECG changes. Thus, in the absence of symptoms, I believe it is important to develop confirmatory evidence of ischemia by some other examination or test. Transient ECG changes that disappear after a myocardial revascularization procedure are highly suggestive of myo-cardial ischemia.

Figure 3-2 shows transient ST-segment changes in an asymptomatic patient during exercise and AECG monitor-ing before revascularization, and absence of these changes after a revascularization procedure.

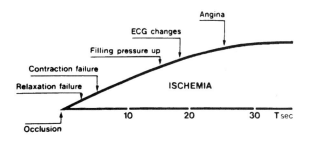

Figure 3-1. *Schematic representation of sequential changes following balloon occlusion of a coronary artery. (Adapted from Sigwart and colleagues [1984].)*

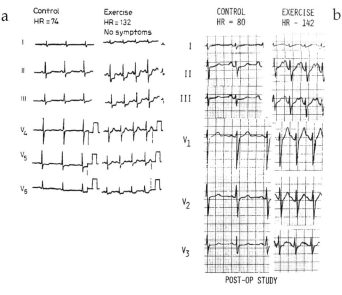

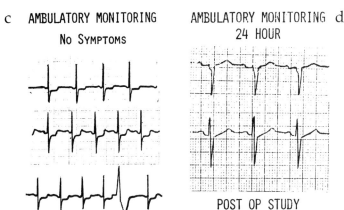

Figure 3-2. *Representative resting and exercise ECGs in an asymptomatic patient preoperatively (a) and postoperatively (b). AECG in the same patient preoperatively (c) and postoperatively (d). The preoperative abnormalities are absent after coronary bypass surgery.*

Auscultation

The simplest examination is cardiac auscultation. The presence of a transient fourth heart sound during transient ECG changes (representing an increase in the diastolic stiffness of the ventricle, a rise in LVEDP, and thus a rise in left atrial pressure) would help confirm the diagnosis of silent myocardial ischemia.

Exercise testing and radionuclides

Exercise testing combined with radionuclides to identify transient perfusion abnormalities provides additional evidence that silent transient electrocardiographic changes are related to myocardial ischemia. I am less confident of the diagnosis of myocardial ischemia when a region of "thallium hypoperfusion" is seen after intravenous persantine or intravenous adenosine. In these latter instances the patient generally has no ECG abnormalities suggestive of ischemia.

Stress testing and left ventricular function

Transient left ventricular wall-motion abnormalities associated with transient ECG changes during either exercise or adrenergic stimulation provide the most convincing evidence that myocardial ischemia is present in patients with or without symptoms. These images can be obtained easily using cardiac ultrasound or radionuclides.

Elhendy and colleagues (1995) infused high-dose dobutamine into patients with anatomically and functionally significant coronary artery disease. The amount of stress-induced left ventricular dysfunction was similar in patients with and without angina. However ST-segment depression was more common in patients with angina and was associated with more extensive ischemia in left ventricular segments that were contracting normally prior to dobutamine infusion.

Glycerol trinitrate and transient ST-segment changes

Glycerol trinitrate, the old standby for relieving myocardial ischemia, still has a clinical role in determining which patient has myocardial ischemia and which patient does not. Shang and Pepine (1977) showed this many years ago when studying young naval personnel with a positive exercise test and proven coronary artery disease. Patients were monitored with AECG recordings. The investigators observed that about three fourths of the episodes of transient ST-segment changes on the AECG were present without accompanying symptoms. In this same patient population, the AECG recordings were repeated and patients were given hourly doses of sublingual nitroglycerin. A critical observation from these studies was that there was a marked reduction in the symptomatic episodes of ST-segment depression as well as episodes of asymptomatic ST-segment depression, strongly suggesting that the asymptomatic episodes were related to myocardial ischemia.

CLINICALLY IMPORTANT MYOCARDIAL ISCHEMIA

It is my belief that clinically important myocardial ischemia, which includes silent myocardial ischemia, is associated with a transient, regional, left ventricular wall-motion abnormality (Pepine et al., 1986). Animal experiments in which coronary arteries are transiently occluded indicate that the first abnormality is an increase in diastolic stiffness of the ventricle, followed by systolic dysfunction (Chierchia et al., 1980). If this does not occur in a patient with transient ST-segment shifts or with thallium or other radionuclide defects should we assume that the patient in not experiencing clinically important myocardial ischemia? If it can be shown that prognosis is related only to a transient wall-motion abnormality due to ischemia, then none of the other observations have clinical relevance. This concept is particularly pertinent in clinical trials in which asymptomatic "myocardial ischemia" is being assessed. To compare study end points or outcome, the definition of asymptomatic myocardial ischemia must be uniform.

WHO HAS SILENT MYOCARDIAL ISCHEMIA?

If asymptomatic cardiac ischemia or silent myocardial ischemia is defined as transient ST-segment shift on an AECG, the majority of patients with any manifestation of symptomatic myocardial ischemia will have silent myocardial ischemia (Conti, 1988). Clinically important silent ischemia occurs in the following patients:

- Stable angina
- Unstable angina
- Variant angina
- Postinfarction angina
- Cardiac arrest survivors
- Cardiac transplant patients
- After coronary angioplasty
- After coronary artery bypass
- Patients with multiple risk factors
- Diabetics

WHY IS MYOCARDIAL ISCHEMIA SILENT?

Several explanations for the absence of symptoms associated with ischemic ECG changes have been proposed. They are generally divided into two categories. Firstly, it is postulated that patients whose ischemia is silent have less ischemic myocardium than during a comparable episode of symptomatic ischemia. The duration of ischemia may be brief in the asymptomatic patient and in some instances the presence of collaterals may limit the extent of ischemia. Secondly, there may be a defective angina warning system. This could be due to nervous system damage, prior myocardial infarction, prior coronary bypass surgery, presence of diabetes mellitus or other neuropathy, surgical denervation, cardiac transplantation, denial by the patient, and variability of pain thresholds in different patients.

How Is Silent Myocardial Ischemia Detected?

Detection of silent myocardial ischemia still remains somewhat of a problem. Although not perfect, the easiest way to detect clinically significant silent ischemia, and perhaps the most cost-effective and least labor-intensive method, is the exercise ECG. Although this seems quite logical, the yield of patients with coronary artery disease is not always high. This is the case because the ECG alone will identify some patients who have ST-segment depression not related to myocardial ischemia. Thus the clinician is faced with the question: What does a "positive" exercise test mean in the symptomless person? Roughly 8% of apparently healthy American men age 35 to 55 will develop ST-segment depression during treadmill exercise (Froelicher et al., 1976). However, only about half of the 8% have proven coronary artery disease. Clinicians must determine into which group their patient falls. Thus some other means to confirm that ECG changes are due to myocardial ischemia must be employed. If the AECG identifies a patient with asymptomatic ST changes, the diagnosis of myocardial ischemia must be confirmed, as is required with exercise testing.

What Is the Clinical Significance of Silent Myocardial Ischemia?

If the presence of myocardial ischemia is established, then the absence of pain during transient ST-segment depression may not have relevance to management or prognosis. Evidence is now accumulating suggesting that prognosis of patients with painless myocardial ischemia may be no different than prognosis of patients who have overt clinical manifestations of myocardial ischemia (Weiner et al., 1988).

Previous studies using AECG monitoring in patients with proven coronary artery disease have shown that high- and low-risk groups can be identified for subsequent coronary-related events (Stern & Tzivoni, 1974). In patients with effort angina and evidence of effort ischemia as determined by AECG during daily life activities, prognosis is poorer than in those who have no ischemia (Deedwania & Carbajal, 1990). The same can be said for every clinical presentation of ischemic heart disease including patients with unstable angina (Gottlieb et al., 1987; Nademanee et al., 1987), myocardial infarction (Theroux et al., 1979; Gerstenblith et al., 1986; Tzivoni et al., 1988), recent PTCA (Kaul et al., 1991), coronary bypass surgery (Weiner et al., 1988; Egstrup, 1988), and survivors of sudden cardiac death (Sharma et al., 1987).

IS THE SILENT ISCHEMIA PATIENT POPULATION UNIFORM?

In the ACIP trial homogeneity of the patient population was studied (Conti et al., 1994). In a group of 618 patients with angiographically proven coronary artery disease, an abnormal exercise stress test, and transient ST-segment abnormalities on a 48-hour AECG, asymptomatic cardiac ischemia varied in the following way. Forty-one percent had no angina by history, 48% had no angina during exercise ECG, and 90% had no angina during 48 hours of AECG monitoring. One hundred seventy-nine patients (29%) had no symptoms by history or during exercise testing or AECG monitoring. Since the cardiac event rates of each asymptomatic cardiac ischemia category may vary considerably, comparison between published trials of anti-ischemic strategies may require more attention to the details of the asymptomatic status of patients being studied.

CAN MYOCARDIAL ISCHEMIA BE SUPPRESSED IN PATIENTS WITH SILENT MYOCARDIAL ISCHEMIA?

Published results of the ACIP trial have shown that, at 12 weeks, ECG evidence of myocardial ischemia determined by AECG decreases regardless of the therapy used, whether it be symptom treatment, ischemia-driven treatment, or revascularization (Knatterud et al., 1994). Table 3-1 summarizes the percentage of patients who had no evidence of ischemia during daily life activities determined by a 48-hour AECG. A significant number of patients had no evidence of ischemia on the week 12 AECG. Both medical therapy arms were almost identical (symptom guided, 38.9%; ischemia guided, 41.3%), but revascularization had more patients without ischemia on the 12-week AECG (54.7%). This difference between revascularization and medical therapy was statistically significant: $p<.001$.

Coronary revascularization also significantly reduced the average number of abnormal ECG leads and average sum of ST depression during exercise-induced myocardial ischemia compared to either medical strategies, as shown in Table 3-2.

The ACIP study has also shown that at 12 weeks patients randomized to revascularization required fewer drugs than those randomized to either medical treatment arm of the trial (Table 3-3).

TABLE 3-1. ISCHEMIA ON AECG DURING DAILY LIFE ACTIVITY

Strategies	Present	Absent
Symptom treatment	61.1%	38.9%
Ischemia treatment	58.7%	41.3%
Revascularization	45.3%	54.7%[a]

[a]$p < .001$.

TABLE 3-2. EXERCISE TEST RESULTS AT 12 WEEKS

Strategies	Average no. abnormal ECG leads	Average sum of ST-segment depression
Symptom treatment	3.5	7.4
Ischemia treatment	3.2	6.8
Revascularization	2.5[a]	5.6[b]

[a]$p < .001$.
[b]$p = .006$.

Thus the ACIP study indicates that over the short term (12 weeks), revascularization therapy reduces or eliminates ischemia better than either form of drug therapy.

Unfortunately, in this trial, drug therapy was titrated upward only at 4 and 8 weeks. Thus therapy was not advanced to the maximum in most patients. Consequently, many patients (60%) continued to have evidence of ischemia on the AECG. In the revascularization group a significant percentage of patients (45%) also had persistent AECG ischemia at 12 weeks. This may have been the result of incomplete revascularization. This pilot study does not address prognosis, since it included only 618 patients from 11 sites. The primary end point of ACIP was the reduction or resolution of myocardial ischemia at 12 weeks. The results of this trial clearly showed that patients could be recruited and that patients could be randomized to one of the three strategies and provide the basis for a future prospective randomized prognosis trial with a large number of patients assessed over a long period of time (e.g., 5,000 patients over 3 to 5 years).

CAN PROGNOSIS BE ALTERED IN PATIENTS WITH SILENT MYOCARDIAL ISCHEMIA?

The answer to this question is not yet known. Recently Pepine and colleagues (1994) have shown that compared with placebo, atenolol reduced ischemia during activities of daily life and was associated with reduced risk for adverse outcome (principally aggravation of angina) in asymptomatic and mildly symptomatic patients compared with placebo. There are no data indicating a reduction in mortality or myocardial infarction rate in patients with silent ischemia treated with drugs or revascularization.

RELATIONSHIP OF SILENT ISCHEMIA TO STUNNING AND HIBERNATION

A stunned myocardium is defined as viable myocardium salvaged by coronary reperfusion that exhibits prolonged postischemic dysfunction after reperfusion (Conti, 1991). In contrast, hibernating myocardium has been defined as ischemic myocardium supplied by a narrowed coronary artery in which ischemic cells remain viable but contraction is chronically depressed.

Both of these conditions require as part of the definition depression of myocardial contraction. In a sense, both of these conditions represent silent myocardial ischemia if the basis for the definition of ischemia is related to transient myocardial depression.

Stunned myocardium has been found in myocardial infarction patients following thrombolysis or angioplasty, unstable angina patients, exercise-induced angina, coronary artery, spasm, platelet aggregation or transient thrombosis of a coronary artery, angioplasty for chronic myocardial ischemia, and immediately following coronary bypass surgery. Hibernating myocardium is found in patients with severe coronary artery stenosis even in asymptomatic patients at rest. Numerous examples of hibernating myocardium have been seen in the cardiac catheterization angiographic laboratories. Everyone will recall a ventricle that is poorly contracting with its blood supply compromised by a severely stenosed coronary artery. Altering blood flow or hemodynamics with intravenous nitroglycerin or intravenous dobutamine tends to improve cardiac function, suggesting ischemic but viable tissue.

Recently Shen and Vatner (1995) performed experiments in conscious pigs using ameroid constrictors to slowly and chronically stenose a coronary artery. Frequent observations of ventricular performance were made before as well as after intermittent occlusion of a coronary artery. Transient coronary occlusion reduced left ventricular systolic thickening 1 day after ameroid constrictor implantation as well as 20 days later. However, at a later time, left ventricular systolic wall thickening was reduced only slightly after transient coronary occlusion. The investigators speculate that perhaps collaterals developed at that time to explain this phenomenon. They conclude that there may be a blurring of definitions between myocardial hibernation and myocardial stunning. They believe that the two conditions may coexist and share the same mechanism. Their present hypothesis is that reduction in regional wall motion reflects consequences of repeated cumulative imbalances between regional oxygen demand and supply resulting in chronic myocardial stunning, a variant of acute myocardial stunning. Chronic myocardial stunning could have been induced by frequent transient episodes of intense imbalance between oxygen supply and demand.

As far as I know, no one has systematically studied ventricular performance in patients categorized as having silent myocardial ischemia as determined by ST-segment shifts during exercise or during AECG recordings. If animal studies are correct (and I assume they are) electrocardiographic change should not occur until after relaxation and contraction abnormalities of the ventricle occur. Thus it is theoretically possible that all of these patients with silent myocardial ischemia have some form of hibernating myocardium. Unfortunately, investigating these patients in the catheterization laboratory does not reveal hibernating myocardium in every case, since the majority of these patients are being treated aggressively for myocardial ischemia with nitrates, beta-blockers, calcium antagonists, aspirin, and often heparin at the time of the cardiac catheterization. Rarely does a patient appear in the catheterization laboratory free of cardiovascular medications.

RELEVANCE TO CLINICIANS

Silent myocardial ischemia is a real phenomenon. Stunned and hibernating myocardium, now commonly recognized, are clear examples of ischemic myocardium without symptoms. As far as I know, no study has shown that any strategy prolongs survival in patients who have evidence of asymptomatic cardiac ischemia. Thus in my opinion no one really knows how to manage the patient with asymptomatic cardiac ischemia based on objective scientific data. Intuition would lead us to believe that the relief or reduction of ischemia is a good thing. Intuition also led us to believe that the relief or reduction of premature ventricular contractions (PVCs) after a myocardial infarction was a good thing. The Cardiac Arrhythmia Suppression Trial revealed that not to be the case (Epstein et al., 1993).

Clearly what is needed is a prognosis trial, but until such a trial is available it seems reasonable to speculate that the goal of therapy in these patients should be to reduce or eliminate myocardial ischemia. This is particularly true in patients with multiple risks factors. Principles of therapy should be the same for patients with symptomatic or asymptomatic myocardial ischemia (i.e., risk factor modification, aggressive drug therapy, angioplasty, or bypass surgery).

REFERENCES

Chierchia S, Brunelli C, Simonetti I, et al. Sequence of events in angina at rest: primary reduction in coronary flow. *Circulation* 1980; 61: 759–768.

Conti CR. Silent myocardial ischemia: prognostic significance and therapeutic implications. *Clin Cardiol* 1988; 11: 807–811.

Conti CR. The stunned and hibernating myocardium: a brief review. *Clin Cardiol* 1991; 14: 708–712.

Conti R, Pratt C, Pepine C, et al. Asymptomatic cardiac ischemia in patients with coronary artery disease: are we all studying the same thing? *Circulation* 1994; 90(4, Part 2): I-560.

Deedwania PC, Carbajal EV. Silent ischemia during daily life is an independent predictor of mortality in stable angina. *Circulation* 1990; 81: 748–756.

Egstrup K. Asymptomatic myocardial ischemia as a predictor of cardiac events after coronary artery bypass grafting for stable angina pectoris. *Am J Cardiol* 1988; 61: 248–252.

Elhendy A, Geleijnse ML, Roelandt JRTC, et al. Stress induced left ventricular dysfunction in silent and symptomatic myocardial ischemia during dobutamine stress test. *Am J Cardiol* 1995; 75: 1112–1115.

Epstein AE, Hallstrom AP, Rogers WJ, et al. Mortality following ventricular arrhythmia suppression by encainide, flecainide, and moricizine after myocardial infarction. The original design concept of the cardiac arrhythmia suppression trial (CAST). *JAMA* 1993; 270(20): 2451–2455.

Froelicher VF, Thompson AJ, Longo MR, et al. Value of exercise testing for asymptomatic men for latent coronary artery disease. *Prog Cardiovasc Dis* 1976; 18: 265–276.

Gerstenblith G, Achuff SE, Mellits ED, Gottlieb SO. Ischemic ST segment changes by ambulatory Holter predicts one year mortality in high risk post infarct patients [abstract]. *Circulation* 1986; 74: II-58.

Gottlieb SO, Weisfeldt ML, Ouwang P, et al. Silent ischemia predicts infarction and death during two-year follow-up of unstable angina. *J Am Coll Cardiol* 1987; 10: 756–760.

Kaul U, Dev V, Manchanda SC, Wasir HS. Silent myocardial ischemia after percutaneous transluminal coronary angioplasty and its prognostic significance. *Clin Cardiol* 1991; 14: 563–566.

Knatterud GL, Bourassa MG, Pepine CJ, et al. Effects of treatment strategies to suppress ischemia in patients with coronary artery disease: 12 week results of the asymptomatic cardiac ischemia pilot (ACIP) study. *J Am Coll Cardiol* 1994; 24: 11–20.

Nademanee K, Intarachot V, Josephson MA, et al. Prognostic significance of silent myocardial ischemia in patients with unstable angina. *J Am Coll Cardiol* 1987; 10: 1–9.

Pepine CJ, Cohn PF, Deedwania PC, et al. Effects of treatment on outcome at asymptomatic and mildly symptomatic patients with ischemia during daily life: the atenolol silent ischemia study (ASIST). *Circulation* 1994; 90(2): 762–768.

Pepine CJ, Feldman RL, Ludbrook P, et al. Left ventricular dyskinesis reversed by intravenous nitroglycerin: a manifestation of silent myocardial ischemia? *Am J Cardiol* 1986; 58: 38B–42B.

Shang SJ, Pepine CJ. Transient ST asymptomatic ST segment depression during daily activity. *Am J Cardiol* 1977; 39: 369–402.

Sharma B, Asinger R, Frances GS, et al. Demonstration of exercise induced painless myocardial ischemia in survivors of out of hospital ventricular fibrillation. *Am J Cardiol* 1987; 59: 740–745.

Shen YT, Vatner SF. Mechanism of impaired myocardial function during progressive coronary stenosis in conscious pigs: hibernation vs. stunning? *Circ Res* 1995; 76: 479–488.

Sigwart U, Grbic M, Payot M, et al. Ischemic events during coronary artery balloon obstruction. In: Rutishauser W, Roskamm H, eds. *Silent myocardial ischemia.* Berlin: Springer-Verlag, 1984: 29–36.

Stern S, Tzivoni D. Early detection of silent ischemic heart disease by 24-hour electrocardiographic monitoring of active subjects. *Br Heart J* 1974; 36: 481–486.

Theroux P, Waters D, Halphen C, et al. Prognostic significance of exercise testing soon after myocardial infarction. *N Engl J Med* 1979; 301: 341–345.

Tzivoni D, Gavish A, Zin D, et al. Prognostic significance of ischemic episodes in patients with previous myocardial infarction. *Am J Cardiol* 1988; 62: 661–664.

Weiner DA, Ryan TJ, McCabe CH, et al. Risk of developing an acute myocardial infarction or sudden coronary death in patients with exercise-induced silent myocardial ischemia. A report from the coronary artery surgery study (CASS) registry. *Am J Cardiol* 1988; 62(17): 1155–1158.

CHAPTER 4

The General Biology
of Ischemic Preconditioning

David P. Jenkins
Derek M. Yellon

DISCOVERY OF ISCHEMIC
PRECONDITIONING

In 1986 Reimer and Jennings were investigating the effects of repetitive brief ischemic episodes in anesthetized dogs and found unexpected results, which led to the concept of endogenous myocardial adaptation to sublethal ischemia resulting in protection against subsequent ischemia. They termed this adaptation *ischemic preconditioning* (Fig 4-1). The aim of their earlier experiments was to separate the effects of high-energy phosphate depletion and catabolite accumulation to investigate the relative importance of each in the mechanism of cell death. By interspersing sublethal ischemic episodes of 10 minutes (to deplete high-energy phosphates) with reperfusion (to wash out catabolites), they expected to observe a progressive fall in ATP with each additional ischemic period. However, they found that after the initial ischemic period, ATP was not depleted any further by subsequent similar ischemic challenges (Reimer et al., 1986). They realized that the first episode of ischemia must have resulted in a change in the tolerance of myocytes to ischemia so that a second similar ischemic insult did not deplete ATP any further.

This concept was extended to include the possibility that this adapted state might persist and actually protect the myocardium against a very severe ischemic insult that would usually result in considerable cell death. The hypothesis was confirmed by subjecting anesthetized dogs to 40 minutes of circumflex artery occlusion, allowing 4 days reperfusion and then measuring infarct size as a percentage of the volume of the circumflex territory at risk (Murry et al., 1986). One group of dogs was preconditioned with four 5-minute periods of ischemia, each separated by 5 minutes of reperfusion immediately before the sustained 40-minute occlusion; the other group received only 40 minutes sustained ischemia and served as the control. The infarct volume in the preconditioned group was only 25% of that seen in the control group ($p < .001$) despite the fact that the preconditioned

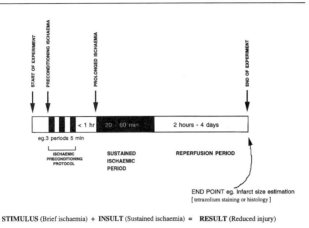

Figure 4-1. Illustration of the concept of ischemic preconditioning. Filled bars represent ischemic periods and open bars represent reperfusion periods. Timing is approximate from the experience in all species.

hearts had actually been subjected to an extra 20 minutes of ischemia. This effect was independent of collateral flow. Ischemic preconditioning can therefore be defined as a rapid adaptation in response to a brief period of ischemia and reperfusion, which results in a delay in cell death during a subsequent prolonged ischemic insult. This chapter will discuss the exciting results from the many experiments investigating the scope and mechanism of ischemic preconditioning. It should be noted, especially when clinical applications are being considered, that pretreatment is nec-

TABLE 4-1. PRECONDITIONING: DEFINITIONS

Term	Definition
Ischemic preconditioning	A rapid adaptation occurring in response to a brief episode of sublethal ischemia that leads to protection against the injury induced by a longer, lethal ischemic episode
Preconditioning protocol	The sequence of brief ischemic and reperfusion periods used to induce ischemic preconditioning
Ischemic insult	The prolonged (sustained) ischemic episode that causes myocardial injury
End points	Markers of myocardial injury measured by experimenters in order to quantitate the degree of injury
Myocardial protection	The reduction in injury induced by preconditioning or another treatment
Adenosine	A nucleoside formed from the breakdown of high-energy phosphates (e.g., ATP, ADP, AMP) that can diffuse out of the myocyte
PKC isoforms	Protein kinases involved in intracellular signaling that phosphorylate (activate) other enzymes, proteins, and channels
K_{ATP} channel	An ion channel, sensitive to ATP levels, regulating potassium transport across the cell and mitochondrial membrane

essary before sustained ischemia. Therefore, if the adaptation is to be exploited as a therapeutic tool it will be limited to situations when ischemia is scheduled as a necessary part of a treatment, for example in cardiac surgery. It must also be remembered that to date no intervention has actually prevented infarction; if ischemic myocardium is not reperfused, myocardial necrosis is inevitable. Preconditioning delays this cell death. Therefore, for a given ischemic challenge there will be less necrosis in preconditioned hearts when compared to control hearts. Some of the terms used in the following sections are explained in Table 4-1.

BIOLOGY OF ISCHEMIC PRECONDITIONING

Following the first report, preconditioning has now been demonstrated by others in dogs (Li et al., 1990), and also observed in pigs (Schott et al., 1990), rabbits (Iwamoto et al., 1991), and rats (Yellon et al., 1992), proving that it is a highly conserved phenomenon. The increasing evidence for ischemic preconditioning occurring in humans is discussed in Chapter 6.

As well as delaying the onset of infarction, which was the original experimental end point and the criterion used to define the adaptation, preconditioning has also been shown to protect against other effects of ischemia/reperfusion injury. Many different models have been used incorporating both in vivo and in vitro hearts from different species and a multitude of end points. Preconditioning has been shown to reduce reperfusion arrhythmias (Shiki et al., 1987), slow energy metabolism during the early stages of ischemia (Murry et al., 1990), improve postischemic recovery of function (Cave et al., 1992), protect the coronary endothelium (Richard et al., 1994), increase the postischemic-developed tension in isolated atrial trabeculae muscles following simulated ischemia (Walker et al., 1995), and increase the resistance of isolated myocytes to hypoxic injury (Armstrong & Ganote, 1994) and simulated ischemia (Ikonomidis et al., 1994). However, it is possible that an underlying limitation of infarction contributes to the protection observed in many of these experiments despite the fact that another end point has been recorded. This notwithstanding, in the majority of studies volume of infarction has been used as the major end point following regional ischemia and reperfusion in dog and rabbit hearts.

TIME COURSE OF ISCHEMIA AND REPERFUSION PERIODS IN PRECONDITIONING

Although the effect of preconditioning is as powerful and more reproducible than previous pharmacological interventions aimed at preserving ischemic myocardium, the phenomenon described in the seminal paper is short lived (Murry et al., 1986).

Decay of protection

If the interval between the brief preconditioning ischemia and the sustained insult is extended any longer than 1 hour in canine hearts, the protection is attenuated and is only half as powerful by 2 hours (Murry et al., 1991). In the smaller animals with faster heart rates (rats and rabbits), the decay in protection after preconditioning is even more rapid. Another interesting and clinically relevant finding is that the window of protection induced by preconditioning can be extended to 2 hours in the in vivo rabbit model if acadesine (a nucleoside that acts as an adenosine-regulating agent) is infused at the time of the preconditioning stimulus and continued for 60 minutes (Tsuchida et al., 1994c). In the group receiving acadesine without preconditioning, infarct size did not differ from that in control hearts. Acadesine is believed to work by increasing tissue adenosine levels during ischemia and this concept is substantiated by the results of the latter study because 8-p-sulphophenyl theophylline (an adenosine antagonist) prevented the extended protection at 2 hours. Of interest, acadesine is a drug that is being evaluated as a means to improved myocardial protection in patients undergoing coronary artery bypass surgery.

It is now accepted that there is also a delayed but longer lasting period of preconditioning protection against infarction and lethal arrhythmia, and this second window of protection will be discussed in detail in Chapter 5. It has been shown that preconditioning is not a once-only phenomenon—protection can be reinstated by a second preconditioning protocol after the advantage conferred by the first has waned (Li and Kloner, 1994; Sack et al., 1993; Yang et al., 1993). However, in a rabbit model allowing multiple repetition of the preconditioning protocol or prolonged adenosine infusion, Downey and colleagues found that tolerance develops after 3 days of preconditioning and the protection against sustained ischemia is lost (Cohen et al., 1994; Tsuchida et al., 1994b).

Limits of protection

The degree of protection from preconditioning is not unlimited and if the duration of the sustained ischemia is extended from 1 to 3 hours of regional ischemia in dog hearts the beneficial effect of preconditioning on infarct size is lost and infarct volume is equal in control and preconditioned hearts (Murry et al., 1986; Flack et al., 1991). Hence it is more accurate to say that necrosis is *delayed* by preconditioning rather than prevented. The delay of necrosis induced by preconditioning was about 20 minutes in the regionally ischemic dog model, assessed by measuring the time to ultrastructural appearance of irreversibility (Murry et al., 1990). However, in the isolated rabbit heart subjected to 15, 20, or 30 minutes of global ischemia, the delay in infarction induced by preconditioning was only 10 minutes (Jenkins et al., 1995).

Induction of protection

The preconditioning protocol used in experiments has varied between investigators and different animal models, but it appears that as long as a minimum degree of ischemia is obtained (whether by a single episode or multiple episodes) and a threshold level of endogenous agonist is reached, then protection will be conferred. A number of preconditioning protocols have been designed (including the 4×5 minutes of the original study) and further animal experiments have demonstrated that one period of 5 minutes is effective. Indeed, in the two most common species studied, the rabbit and the dog, a single 5-minute period of ischemia has been found to precondition (Jenkins et al., 1995; Gross & Auchrampach, 1992). In rabbits it has been shown that a single period of 2-minute ischemia is not enough to induce preconditioning, but that in the presence of acadesine 2-minute ischemia is enough (Tsuchida et al., 1993). Dipyridamole, a nucleoside transport inhibitor that increases interstitial adenosine during ischemia, has a similar effect in rabbits. When rabbits were treated with 0.25 mg/kg dipyridamole, marginal protection from 2-minute preconditioning ischemia was potentiated and infarction following 30-minute regional ischemia was significantly reduced (Miura et al., 1992). The longest ischemic protocol used to precondition (two periods of 10-minute regional ischemia separated by 30 minutes of reperfusion) has been reported in pigs (Schott et al., 1990).

It is not necessary to abolish coronary flow completely in order to precondition. Ovize and colleagues (1992a) showed that variations in coronary flow, mimicking conditions in human coronary artery disease, can precondition the dog heart. More surprisingly the same group found that preconditioning of the circumflex coronary bed in the dog reduced infarction in the left anterior descending coronary bed (Przyklenk et al., 1993). This "remote" preconditioning in the dog heart was subsequently thought to be due to the effect of stretch via stretch-activated (gadolinium-sensitive) ion channels (Ovize et al., 1994). This finding has important implications for experimental methodology since many isolated muscle and myocyte preparations may involve some stretching. Others have shown that it is possible to precondition using hypoxia (Lasley et al., 1993; Shizukuda et al., 1992), but it should be remembered that the latter protocols are very different from those described in the original definition of ischemic preconditioning.

The minimum length of time necessary to reperfuse before the sustained ischemia has only been assessed in one study. In the rat model of regional ischemia in vivo, 30 seconds of reperfusion is not enough but 1 minute is sufficient (Alkhulaifi et al., 1993). It is theoretically possible that this interval is necessary to wash out catabolites or to allow time for signal transduction within the myocyte, but the latter explanation is more likely in the light of the discovery that preconditioning is possible in the pig with a protocol of 30 minutes of coronary flow reduction immediately before complete occlusion with no reperfusion (Koning et al., 1994). It is possible that the optimum protocol for preconditioning is species and model dependent, and will vary with the degree of collateralization, heart size, heart rate, and myocardial temperature.

PROTECTION AGAINST ARRYTHMIA

There is increasing literature on the effect of prior brief ischemia on ischemia- and reperfusion-induced arrhythmia. The fact that pretreatment with brief ischemia delayed ischemia-induced ventricular arrhythmia had been known for years and predates the preconditioning era. Shiki and Hearse (1987) demonstrated that preconditioning reduced reperfusion-induced arrhythmia following regional myocardial ischemia in vivo in rats and that the time course of this effect was similar to that seen for the infarct-delaying property. Vegh and colleagues (1990, 1992) were the first to specifically study the effect of preconditioning on ischemia-induced arrhythmia in dogs and demonstrated a profound protection against lethal ventricular arrhythmia. Later Lawson demonstrated that, in the rat, preconditioning caused an absolute reduction in ischemic-induced arrhythmia rather than a delay in appearance (Lawson et al., 1993). It was also demonstrated that the protection against ischemia- and reperfusion-induced arrhythmia was dose dependent, with more cycles of preconditioning resulting in better protection (Lawson et al., 1993b). At the time, it was thought that this was a major difference between the protection against arrhythmia and infarction, but it is now recognized that multiple cycles of preconditioning ischemia probably give better protection against infarction. Some confusion has resulted from the results of experiments designed with infarct size as the major end point reporting arrhythmia as well, and in general separate experiments and protocols should be designed specifically with arrhythmia as the main end point. This is one of the reasons why the results of experiments investigating the mechanism of the infarct-sparing property of preconditioning may not be relevant to its antiarrhythmic properties.

ISCHEMIC PRECONDITIONING AND POSTISCHEMIC VENTRICULAR FUNCTION

The evidence for a beneficial effect of preconditioning is more complicated when recovery of contractile function is used as the end point rather than infarct size. This is largely due to the differences in models used and parameters measured, and the fact that postischemic ventricular function is dependent on both the amount of irreversible injury (necrosis) and the degree of reversible injury in surviving myocytes (stunning). Stunning can be defined as a depression of contractile performance in viable myocardium seen on reperfusion following ischemia, which is fully reversible with continued reperfusion. Although by definition stunning is fully reversible, it is of clinical relevance and probably accounts for some of the reduced contractility observed in some patients recovering from cardiac surgery and acute myocardial infarction.

It is clear that ischemic preconditioning in isolated perfused rat hearts prior to a period of global ischemia results in better recovery of postischemic ventricular function (Asimakis et al., 1992; Cave et al., 1992; Lasley et al., 1993). What is unclear is to what degree the postischemic ventricular dysfunction measured in these models is a manifestation of myocyte necrosis or a result of stunning, because the ischemic insult used in many isolated heart experiments would be long enough to cause some necrosis. In these preparations the experiment can never be continued long enough to show complete recovery after ischemia and so the definition of stunning is not fulfilled; hence, to be accepted as a true stunning model, necrosis should be absent. Therefore, it is difficult to decide from the postischemic ventricular function results reported whether preconditioning reduces necrosis, stunning, or both in these models. Studies in isolated rabbit hearts have revealed that when postischemic functional recovery and infarct size are evaluated in the same hearts preconditioning reduces infarction without necessarily improving overall recovery of ventricular function (Sandhu et al., 1993). Further studies have demonstrated that the measurable improvement in recovery of preconditioned hearts following regional or global ischemia in vitro correlates with the infarct size limitation, suggesting that most of the benefit is the result of a reduced infarction (Jenkins et al., 1995; Walker et al., 1993). When left ventricular function is plotted against infarct volume the regression lines demonstrate that for a given infarct volume the postischemic ventricular function in preconditioned hearts is no different from that in controls (Jenkins et al., 1995).

Other experiments have attempted to measure ventricular function in in vivo models of regional myocardial infarction. One study designed to monitor regional wall motion in vivo using ultrasonic crystals implanted in the mid myocardium of rabbits showed improved postischemic segment shortening on reperfusion in preconditioned hearts, but these hearts also had significantly smaller infarcts (3.0 ± 1.6% vs. 28.8 ± 7.0%) compared with controls (Cohen et al., 1991). Thus in this study the improvement in regional wall motion was influenced by the amount of necrosis. Many of the experiments reported in dogs and pigs have provided confusing results with some suggesting improved function and others no change, but the position of the ultrasonic crystals has varied. It is therefore not surprising that experiments employing ultrasonic crystals to monitor segment shortening in models of regional infarction give conflicting results because the effects of ischemia vary as one moves from endocardium to epicardium.

Some studies have employed an alternative protocol to investigate ventricular function using shorter, regional ischemic insults, which cause true stunning without necrosis. Ovize and coworkers (1992b) used a 15-minute regional ischemic insult in anesthetized dogs, and postischemic ventricular function (determined by ultrasonic crystals measuring systolic shortening) was not improved with 2.5 or 5 minutes of preconditioning. In apparent contrast one study has shown less stunning occurring during successive, 5-minute regional ischemic periods in rabbits (Bunch et al., 1992).

Taking all the results together it is more likely that the preconditioning induced improvement in postischemic ventricular function (at least following longer ischemic periods) is the result of reduction in myocyte necrosis rather than a true attenuation of stunning.

METABOLIC STUDIES

Originally it was the unexpected metabolic changes occurring during repetitive ischemia and reperfusion that led to the concept of preconditioning. Since then the metabolic changes have been examined in more detail. Murry and colleagues (1990) demonstrated that the preconditioning protocol (ischemia) lowered myocardial ATP levels, but following this the decline in ATP during the first 20 minutes of a 40-minute sustained ischemic period in anesthetized dogs was much less rapid in the preconditioned myocardium than in the control. They found that the ATP content of the preconditioned hearts was significantly higher after 10 minutes of sustained ischemia (12.4 ± 0.5 µmol/g) than in controls (9.1 ± 0.8 µmol/g). However, at the end of 40 minutes of sustained ischemia the ATP content was equally low in both groups. In the same study they found reduced lactate production in preconditioned myocardium during ischemia, suggesting reduced anaerobic glycolysis and, hence, evidence for reduced utilization preserving ATP rather than increased production; this has been confirmed by others (Wolfe et al., 1993).

Since then there have been numerous reports demonstrating a similar, slower decline in high-energy phosphate content in preconditioned tissue during the early phase of sustained ischemia in dogs and pigs (Flack et al., 1991; Jennings et al., 1991; Kida et al., 1991; Miyamae et al., 1993), and also in patients during cardiac surgery (Yellon et al., 1993). This effect appears to be less dramatic in studies using rats (Banerjee et al., 1993; Steenbergen et al., 1993; Volovsek et al., 1992; Vuorinen et al., 1995; Wolfe et al., 1993) and most report equally low levels by the end of a 30-minute sustained ischemic period. There is also evidence for improved recovery of ATP during reperfusion in preconditioned hearts (Albuquerque et al., 1994; Banerjee et al., 1993; Flack et al., 1991; Miyamae et al., 1993; Vuorinen et al., 1995; Wolfe et al., 1993), but this increased recovery is not significant in all studies (Schott et al., 1990) and was not apparent in some (Cave et al., 1992; Ovize et al., 1992b). A recent report comparing ischemic preconditioning with cardioplegia and controls in isolated, blood-perfused rat hearts demonstrated that preconditioning actually accelerated the decline in ATP during sustained ischemia (Kolocassides et al., 1995). This finding is consistent with the earlier onset of ischemic contracture observed after preconditioning in the globally ischemic rat heart, but is contradictory to reports in other species and is difficult to reconcile with the fact that the same preconditioning protocol protects the rat heart from ischemic injury in terms of postischemic functional recovery.

In isolated dog hearts it has been shown that adenosine infusion (0.35–1.0 mg/ml for 7–12 min) into the circumflex arterial bed prior to ischemia slowed the rate of ATP depletion during the first 20 minutes of total ischemia compared to that in a control arterial bed (Vander Heide et al., 1993). Recently the metabolic effects of transient adenosine infusion have been compared directly to those of ischemic preconditioning in in vivo pig hearts subjected to 15 minutes of regional ischemia (Yokota et al., 1995). Both ischemic preconditioning and adenosine pretreatment resulted in significant preservation of ATP during ischemia, and equally significant recovery in ATP content during reperfusion. The latter studies demonstrate that the metabolic effects of adenosine treatment, infused prior to ischemia in the dog and pig are the same as those of ischemic preconditioning.

Studies using NMR imaging to follow the metabolic changes during ischemia and reperfusion have been able to estimate intracellular pH and ATP noninvasively and repeatedly. These experiments show that preconditioning reduces acidosis during ischemia (Wolfe et al., 1993) and that this effect correlates better with functional recovery of isolated hearts than the preservation of ATP (Albuquerque et al., 1994). Vuorinen and colleagues (1995) recently reported ATP content and intracellular pH measurements using NMR imaging in isolated rat hearts and, like the latter study, they found significantly less intracellular acidosis at the end of 21 minutes of ischemia in preconditioned hearts, but unlike Albuquerque and coworkers they also observed a reduced rate of ATP decline during early ischemia in preconditioned hearts and improved recovery of ATP levels during reperfusion. It should be noted that these latter results obtained in the rat may not necessarily be true for all species. The most recent report has demonstrated that the preservation of pH seen in preconditioned rat hearts by NMR imaging was not due to better buffering capacity, but to reduced proton generation (Albuquerque et al., 1995).

It is not understood how the time course of ATP changes is linked to the infarct-delaying effect of preconditioning, especially since the difference in ATP content between control and preconditioned hearts is small and temporary and all hearts have equally low levels of ATP at the end of the long ischemic period. However, it is now recognized that ATP is compartmentalized within the cell and at present we are only able to measure gross tissue content, so the results and interpretation are necessarily crude. The importance of the ATP changes in relation to the mechanism of preconditioning has been questioned because of the results from the rat NMR imaging experiments, but the characteristic ATP changes are certainly associated with preconditioning in larger animals even if they have not been proven to be causal to the infarct limitation. Although the concept of a critical ATP content for cell viability is probably too simplistic (Opie, 1993), the principle that energy conservation and limitation of acidosis can delay myocyte necrosis is logical. Therefore, one might expect that any hypothesis proposed to explain the subcellular mechanism of preconditioning should in some way be linked to these metabolic changes. However, one of the greatest problems is that the final cause of cell death is not understood and it is difficult to decipher which of the many factors involved are associations and which are actually causal (Opie, 1993).

MECHANISM OF PRECONDITIONING

Preconditioning is not simply explained by the brief ischemia opening up collateral vessels, as the protection is present for any given collateral flow in dogs (Murry et al.,

1986), is present in species without significant collateral flow (Schott et al., 1990), and is evident in isolated hearts subjected to global ischemia (Asimakis et al., 1992). The ability to precondition isolated hearts perfused with crystalloid buffer rather than blood also means that blood is not necessary to precondition (Jenkins et al., 1995; Sandhu et al., 1993). Another early suggestion to explain the effect of preconditioning can also be dismissed. It is known that brief regional ischemia can lead to localized stunning and it was thought that the resulting reduced metabolic demand in the stunned myocardium could lead to less necrosis during sustained ischemia. However, preconditioning and stunning have been dissociated since their time courses are different (Murry et al., 1991), the degree of stunning by different ischemic protocols does not correlate with the degree of subsequent protection (Miura et al., 1991), and reversing any stunning caused by the preconditioning protocol with dobutamine failed to prevent preconditioning (Matsuda et al., 1993).

Any hypothesis proposed to explain the protective mechanism of ischemic preconditioning should be able to incorporate the known facts: The process is triggered by ischemia itself, the change induced is rapid and the initial effect is short lived, the phenomenon occurs at the level of the myocyte and appears to be independent of other cellular elements, the process is associated with a reduced intracellular acidosis during ischemia and/or a reduced rate of ATP depletion, and the end result is a delay in cell death. After discarding the original physical theories (localized stunning and increased collateral flow) as explanations for reduced energy demand and therefore myocardial salvage during ischemia, attention has turned to the changes occurring within the myocyte.

Much of the data discussed here have been obtained from experiments using regional myocardial ischemia in vivo in dogs, pigs, and rabbits with infarct size—determined by histology or tetrazolium staining—as the end point, expressed as a percentage of the volume of myocardium made ischemic. Because of our limited ability to measure components of the subcellular signal transduction systems directly, much of the evidence implicating given enzymes or channels is necessarily indirect. In most experiments two methods of investigation have dominated. Exogenously applied agonists or activators have been used in attempts to induce similar protection to preconditioning and/or antagonists, or inhibitors have been infused in attempts to prevent ischemic preconditioning. Another factor that should be remembered is that the ischemic insults employed in many of the experimental models are designed specifically for the model in question and an intervention that produces a dramatic effect in one experiment may not be so beneficial when the ischemic time is shorter or longer. The mechanism of the antiarrhythmic effect of preconditioning seen in rat and dog hearts may well be different and is discussed elsewhere (Parratt, 1994; Parratt & Kane, 1994).

Adenosine

Adenosine (an endogenous nucleoside resulting from the breakdown of high-energy phosphates in myocytes during ischemia) was originally considered to be one of the most likely candidates to initiate preconditioning because it was known to be formed during ischemia and was already known to protect the myocardium. Downey and colleagues were the first to investigate the role of adenosine in preconditioning. They used an in vivo rabbit model of regional ischemia, to show that antagonists of adenosine receptors (8-p-sulphophenyl theophylline and PD1151199) could prevent ischemic preconditioning and intracoronary infusion of adenosine or the A1 receptor agonist R-phenyl-isopropyladenosine (R-PIA) could reduce infarct size, measured by tetrazolium staining, to the same extent as ischemic preconditioning (Liu et al., 1991). This work on the infarct-limiting mechanism of preconditioning has been confirmed, using histology to measure infarct size in the rabbit (Tsuchida et al., 1992; Tsuchida et al., 1993).

The fact that agents that augment endogenous adenosine levels (acadesine and dipyridamole) lower the threshold for ischemic preconditioning and extend the window of protection is further evidence for the importance of adenosine. Adenosine has also been shown to slow metabolism during the first 20 minutes of sustained ischemia in the dog in a similar way to ischemic preconditioning (Vander Heide et al., 1993). The latter work not only links adenosine to the metabolic sparing effects of ischemic preconditioning, but confirms its importance in the dog, as does a more recent piece of work (Yao & Gross, 1994a). However, in the study by Yao and Gross a 10-minute intracoronary infusion of adenosine was as effective as 10 minutes of ischemia and 10 minutes of reperfusion. But when the reperfusion interval was extended to 60 minutes, ischemic preconditioning significantly reduced infarction but adenosine did not. Likewise, inhibition of adenosine deaminase with pentostatin raised interstitial adenosine levels in the dog, but did not reduce infarction (Silva et al., 1995). Therefore, it is probable that in some species other endogenous initiators are involved in the preconditioning response. Adenosine and R-PIA given by intermittent coronary infusion reduce infarction in the pig heart (Van Winkle et al., 1994). However, there is evidence against adenosine initiating preconditioning in all species; the protection of ischemic preconditioning against infarction and postischemic recovery of function does not appear to be blocked by adenosine antagonists in the isolated rat heart (Li and Kloner, 1993; Cave et al., 1993). The evidence for involvement of adenosine in other species is strong, but the actual receptor subtype has recently been questioned. The adenosine receptors were originally classified into A1 and A2 according to their relative selectivity for adenosine analogs, and recently a third subtype has been recognized—the A3 receptor. The original in vivo rabbit experiments suggested that adenosine triggered preconditioning via the A1 receptor (Liu et al., 1991), but in an isolated rabbit myocyte preparation the specific A1 antagonist 1,3-dipropyl-8-cyclopentylxanthine (DPCPX) did not attenuate ischemic preconditioning, but the A1/A3 receptor antagonist BW 1433U did (Armstrong & Ganote, 1994). In a parallel series of experiments by Downey's group the same result was obtained in isolated rabbit hearts (Liu et al., 1994a). It is possible that both A1 and A3 receptors are involved in preconditioning, but it should be remembered that this evidence is indirect and the presence of A3 receptors in ventricular muscle is not yet confirmed.

Noradrenaline

In the rat it was thought that noradrenaline rather than adenosine might be the most important endogenous initiator of preconditioning via 1-adrenergic receptors. In the isolated rat heart subjected to global ischemia Banerjee and colleagues (1993) demonstrated that phenylepherine or noradrenaline could precondition and phentolamine blocked ischemic preconditioning with recovery of postischemic function as the end point. These findings were confirmed in a subsequent study examining ventricular function in isolated rat hearts where it was demonstrated that stimulation of α_{1B} receptors caused preconditioning and that this led to activation of a pertussis toxin-sensitive G-protein and PKC (Hu & Nattel, 1995). The latter intracellular signaling pathways are discussed in more detail later. However, another study has examined catecholamine-induced preconditioning in the rat with infarct size as the end point and the conclusions are different. In isolated rat hearts subjected to regional ischemia it has been found that blockade of receptors with phenoxybenzamine does not prevent the infarct size reduction of ischemic preconditioning, but that inhibition of PKC with polymixin or chelerythrine does prevent the protection (Bugge & Ytrehus, 1995). Grover has recently demonstrated that endogenous catecholamines are not necessary for ischemic preconditioning since hearts from reserpinized animals could be preconditioned (Weselcouch et al., 1995). Therefore, at present, the role of noradrenaline as the main endogenous initiator of preconditioning in the rat is not certain and the discrepant results between models remains unexplained.

Signal transduction

The adenosine hypothesis has been extended by Downey's group by investigating the intracellular signaling pathways. The next logical step was to investigate the G-proteins (named because of their guanine nucleotide binding property). G-proteins can interact with many different cell surface receptors and act as a link between receptor occupancy and intracellular signaling for these coupled receptors. The G-proteins have important regulating properties and exist in two forms: stimulatory (G_S) and inhibitory (G_i), which are sensitive to two different bacterial toxins, cholera and pertussis respectively, allowing differentiation between the two in experiments. Downey's group found that a pertussis toxin, which inactivates G_i protein, could abolish preconditioning in the in vivo rabbit heart and that other receptors coupled to G-proteins (e.g., muscarinic) could initiate preconditioning (Thornton et al., 1993a).

Next, the G-protein-coupled effector systems within the cell were examined. G-proteins interact with two major intracellular pathways: the adenylate cyclase/cAMP system and the phospholipase/inositol tris-phosphate/diacylglycerol system (as well as with guanylate cyclase and directly with ion channels). Most investigations of the signaling mechanism involved in preconditioning have concentrated on the latter system simply because the pharmacological tools to manipulate the components are available. Briefly, in this system G-proteins act on a membrane-bound enzyme (phospholipase C), which splits a phospholipid (phosphatidylinositol) into second messengers (diacylglycerol and inositol tris-phosphate). Inositol tris-phosphate is involved in the regulation of calcium release from intracellular stores and has not been specifically explored in preconditioning experiments, but diacylglycerol regulates a protein kinase C (PKC) and this part of the pathway has been explored further.

Protein kinase C was discovered in the late 1970s and received little attention until it was realized that it was activated by the tumor-promoting phorbol esters. The structural similarity between these phorbol esters and diacylglycerol was recognized and the links realized. It is now known that other phospholipases produce diacylglycerol (phospholipase D) and thus activate PKC, and so PKC activation is not limited to G-protein-coupled receptors. Molecular cloning has demonstrated that PKC exists in up to nine different isoforms that can be divided into two main groups according to their calcium sensitivity. Active PKC isoforms phosphorylate the serine and threonine residues of many intracellular and membrane proteins and thus have an enormous range of diverse physiological effects and also interact with other kinase systems. Downey was the first to report that PKC activation is necessary for ischemic preconditioning in the rabbit heart because inhibition of PKC with polymyxin or staurosporin prevented ischemic preconditioning, and activation with phorbol esters resulted in protection (Ytrehus et al., 1994). It was thought that translocation of PKC from cytosol to membrane (which is blocked by the action of colchicine on microtubules) during sustained ischemia might be an important event (Liu et al., 1994b). The time course of this sequence would fit with that of ischemic preconditioning, but it has been difficult to actually demonstrate translocation because PKC, as explained here, exists in multiple isoforms that translocate to different cellular sites with variable time courses. At present, progress on understanding the contribution of PKC is a little limited by the absence of specific activators and inhibitors for its different isoforms and therefore pharmacological interventions are necessarily crude. Also, activation of PKC using compounds like phorbol esters may have very different cellular consequences compared to the physiological activation by diacylglycerol because the binding affinity of the esters is far greater and they are not metabolized.

Recently Sakamoto and associates (1995) have reported that R-PIA-induced protection in rabbits (via adenosine A1/A3 receptors) can be blocked by staurosporine or polymyxin B (both PKC inhibitors). This confirms the previously reported results and is the first direct proof that the protection initiated by adenosine is mediated by activation of PKC.

Evidence is accumulating in other species for the importance of PKC in preconditioning. Yellon's group has recently shown that chelerytherine (another PKC inhibitor) blocks ischemic preconditioning in an in vivo rat model (Speechly-Dick et al., 1994), a species in which adenosine itself does not appear to be an important initiator. This work has been confirmed in the in vivo rat model using the PKC inhibitor calphostin C (Li & Kloner, 1995) and in the isolated rat heart using chelerytherine (Mitchell et al., 1995). Banerjee and colleagues (1993) have also been able to demonstrate translocation of PKC isoforms in the rat. However, so far there is little evidence for the involvement of PKC in ischemic preconditioning in canine models. In the only study to investigate PKC in the dog model preconditioning-induced reduction in infarction was not prevented by the PKC inhibitors H-7 and polymyxin B. In addition there was no evidence of PKC translocation to the cell membrane when the cells were stained with a fluorescent probe for PKC (Przyklenk et al., 1995).

It might follow that the stimulation of any receptor that eventually activates PKC should result in preconditioning. Downey's group has accumulated considerable evidence in support of this theory in the rabbit including alpha adrenergic agonists (Tsuchida et al., 1994a), angiotensin II (Liu et al., 1995), and bradykinin (Goto et al., 1995). In the latter study this concept was developed by demonstrating that there is redundancy in the pathways leading to PKC activation, and in the rabbit both adenosine and bradykinin are physiologically important. Blocking adenosine or bradykinin receptors prevented the infarct-limiting effect of one 5-minute cycle of preconditioning ischemia, but when the preconditioning stimulus was increased to four cycles, blockade of one receptor population was not enough to prevent preconditioning. Downey's results suggest that brief ischemia leads to the release of a number of agonists (adenosine, noradrenaline, bradykinin) and that if a threshold level of PKC stimulation is reached, protection will result. Increased release of one agonist, stimulated by additional preconditioning cycles, can compensate for lack of another and the relative importance of each may vary between species.

K_{ATP} channels

The other major hypothesis for the mechanism of preconditioning involves K_{ATP} channels. It had been known for years that ischemia caused rapid shortening of the action potential duration as a result of a potassium efflux, but it was only in 1983 that the cause of this action was discovered. Noma (1983) reported the presence of potassium channels in ventricular myocytes that were regulated by the intracellular ATP concentration. It is known that these channels are numerous in the cell membrane and are normally in the closed state but open rapidly in response to the declining energy status of the cell during ischemia and hypoxia. It is now realized that there are many regulators of the channel and the ADP/ATP ratio is more important than the ATP concentration alone. The actual function of these channels remains unknown but it has been postulated that they have a cardioprotective action even though they are known to exist in other tissues. It is thought that the opening of K_{ATP} channels during ischemia leads to increased potassium conductance and shortening of the action potential duration, which limits calcium entry, depressing contractility and decreasing energy metabolism.

In dogs, Gross and Auchampach (1992) found that glibenclamide (a blocker of K_{ATP} channels) could abolish the infarct size limitation of preconditioning. This has been repeated with a more specific, ischemia-sensitive K_{ATP} channel blocker, 5-hydroxydecanoate (Auchampach et al., 1992) and was also shown in pigs (Schulz et al., 1994). There is also substantial evidence in the rat and dog heart to confirm the hypothesis that K_{ATP} channel-opening drugs are cardioprotective (Auchampach et al., 1994; Grover et al., 1990; Hearse, 1995). Recently in a model of superfused human atrial trabeculae it was found that the recovery from simulated ischemia was enhanced in ischemic preconditioning and cromakalim-treated muscles, and that this protection was abolished by glibenclamide (Speechly-Dick et al., 1995).

Interestingly, some investigators have tried to connect the adenosine and K_{ATP} channel hypotheses by examining the cardioprotective actions of adenosine in the presence of K_{ATP} channel blockers. It has been suggested that the K_{ATP} channel may be the "end effector" of preconditioning and there is evidence indicating that opening of the channel is a "downstream" event to receptor-mediated initiation. In pigs it has been shown that ischemia, adenosine, and R-PIA all reduced regional infarct size and when the K_{ATP} channel blocker 5-hydroxydecanoate was added to R-PIA this protection was lost (Van Winkle et al., 1994). In dogs Yao and Gross (1994b) were able to show that adenosine reduced infarct size to a similar degree as preconditioning with ischemia, and that K_{ATP} channel blockers prevented this effect. These studies provide good evidence that adenosine-induced cardioprotection may involve the opening of K_{ATP} channels. It may be that preconditioning ischemia by releasing adenosine or by PKC activation leads to earlier or greater K_{ATP} channel opening during sustained ischemia. In the superfused human atrial trabeculae model Yellon's group found that the protection induced by PKC activation was blocked by glibenclamide (Speechly-Dick et al., 1995). This is the first evidence to suggest that K_{ATP} channel opening may be a downstream event to PKC activation. Whether the threshold for opening of K_{ATP} channels or the proportion opening or the consequences of opening is altered is not resolved, and the time course and channel state during preconditioning and sustained ischemia is unknown.

However, in contrast to the apparently universal nature of ischemic preconditioning, the evidence for the importance of K_{ATP} channels in ischemic preconditioning in small animal models is conflicting. In the first study in rabbits, Downey and colleagues found that in animals anesthetized with pentobarbitone, glibenclamide (which closes the channel) increased infarct size in control hearts but did not prevent the infarct-delaying action of ischemic preconditioning (Thornton et al., 1993b). However, when Toombs and colleagues (1993) investigated rabbits anesthetized with ketamine/xylazine, the protective effect of ischemic preconditioning was blocked by glibenclamide and this was later substantiated by Downey (Walsh et al., 1994). This difference in results has been attributed to the anesthetic, as in all other respects the models were similar, and this hypothesis has been confirmed recently. Miura and associates (1995) demonstrated that it was the xylazine component that resulted in gliben-clamide blocking ischemic preconditioning. Hence, it appears that the results of in vivo experiments can be influenced by the choice of anesthetic. In fact, in a study comparing ischemic preconditioning in in vivo rabbit models anesthetized with different compounds it was demonstrated that the infarct-delaying properties of preconditioning were much greater with pentobarbitone anesthesia than with ketamine/xylazine (Haessler et al., 1994). Paradoxically many of the canine experiments reporting the significance of the K_{ATP} channel in preconditioning used pentobarbitone anesthesia.

Recently it has been reported that although K_{ATP} channel openers were thought to exert their cardioprotective actions by accelerating channel opening during early ischemia, low doses of bimakalim or nicorandil (other channel openers) were cardioprotective without the action potential duration-shortening actions of the higher doses (Grover et al., 1995; Yao and Cross, 1994b). Although it is not understood how K_{ATP} channel-opening drugs could be cardioprotective without shortening the action potential duration, this result is of potential importance because action potential shortening is theoretically a disadvantage, as it may potentiate arrhythmia. The link between K_{ATP} channels and high-energy phosphate changes has recently been explored in a preparation of a guinea pig-perfused ventricle, confirming that pinacidil inhibited ATP depletion during ischemia (McPherson et al., 1993). However, there remain many unanswered questions. The lack of any correlation between shortening of action potential duration and cardioprotection for the channel openers has brought into question the action of the so-called K_{ATP} channel-opening drugs. It should be remembered that the site of action of these compounds is not really known; they may be acting on mitochondrial K_{ATP} channels as well as sarcolemmal channels, and it may be that sarcolemmal channel opening and potassium efflux is just an epiphenomenon.

A simplified diagram illustrating the probable mechanism(s) of ischemic preconditioning is shown in Figure 4-2.

SUMMARY

This chapter has reviewed the biology of ischemic preconditioning. Ischemic preconditioning can be defined as a rapid adaptation in response to a brief period of ischemia and reperfusion, which results in a delay in cell death during a subsequent, prolonged ischemic insult. This endogenous adaptation seems to be a highly conserved phenomenon and is observed in all species, and although it is reproducible in many experimental models of ischemia/reperfusion injury, the duration of protection against ischemia is only a few hours. Preconditioning delays myocardial necrosis and reduces arrhythmia, and is associated with reduced intracellular acidosis and preservation of high-energy phosphates. As

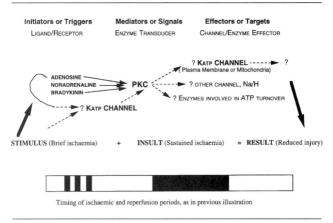

Figure 4-2. Schematic diagram for the potential mechanism of ischemic preconditioning in terms of an initiator-mediator-effector sequence. As indicated, the exact place of K_{ATP} is not certain. Compounds shown in bold type have been proved to be involved in at least two species.

yet, the signal transduction pathways in preconditioning are not finally resolved. In rats and rabbits there is substantial evidence in favor of PKC as an essential step, but there is no evidence for activation of PKC in the dog. However, there is increasing evidence for the importance of K_{ATP} channels in dogs. It is known that activated PKC is important in other species, but it is not known which protein or channel is phosphorylated by PKC. Similarly it is known that K_{ATP} channels are essential in some species but it is unclear whether their role is in initiation of preconditioning or mediation.

Therefore there is much left to discover about the infarction-delaying mechanism of preconditioning and in particular whether there is some step in the signal transduction pathway that is common to all species. It may be that a better understanding of the mechanism of preconditioning will result in a greater appreciation of the ultimate cause of myocyte death in ischemia. However, we have learned that adenosine receptors and K_{ATP} channels are intimately related to preconditioning, and cardioprotective drugs to stimulate the receptor and open the channel respectively are available for use in humans. Therefore, the protective potential of preconditioning may be explored in patients even without a full knowledge of the initiator-mediator-effector sequence for each species.

REFERENCES

Albuquerque CP, Gerstenblith G, Weiss RG. Importance of metabolic inhibition and cellular pH in mediating preconditioning contractile and metabolic effects in rat hearts. *Circ Res* 1994; 74: 139–150.

Albuquerque CP, Gerstenblith G, Weiss RG. Myocardial buffering capacity in ischemia preconditioned rat hearts. *J Mol Cell Cardiol* 1995; 27: 777–781.

Alkhulaifi AM, Pugsley WB, Yellon DM. The influence of the time period between preconditioning ischemia and prolonged ischemia on myocardial protection. *Cardioscience* 1993; 4: 163–169.

Armstrong S, Ganote CE. Adenosine receptor specificity in preconditioning of isolated rabbit cardiomyocytes: evidence of A3 receptor involvement. *Cardiovasc Res* 1994; 28: 1049–1056.

Asimakis GK, Inners-McBride K, Medellin G, Conti VR. Ischemic preconditioning attenuates acidosis in isolated rat heart. *Am J Physiol* 1992; 263: H887–H894.

Auchampach JA, Grover GJ, Gross GJ. Blockade of ischemic preconditioning in dogs by the novel ATP dependent potassium channel antagonist sodium 5-hydroxydecanoate. *Cardiovasc Res* 1992; 26: 1054–1062.

Auchampach JA, Maruyama M, Gross GJ. Cardioprotective actions of potassium channel openers. *Eur Heart J* 1994; 15: 89–94.

Banerjee A, Locke-Winter C, Rogers KB, et al. Preconditioning against myocardial dysfunction after ischemia and reperfusion by an alpha1-adrenergic mechanism. *Circ Res* 1993; 73: 656–670.

Bugge E, Ytrehus K. Ischemic preconditioning is protein kinase C dependent but not through stimulation of adrenergic or adenosine receptors in the isolated rat heart. *Cardiovasc Res* 1995; 29: 401–406.

Bunch FT, Thornton J, Cohen MV, Downey JM. Adenosine is an endogenous protectant against stunning during repetitive ischemic episodes in the heart. *Am Heart J* 1992; 124: 1440–1446.

Cave AC, Collis CS, Downey JM, Hearse DJ. Improved functional recovery by ischemic preconditioning is not mediated by adenosine in the globally ischemic rat heart. *Cardiovasc Res* 1993; 27: 663–668.

Cave AC, Hearse DJ. Ischemic preconditioning and contractile function: studies with normothermic and hypothermic global ischemia. *J Mol Cell Cardiol* 1992; 24: 1113–1123.

Cohen MV, Liu GS, Downey JM. Preconditioning causes improved wall motion as well as smaller infarcts after transient coronary occlusion in rabbits. *Circulation* 1991; 84: 341–349.

Cohen MV, Yang XM, Downey JM. Conscious rabbits become tolerant to multiple episodes of ischemic preconditioning. *Circ Res* 1994; 74: 998–1004.

Flack JE, Kimura Y, Engelman RM, et al. Preconditioning the heart by repeated stunning improves myocardial salvage. *Circulation* 1991; 84(Suppl III): III369–III374.

Goto M, Liu Y, Yang X-M, et al. Role of bradykinin in protection of ischemic preconditioning in rabbit hearts. *Circ Res* 1995; 77: 611–621.

Gross GJ, Auchampach JA. Blockade of ATP-sensitive potassium channels prevents myocardial preconditioning in dogs. *Circ Res* 1992; 70: 223–233.

Grover GJ, D'Alonzo AJ, Hess T, et al. Glyburide-reversible cardioprotective effect of BMS-180448 is independent of action potential shortening. *Cardiovasc Res* 1995; 30: 731–738.

Grover GJ, Dzwonczyk S, Parham CS, Sleph PG. The protective effects of cromakalim and pinacidil on reperfusion function and infarct size in isolated perfused rat hearts and anesthetized dogs. *Cardiovasc Drug Ther* 1990; 4: 465–474.

Haessler R, Kuzume K, Chien GL, et al. Anesthetics alter the magnitude of infarct limitation by ischemic preconditioning. *Cardiovasc Res* 1994; 28: 1574–1580.

Hearse DJ. Activation of ATP-sensitive potassium channels: a novel pharmacological approach to myocardial protection? *Cardiovasc Res* 1995; 30: 1–17.

Hu K, Nattel S. Mechanisms of ischemic preconditioning in rat hearts. *Circulation* 1995; 92: 2259–2265.

Ikonomidis JS, Tumiati LC, Weisel RD, et al. Preconditioning human ventricular cardiomyocytes with brief periods of simulated ischemia. *Cardiovasc Res* 1994; 28: 1285–1291.

Iwamoto T, Miura T, Adachi T, et al. Myocardial infarct size-limiting effect of ischemic preconditioning was not attenuated by oxygen free-radical scavengers in the rabbit. *Circulation* 1991; 83: 1015–1022.

Jenkins DP, Pugsley WB, Yellon DM. Ischemic preconditioning in a model of global ischemia: infarct size limitation but no reduction of stunning. *J Mol Cell Cardiol* 1995; 27: 1623–1632.

Jennings RB, Murry CE, Reimer KA. Energy metabolism in preconditioned and control myocardium: effect of total ischemia. *J Mol Cell Cardiol* 1991; 23: 1449–1458.

Kida M, Fujiwara H, Ishida M, et al. Ischemic preconditioning preserves creatine phosphate and intracellular pH. *Circulation* 1991; 84: 2495–2503.

Kolocassides KG, Galinanes M, Hearse DJ. Preconditioning accelerates contracture and ATP depletion in blood-perfused rat hearts. *Am J Physiol* 1995; 269: H1415–H1420.

Koning MMG, Simonis LAJ, de Zeeuw S, et al. Ischemic preconditioning by partial occlusion without intermittent reperfusion. *Cardiovasc Res* 1994; 28: 1146–1151.

Lasley RD, Anderson GM, Mentzer RM. Ischemic and hypoxic preconditioning enhance postischemic recovery of function in the rat heart. *Cardiovasc Res* 1993; 27: 565–570.

Lawson CS, Avkiran M, Shattock MJ, et al. Preconditioning and reperfusion arrhythmias in the isolated rat heart: true protection or temporal shift in vulnerability? *Cardiovasc Res* 1993a; 27: 2274–2281.

Lawson CS, Coltart DJ, Hearse DJ. "Dose"-dependency and temporal characteristics of protection by ischemic preconditioning against ischemia-induced arrhythmias in rat hearts. *J Mol Cell Cardiol* 1993b; 25: 1391–1402.

Li GC, Vasquez JA, Gallagher KP, Lucchesi BR. Myocardial protection with preconditioning. *Circulation* 1990; 82: 609–619.

Li Y, Kloner RA. The cardioprotective effects of ischemic "preconditioning" are not mediated by adenosine receptors in rat hearts. *Circulation* 1993; 87: 1642–1648.

Li Y, Kloner RA. Cardioprotective effects of ischemic preconditioning can be recaptured after they are lost. *J Am Coll Cardiol* 1994; 23: 470–474.

Li Y, Kloner RA. Does protein kinase C play a role in ischemic preconditioning in rat hearts? *Am J Physiol* 1995; 268: H426–431.

Liu GS, Richards SC, Olsson RA, et al. Evidence that the adenosine A3 receptor may mediate the protection afforded by preconditioning in the isolated rabbit heart. *Cardiovasc Res* 1994a; 28: 1057–1061.

Liu GS, Thornton J, Van Win, et al. Protection against infarction afforded by preconditioning is mediated by A1 adenosine receptors in rabbit heart. *Circulation* 1991;84:350–356.

Liu Y, Tsuchida A, Cohen MV, Downey JM.Pretreatment with angiotensin II activates protein kinase C and limits myocardial infarction in isolated rabbit hearts. *J Mol Cell Cardiol* 1995; 27: 883–892.

Liu Y, Ytrehus K, Downey JM. Evidence that translocation of protein kinase C is a key event during ischemic preconditioning of rabbit myocardium. *J Mol Cell Cardiol* 1994b; 26: 661–668.

Matsuda M, Catena TG, Vander Heide RS, et al. Cardiac protection by ischemic preconditioning is not mediated by myocardial stunning. *Cardiovasc Res* 1993; 27: 585–592.

McPherson CD, Pierce GN, Cole WC. Ischemic cardioprotection by ATP-sensitive K channels involves high-energy phosphate preservation. *Am J Physiol* 1993; 265: H1809–H1818.

Mitchell MB, Meng X, Ao L, et al. Preconditioning of isolated rat heart is mediated by protein kinase C. *Circ Res* 1995; 76: 73–81.

Miura T, Goto M, Miki T, et al. Glibenclamide, a blocker of ATP-sensitive potassium channels, abolishes infarct size limitation by preconditioning in rabbits anesthetized with xylazine/pentobarbital but not with pentobarbital alone. *J Cardiovasc Pharmacol* 1995; 25: 531–538.

Miura T, Goto M, Urabe K, et al. Does myocardial stunning contribute to infarct size limitation by ischemic preconditioning? *Circulation* 1991; 84(6): 2504–2512.

Miura T, Ogawa T, Iwamoto T, et al. Dipyridamole potentiates infarct size-limiting effect of ischemic preconditioning. *Circulation* 1992; 86: 979–985.

Miyamae M, Fujiwara H, Kida M, et al. Preconditioning improves energy metabolism during reperfusion but does not attenuate myocardial stunning in porcine hearts. *Circulation* 1993; 88: 223–234.

Murry CE, Jennings RB, Reimer KA. Preconditioning with ischemia: a delay of lethal cell injury in ischemic myocardium. *Circulation* 1986; 74: 1124–1136.

Murry CE, Richard VJ, Jennings RB, Reimer KA. Myocardial protection is lost before contractile function recovers from preconditioning. *Am J Physiol* 1991; 260: H796–H804.

Murry CE, Richard VJ, Reimer KA, Jennings RB. Ischemic preconditioning slows energy metabolism and delays ultrastructural damage during a sustained ischemic episode. *Circ Res* 1990; 66(4): 913–931.

Noma A. ATP-regulated K channels in cardiac muscle. *Nature* 1983; 305: 147–148.

Opie LH. The mechanism of cell death in ischemia. *Eur Heart J* 1993; 14(Suppl G): 31–33.

Ovize M, Kloner RA, Hale SL, Przyklenk K. Coronary cyclic flow variations "precondition" ischemic myocardium. *Circulation* 1992a; 85: 779–789.

Ovize M, Kloner RA, Przyklenk K. Stretch preconditions the myocardium. *Am J Physiol* 1994; 266: H137–H146.

Ovize M, Przyklenk K, Hale SL, Kloner RA. Preconditioning does not attenuate myocardial stunning. *Circulation* 1992b; 85: 2247–2254.

Parratt JR. Protection of the heart by ischemic preconditioning: mechanisms and possible pharmacological exploitation. *TIPS* 1994; 15: 19–25.

Parratt JR, Kane KK. K_{ATP} channels in ischemic preconditioning. *Cardiovasc Res* 1994; 28: 783–787.

Przyklenk K, Bauer B, Ovize M, et al. Regional ischemic preconditioning protects remote virgin myocardium from subsequent sustained coronary occlusion. *Circulation* 1993; 87: 893–899.

Przyklenk K, Sussman MA, Simkhovich BZ, Kloner RA. Does ischemic preconditioning trigger translocation of protein kinase C in the canine model? *Circulation* 1995; 92: 1546–1557.

Reimer KA, Murry CE, Yamasawa I, et al. Four brief periods of ischemia cause no cumulative ATP loss or necrosis. *Am J Physiol* 1986; 251: H1306–H1315.

Richard V, Kaeffer N, Tron C, Thuillez C. Ischemic preconditioning protects against coronary endothelial dysfunction induced by ischemia and reperfusion. *Circulation* 1994; 89: 1254–1261.

Sack S, Mohri M, Arras M, et al. Ischemic preconditioning—time course of renewal in the pig. *Cardiovasc Res* 1993; 27: 551–555.

Sakamoto J, Miura T, Goto M, Iimura O. Limitation of myocardial infarct size by adenosine A1 receptor activation is abolished by protein kinase C inhibitors in the rabbit. *Cardiovasc Res* 1995; 29: 682–688.

Sandhu R, Diaz RJ, Wilson GJ. Comparison of ischemic preconditioning in blood and buffer perfused isolated heart models. *Cardiovasc Res* 1993; 27: 602–607.

Schott RJ, Rohmann S, Braun ER, Schaper W. Ischemic preconditioning reduces infarct size in swine myocardium. *Circ Res* 1990; 66(4): 1133–1142.

Schulz R, Rose J, Heusch G. Involvement of activation of ATP-dependent potassium channels in ischemic preconditioning in swine. *Am J Physiol* 1994; 267: H1341–H1352.

Shiki K, Hearse DJ. Preconditioning of ischemic myocardium: reperfusion-induced arrhythmias. *Am J Physiol* 1987; 253: H1470–H1476.

Shizukuda Y, Mallet RT, Lee S-C, Downey HF. Hypoxic preconditioning of ischemic canine myocardium. *Cardiovasc Res* 1992; 26: 534–542.

Silva PH, Dillon D, Van Wylen DG. Adenosine deaminase inhibition augments interstitial adenosine but does not attenuate myocardial infarction. *Cardiovasc Res* 1995; 29: 616–623.

Speechly-Dick ME, Grover GJ, Yellon DM. Does ischemic preconditioning in the human involve protein kinase C and the ATP-dependent K channel? *Circ Res* 1995; 77: 1030–1035.

Speechly-Dick ME, Mocanu MM, Yellon DM. Protein kinase C. Its role in ischemic preconditioning in the rat. *Circ Res* 1994; 75: 586–590.

Steenbergen C, Perlman ME, London RE, Murphy E. Mechanism of preconditioning. Ionic alterations. *Circ Res* 1993; 72(1): 112–125.

Thornton JD, Liu GS, Downey JM. Pretreatment with pertussis toxin blocks the protective effects of preconditioning: evidence for a G-protein mechanism. *J Mol Cell Cardiol* 1993a; 25: 311–320.

Thornton JD, Thornton CS, Sterling DL, Downey JM. Blockade of ATP-sensitive potassium channels increases infarct size but does not prevent preconditioning in rabbit hearts. *Circ Res* 1993b; 72: 44–49.

Toombs CF, Moore TL, Shebuski RJ. Limitation of infarct size in the rabbit by ischemic preconditioning is reversible with glibenclamide. *Cardiovasc Res* 1993; 27: 617–622.

Tsuchida A, Liu GS, Wilborn WH, Downey JM. Pretreatment with the adenosine A1 selective agonist, 2-chloro-N6-cyclopentyladenosine (CCPA), causes a sustained limitation of infarct size in rabbits. *Cardiovasc Res* 1993; 27: 652–656.

Tsuchida A, Liu Y, Liu GS, et al. Adrenergic agonists precondition rabbit ischemic myocardium independent of adenosine by direct activation of protein kinase C. *Circ Res* 1994a; 75: 576–585.

Tsuchida A, Miura T, Miki T, et al. Role of adenosine receptor activation in myocardial infarct size limitation by ischemic preconditioning. *Cardiovasc Res* 1992; 26: 456–461.

Tsuchida A, Thompson R, Olsson RA, Downey JM. The anti-infarct effect of an adenosine A1-selective agonist is diminished after prolonged infusion as is the cardioprotective effect of ischemic preconditioning in rabbit heart. *J Mol Cell Cardiol* 1994b; 26: 303–311.

Tsuchida A, Yang X, Burckhartt B, et al. Acadesine extends the window of protection afforded by ischemic preconditioning. *Cardiovasc Res* 1994c; 28: 379–383.

Vander Heide RS, Reimer KA, Jennings RB. Adenosine slows ischemic metabolism in vitro: relationship to ischemic preconditioning. *Cardiovasc Res* 1993; 27: 669–673.

Van Winkle DM, Chien GL, Wolff RA, et al. Cardioprotection provided by adenosine receptor activation is abolished by blockade of the K_{ATP} channel. *Cardiovasc Res* 1994; 28: 1337–1341.

Vegh A, Komoro S, Szekeres L, Parratt JR. Antiarrhythmic effects of preconditioning in anesthetized dogs and rats. *Cardiovasc Res* 1992; 26: 487–495.

Vegh A, Szekeres L, Parratt JR. Protective effects of preconditioning of the ischemic myocardium involve cyclo-oxygenase products. *Cardiovasc Res* 1990; 24: 1020–1023.

Volovsek A, Subramanian R, Reboussin D. Effects of duration of ischemia during preconditioning on mechanical function, enzyme release and energy production in the isolated working heart. *J Mol Cell Cardiol* 1992; 24: 1011–1019.

Vuorinen K, Ylitalo K, Peuhkurinen K, et al. Mechanisms of ischemic preconditioning in rat myocardium. *Circulation* 1995; 91: 2810–2818.

Walker DM, Walker JM, Yellon DM. Global myocardial ischemia protects the myocardium from subsequent regional ischemia. *Cardioscience* 1993; 4: 263–266.

Walker DM, Walker JM, Pugsley WB, Pattison CW, Yellon DM. Preconditioning in isolated superfused human muscle. *J Mol Cell Cardiol* 1995; 27: 1349–1357.

Walsh RS, Tsuchida A, Daly JJF, et al. Ketamine-xylazine anesthesia permits a K_{ATP} channel antagonist to attenuate preconditioning in rabbit myocardium. *Cardiovasc Res* 1994; 28: 1337–1341.

Weselcouch EO, Baird AJ, Sleph PG, et al. Endogenous catecholamines are not necessary for ischemic preconditioning in the isolated perfused rat heart. *Cardiovasc Res* 1995; 29: 126–132.

Wolfe CL, Sievers RE, Visseren FLJ, Donnelly TJ. Loss of myocardial protection after preconditioning correlates with the time course of glycogen recovery within the preconditioned segment. *Circulation* 1993; 87: 881–892.

Yang XM, Arnoult S, Tsuchida A, et al. The protection of ischemic preconditioning can be reinstated in the rabbit heart after the initial protection has waned. *Cardiovasc Res* 1993; 27: 556–558.

Yao Z, Gross GJ. A comparison of adenosine-induced cardioprotection and ischemic preconditioning in dogs. *Circulation* 1994a; 89: 1229–1236.

Yao Z, Gross GJ. Effects of the K_{ATP} channel opener bimakalim on coronary blood flow, monophasic action potential duration and infarct size in dogs. *Circulation* 1994b; 89: 1769–1775.

Yellon DM, Alkhulaifi AM, Browne EE, Pugsley WB. Ischemic preconditioning limits infarct size in the rat heart. *Cardiovasc Res* 1992; 26: 983–987.

Yellon DM, Alkhulaifi AM, Pugsley WB. Preconditioning the human myocardium. *Lancet* 1993; 342: 276–277.

Yokota R, Fujiwara H, Miyamae M, et al. Transient adenosine infusion before ischemia and reperfusion protects against metabolic damage in pig hearts. *Am J Physiol* 1995; 268: H1149–H1157.

Ytrehus K, Liu Y, Downey JM. Preconditioning protects ischemic rabbit heart by protein kinase C activation. *Am J Physiol* 1994; 266: H1145–H1152.

CHAPTER 5

Late Adaptive Responses to Sublethal Ischemia: A Second Window of Protection after Preconditioning

Gary F. Baxter
Derek M. Yellon

Ischemic preconditioning of myocardium induces two distinct phases of myocardial protection. The extremely rapid appearance of an ischemia-tolerant state is one of the most striking features of classic preconditioning, but it is well recognized that the protected state is short lived and, depending on the experimental model, no protection is observed 1 to 3 hours after the ischemic preconditioning stimulus (see Chapter 4). There is now increasing experimental evidence for a delayed phase of protection termed the *second window of protection* or *late preconditioning* (Yellon & Baxter, 1995) which appears long after the early protection associated with classic preconditioning has disappeared (Fig 5-1). The second window of protection, as we shall see, is a period of enhanced tolerance to ischemia/reperfusion injury that develops many hours after a sublethal ischemic stimulus. Typically, the second window of protection is observed 24 hours after preconditioning. This form of adaptive cytoprotection is much more prolonged than the protection associated with classic preconditioning. The ischemia-tolerant phenotype is associated with the appearance of new protein activity, probably as a result of genomic modifications. In this chapter, we describe the background leading up to the discovery of the phenomenon, discuss the characteristics and possible mechanisms of protection, and speculate on the relevance of the second window to ischemic heart disease in humans.

THE TISSUE STRESS RESPONSE AS A BASIS FOR THE SECOND WINDOW OF PROTECTION

A complex series of intracellular perturbations occurs during even brief periods of ischemia. Ischemia (and subsequent reperfusion) imposes hypoxic, metabolic, osmotic, and

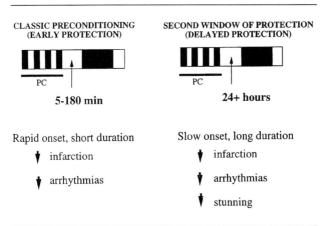

CLASSIC PRECONDITIONING
(EARLY PROTECTION)

PC

5-180 min

SECOND WINDOW OF PROTECTION
(DELAYED PROTECTION)

PC

24+ hours

Rapid onset, short duration

⬇ infarction

⬇ arrhythmias

Slow onset, long duration

⬇ infarction

⬇ arrhythmias

⬇ stunning

Figure 5-1. Preconditioning (PC) of myocardium with brief, intermittent periods of ischemia induces two distinct patterns of protection. An early phase of enhanced tolerance to ischemia/reperfusion injury (classic preconditioning) is apparent within a few minutes but disappears in 1 to 2 hours. A delayed phase of protection (the second window of protection) develops more gradually and is observed 24 hours after preconditioning. This phase of enhanced tolerance to ischemia/reperfusion injury may be sustained over 2 or 3 days.

chemical stresses on the cell that result very rapidly in biochemical and biophysical changes. An important response to a variety of stresses is the *stress response* (or *heat shock response*) (Lindquist, 1986; Minowada & Welch, 1995). This response involves alterations in the patterns of protein activity, intracellular localization, and synthesis, with the result that there is (1) preservation of essential cell functions during and immediately after the period of stress, and (2) induction of a transient tolerant state so that the cell is better able to withstand a subsequent stress. Two classes of intracellular proteins are known to be modified during the stress response: the heat shock proteins (HSPs, also known as *stress proteins*) and endogenous antioxidant enzymes. The independent discovery of the second window of protection by two groups (Kuzuya et al., 1993; Marber et al., 1993) was framed by a series of studies examining the effects of the myocardial stress response on these two classes of proteins. In order to set the scene for discussion of the second window we feel it is necessary to say something about these two types of proteins.

Stress response and cytoprotective proteins

Heat shock proteins (HSPs) are a family of proteins that are known to be preferentially expressed or posttranslationally modified during and after metabolic and other stresses, including hyperthermia ("heat shock") and ischemia. These proteins are often described according to their molecular weight (e.g., 70 kDa HSP [HSP70], 60 kDa HSP [HSP60], 27 kDa HSP [HSP27]). Some of these proteins are expressed constitutively and others are specifically stress inducible. They have many diverse functions in the general maintenance of cellular integrity (functions often referred to as housekeeping roles). These functions may include important roles in the control of protein synthesis, folding and degradation, and some HSPs are associated with specific organelles (e.g., HSP60 and the mitochondrion, and HSP27 and the cytoskeleton). It is known that during the 24 hours following heat stress, hearts acquire a tolerance to subsequent ischemia/reperfusion, an example of a phenomenon called *cross-tolerance* (Yellon et al., 1993). This acquired tolerance to ischemia/reperfusion as part of the stress response is thought to be associated with increased activity and/or content of specific stress-induced or stress-activated proteins. For example, whole-body hyperthermia increases myocardial HSP70i content and myocardial protection can be observed 24 hours after hyperthermia (Currie et al., 1988, 1993; Yellon et al., 1992).

Apart from HSPs, other proteins display altered activity or content after hyperthermia and other stresses. Endogenous antioxidant proteins play a fundamental role in maintaining cell homeostasis in the face of intracellular free radical production. Free radicals are extremely reactive oxygen or oxygen-conjugated species that react avidly with many biological molecules, including structural molecules such as membrane phospholipids and membrane-bound proteins, and nuclear material such as deoxyribonucleic acid (DNA) and ribonucleic acid (RNA). Free radicals are produced constantly during normal cell activity and they are inactivated by a variety of enzymes and "scavenger" molecules. During oxidative stresses, such as hyperthermia or ischemia/reperfusion, increased production of free radicals can be detected, but cells may adapt biochemically   by increasing the activity of the enzymes that inactivate free radicals or by modifying their reactivity. Increases in endogenous antioxidant protein activity, notably catalase and superoxide dismutase (SOD), have been observed in many studies investigating the biology of cellular adaptation to stress.

Discovery of the second window of protection

Work in our laboratory has been directed for several years at examining the hypothesis that the inducible 70 kDa heat shock protein (HSP70i) is a cytoprotective protein that, when present in sufficient quantity, is able to confer resistance to ischemia/reperfusion injury (Yellon et al., 1993). Although hyperthermia is a classic stimulus for HSP induction, it has been known for some time that ischemia can increase the expression of HSP70i messenger RNA (mRNA) and protein in myocardium (Dillmann et al., 1986; Knowlton et al., 1991; Mehta et al., 1988), and this appeared to offer a pathophysiologically relevant method of inducing HSP70i in the heart. An experiment was conducted using a rabbit model of preconditioning with four 5-minute coronary artery occlusions and subsequent recovery (Marber et al., 1993). Twenty-four hours following this preconditioning stimulus, the animals were subjected to a 30-minute coronary occlusion and infarct size was determined. The percentage of infarcted myocardium within the risk zone (% infarct/risk ratio [I/R]) was reduced from 52% to 29%, a 44% relative reduction in infarct size. This protection was very similar to the protection that was observed in a separate group of animals following prior heat stress (a treatment well known to induce myocardial protection 24 hours later) in which there was a 42% relative reduction in I/R.

At the same time, another group of workers observed that repetitive brief ischemia with reperfusion caused an increase in the endogenous antioxidant capacity of canine myocardium and that this conferred enhanced tolerance to subsequent ischemia. Hoshida and colleagues (1993) initially showed that four 5-minute coronary occlusions in the dog produced a modest but statistically significant increase in the activity of the mitochondrial form of SOD that is conjugated to manganese (manganese-SOD). This work was followed by a report of a study from the same group describing the time course of infarct limitation in dogs between 3 and 24 hours after preconditioning (Kuzuya et al., 1993). The preconditioning protocol was identical to that used in their earlier study examining alterations in manganese-SOD and very similar to that used by us (Marber et al., 1993), namely four 5-minute coronary occlusions each separated by 5 minutes of reperfusion. There were four phases to their infarct studies. The first stage demonstrated classic preconditioning with a 63% reduction of infarction produced by a 90-minute coronary occlusion. Three hours after preconditioning there was a nonsignificant 17% difference between I/R in preconditioned and control groups. At 12 hours following preconditioning there was a nonsignificant 27% reduction in I/R. Twenty-four hours following preconditioning ischemia, I/R was 46% lower in preconditioned versus control hearts, a difference that was statistically significant.

CHARACTERISTICS OF THE SECOND WINDOW OF PROTECTION

Since the publication of these two initial studies, several additional studies have been published in the last 3 years that examine this phenomenon in a variety of species and experimental models. These are described here and summarized in Table 5-1.

Protection against ischemic necrosis

The delayed anti-infarct effect, originally described by Marber and colleagues (1993) in the rabbit and Kuzuya and associates (1993) in the dog has subsequently been confirmed in further open-chest rabbit studies that are discussed in more detail later (Baxter et al., 1994a; 1995a; 1995b) and also in chronically instrumented conscious rabbits (Yang et al., 1996). The rat is another species in which a second window of protection has been described. Recently, Yamashita and colleagues (1995) have shown that preconditioning with two 3-minute coronary occlusions, each separated by 5 minutes of reperfusion, protected against a 30-minute occlusion 24 hours later. I/R was reduced from 62% in sham-operated animals to 41% in preconditioned animals.

TABLE 5-1 SUMMARY OF SECOND WINDOW OF PROTECTION STUDIES

Species	Model	Preconditioning protocol	Index ischemia	Interval (hr)	Outcome	Reference
In vivo studies						
Dog	Infarction	4 × 5-min LAD occlusions	90-min LAD occlusion	24	Reduced I/R	Kuzuya et al., 1993
Rabbit	Infarction	4 × 5-min coronary occlusions	30-min occlusion	24	Reduced I/R	Marber et al., 1993
Rabbit	Infarction	4 × 5-min coronary occlusions	30-min occlusion	24	Reduced I/R	Baxter et al., 1994a
Pig	Infarction	4 × 5-min LAD occlusions	60-min occlusion	24	No reduction in I/R	Strasser et al., 1994
Rabbit	Infarction	4 × 5-min coronary occlusions	30-min occlusion	24	No reduction in I/R	Tanaka et al., 1994
Dog	Arrhythmias	4 × 5-min periods of rapid pacing	25-min LAD occlusion and reperfusion	20–24	Reduced VT, VF, and mortality	Vegh et al., 1994
Pig[a]	Stunning	10 × 2-min LAD occlusions	10 × 2-min LAD occlusions	24	More rapid recovery of contractility	Sun et al., 1995
Rabbit	Infarction	4 × 5-min coronary occlusions	30-min occlusion	24	Reduced I/R	Baxter et al., 1995a
Rabbit	Infarction	4 × 5-min coronary occlusions	30-min occlusion	24–72	Reduced I/R	Baxter et al., 1995b
Dog	Arrhythmias	4 × 5-min periods of rapid pacing	25-min LAD occlusion and reperfusion	24–48	Reduced VT and VF	Kaszala et al., 1995
Pig[a]	Stunning	10 × 2-min LAD occlusions	10 × 2-min LAD occlusions	24–72	More rapid recovery of contractility	Tang et al., 1995
Pig[a]	Infarction	10 × 2-min or 25 × 2-min LAD occlusions	40-min LAD occlusion	24	No reduction in I/R	Qiu et al., 1995

Rat	Infarction	2 × 5-min L coronary occlusions	30-min L coronary occlusion	24	Reduced I/R	Yamashita et al., 1995
Rabbit[a]	Infarction	4 × 5-min coronary occlusions	30-min coronary occlusion	24	Reduced I/R	Yang et al., 1996
In vitro studies						
Rat myocytes	CK release	60-min hypoxia	180-min hypoxia	24	Reduced CK release	Yamashita et al., 1994
Rat myocytes	LDH release cell death	20-min simulated ischemia	120-min simulated ischemia	24	Reduced LDH; more cell survival	Cumming et al., 1996a

[a] Studies conducted in conscious (nonanesthetized) animals.

LAD = left anterior descending coronary artery; I/R = infarct-to-risk ratio; VT = ventricular tachycardia; VF = ventricular fibrillation; CK = creatine kinase; LDH = lactate dehydrogenase.

Protection against ischemia/reperfusion arrhythmias

There is evidence that the delayed protection conferred by preconditioning extends to other indices of ischemic and postischemic myocardial dysfunction. Recently Vegh's group (1994) reported a delayed antiarrhythmic effect following preconditioning. Four 5-minute periods of ventricular rapid pacing in the dog induced a biphasic pattern of protection against coronary occlusion- and reperfusion-induced tachyarrhythmias, with a second window of protection around 20 to 24 hours after the pacing stimulus. It is germane to this discussion that in an investigation of the second window in a conscious rabbit model we observed abolition of coronary occlusion-induced ventricular fibrillation 24 hours after preconditioning (Yang et al., 1996). In control rabbits ventricular fibrillation occurred in 3 out of 7 animals during the prolonged coronary occlusion whereas 0 out of 7 preconditioned animals fibrillated ($p < 0.1$).

Protection against myocardial stunning

A second window of protection against myocardial stunning has recently been described by Bolli's group (Sun et al., 1995). This novel finding is particularly interesting since it describes an index of protection in the second window that is not seen in the early window, there being no conclusive evidence that classic preconditioning confers protection against myocardial stunning in the absence of tissue necrosis. These workers used chronically instrumented conscious pigs to investigate postischemic myocardial dysfunction following ten 2-minute coronary artery occlusions. This protocol induced severe postischemic stunning (determined by systolic thickening measurement) lasting 3 to 4 hours. However, when the protocol was repeated in the same animals 24 hours later it was found that the postischemic recovery of thickening fraction was significantly accelerated compared with recovery following the initial protocol. Thus it would appear that the first stunning protocol preconditioned against a subsequent stunning protocol 24 hours later.

Protection against hypoxia and simulated ischemia in isolated myocytes

Evidence for a delayed effect of preconditioning in vitro has been obtained in isolated cardiomyocyte studies. Yamashita and colleagues (1994) established that hypoxic preconditioning of rat neonatal cardiomyocytes conferred resistance to a subsequent, more prolonged hypoxic period 24 hours later: There was reduced CK release in myocytes preconditioned 24 hours earlier by exposure to a brief hypoxic period. More recently work in our laboratory has examined a model of delayed protection in neonatal rat cardiomyocytes following preconditioning with 10 mM deoxyglucose and 20 mM lactate (Cumming et al., 1996a). Metabolic preconditioning with simulated ischemia, 24 hours before a long, simulated ischemic period, resulted in less cell death (56% cell death in preconditioned cells vs. 69% in nonpreconditioned cells).

Lactate dehydrogenase release following the "lethal" ischemic period was also attenuated in the cells preconditioned 24 hours earlier.

Time course of the second window of protection

The slow onset of the second window of protection, originally shown in the study of Kuzuya and coworkers (1993), suggested that it was likely to be of greater duration than classic preconditioning protection. Recent work from our laboratory suggests that the delayed anti-infarct effect of preconditioning in the rabbit extends over a period of 3 days (Baxter et al., 1995b). Interestingly, the magnitude of the infarct-limiting effect in the rabbit increases as the interval between preconditioning and acute myocardial infarction is extended beyond 24 hours and is maximal 48 to 72 hours after preconditioning. By 96 hours after preconditioning, however, no protection against infarction is seen. In an investigation of the time course of the rapid pacing-induced delayed protection against arrhythmias, Vegh and associates have extended the interval between the pacing stimulus and coronary occlusion up to 72 hours and found that protection against fibrillation (and hence mortality) was almost completely lost by 48 hours (Kaszala et al., 1995). However, there was evidence that even 72 hours later some attenuation of parameters such as electrical inhomogeneity was present. With regard to the time course of the second window against myocardial stunning in the pig, Sun and coworkers (1995) initially reported that the antistunning effect could be renewed by preconditioning again after 24 hours so that protection was seen 48 hours after the first stunning protocol. No protection was observed after a 10-day interval between the preconditioning protocol and the subsequent stunning protocol. More recently this group has examined the time course of this delayed antistunning phenomenon more specifically (Tang et al., 1995). They have shown that the systolic wall-thickening deficit was reduced when the second stunning protocol was induced 12, 24, and 72 hours after the first stunning protocol, but no protection was observed 6 days after preconditioning.

Failure to observe the second window of protection

Some studies designed to examine the existence of late protection following preconditioning have reported negative findings. Arguably, the first of these was contained in a report by Shiki and Hearse (1987) of a study of preconditioning against reperfusion-induced arrythmias in the rat heart. The interval between the first coronary occlusion and the second (or index) coronary occlusion was extended to 24 hours, at which time no reduction in arrhythmia incidence or severity was seen. In a study undertaken specifically to confirm the second window of protection against infarction in the rabbit, Tanaka and associates (1994) demonstrated the protective effects of classic preconditioning in this model (a

72% reduction in infarct size), but no protection was observed 24 or 48 hours later. Reasons for the absence of protection, in contrast to our own studies (Baxter et al., 1994a, 1995a, 1995b; Marber et al., 1993), are not immediately apparent. Differences in surgical technique may explain the discrepancy. Nevertheless, a study that we undertook in chronically instrumented conscious rabbits, in which a 33% reduction in infarct size was observed in preconditioned animals, tends to suggest that the second window of protection in this species *can occur* independently of any confounding effects of surgery or anesthetic (Yang et al., 1996). A further two studies, presented in preliminary form, have examined preconditioning protocols in pig myocardium and have not seen statistically significant limitation of infarction 24 hours later. In the first of these studies, Strasser and associates (1994) reported that four 5-minute cycles of ischemia failed to elicit protection against a sustained 60-minute coronary occlusion 24 hours later (I/R was 71.3% in controls vs. 60.4% in preconditioned, p was not significant). We think it likely that the duration of this sustained ischemic insult in a noncollateralized species may have been too severe to permit demonstration of a protective effect. A more recent study in the pig has been more carefully designed to examine the possibility of a second window of protection. Qiu and associates (1995) examined the effects of repeated brief coronary occlusions (10×2 minutes) in conscious pigs 24 hours before a 40-minute occlusion. In the preconditioned group a nonsignificant 26% relative reduction in I/R was observed (I/R 45.1% vs. 33.3%). A further group of animals preconditioned with 25×2-minute occlusions did not display further enhancement of ischemic tolerance at 24 hours and these workers have concluded that a second window of protection against infarction does not occur in the pig. However, as was discussed earlier, it is possible that 24 hours after preconditioning may not be the ideal time for examination of the delayed phase of protection against infarction in the pig; maximum infarct limitation may be observed at a time point beyond 24 hours, as is the case in the rabbit.

MECHANISMS OF DELAYED PROTECTION

At the beginning of this chapter we stated our belief that the second window of protection is closely related to the stress response in myocardium and is associated with the appearance of cytoprotective proteins (Fig 5-2). The appearance of a large number of new gene products including proto-oncogenes and regulatory proteins, as well as the posttranslational modification of proteins, would be anticipated after sublethal ischemia as part of the stress response and also as a consequence of the activation of various signaling pathways triggered by the local release of paracrine mediators during preconditioning. Associations between enhanced myocardial tolerance and stress-induced cytoprotective protein activity, the gradual onset of the second window of protection (Kuzuya et al., 1993), and the prolonged period of protection (Baxter et al., 1995b; Tang et al., 1995) suggest that

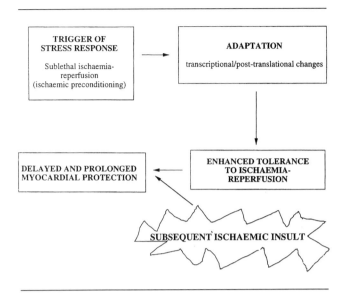

Figure 5-2. *The development of the second window of protection after preconditioning is a form of subacute adaptation that occurs over many hours and shares some of the features of the cell stress response. Sublethal ischemia/reperfusion insult (preconditioning) triggers a complex signal cascade that culminates in changes in the activity and content of cytoprotective proteins through regulation at the transcriptional and posttranslational levels. This process of "adaptation" results in a temporary state of increased tolerance to ischemia/reperfusion.*

the phenomenon is related to changes in patterns of protein activity in the preconditioned myocardium. Almost certainly, de novo protein synthesis will be stimulated by ischemic preconditioning, but so far there is no evidence from studies with transcriptional and translational inhibitors in vivo to support directly the concept that the second window of protection involves genomic modifications. Nevertheless, as we have already mentioned, antioxidant proteins and HSPs have been associated with late preconditioning and may, for the moment, be considered as candidate mediators of protection. We now discuss the evidence for these proteins as potential mediators of protection and draw attention to some other possible mechanisms.

Heat shock proteins (stress proteins) as mediators of delayed protection

Several lines of evidence suggest that HSP70i is a cytoprotective protein conferring tissue tolerance to ischemia/reperfusion injury. For example, recent studies with transgenic mice that overexpress HSP70i (Marber et al., 1995b; Plumier et al., 1995) and studies involving transfection of the gene encoding for HSP70 into isolated myogenic cells (Heads et al., 1995b; Mestril et al., 1994) and cardiac myocytes (Cumming et al., 1996b) show convincingly that the protein *directly confers protection* against ischemic injury. Several reports have suggested that transient ischemia in whole animals and isolated cells induces HSPs. Dillmann's group showed that ischemia in canine myocardium caused increases in mRNA for HSP70 (Dillmann et al., 1986; Mehta et al., 1988). Knowlton and colleagues (1991) reported that four 5-minute coronary occlusions followed by reperfusion in the rabbit led to an increase in HSP70i mRNA and a qualitative increase in protein immunoreactivity 24 hours later. Work in our own laboratory, employing both in vitro and in vivo techniques, has been directed at exploring the complex relationships between the induction of several HSPs by ischemic preconditioning and the subsequent second window of protection. In our group's initial report of the second window of protection (Marber et al., 1993) it was shown that elevation of HSP70i (determined by Western blot analysis) occurred in rabbit myocardium 24 hours following either hyperthermia or preconditioning and at this time point protection against infarction was conferred by each treatment. Additionally, ischemic preconditioning, but not hyperthermia, induced HSP60. However, this particular preconditioning protocol (four 5-minute coronary occlusions) may not consistently induce HSP70i. For example, in subsequent studies with the protocol, we have observed only modest HSP70i induction in rabbits preconditioned in the conscious state (Yang et al., 1996) and no induction of HSP70i mRNA (unpublished results) or protein (Heads et al., 1995a) in rabbits preconditioned in the anesthetized state, even though the preconditioning protocol reliably confers a second window of protection. In contrast, Tanaka and coworkers (1994) have reported induction of HSP70i in rabbit myocardium 24 and 48 hours after four 5-minute coronary occlusions, without observing a second window of protection. It seems then that HSP70i induction following ischemic preconditioning may not be as robust in this experimental animal model as was initially observed. It may well be the case that elevation of HSP70i content is not responsible for mediation of the second window of protection, but we cannot exclude the possibility that subtle alterations in the protein's regulation may be relevant, such as translocation of both the constitutive and inducible isoforms to selected cell "compartments." Additionally, the regulation of other HSPs in response to ischemia, which have not so far been widely investigated (especially HSP27), may be fundamental to ischemia-induced delayed myocardial protection and protection induced by other agents. The adenosine A_1 receptor agonist CCPA induces delayed protection against ischemia (discussed in detail later) and although this agent does not induce HSP70i, changes in the phosphorylation state and/or translocation of HSP27, as well as induction of manganese-SOD may follow adenosine A_1 receptor activation (Heads et al., 1995a).

Endogenous antioxidant enzymes as mediators of delayed protection

There is some evidence from in vivo animal studies that SOD activity may be elevated 24 hours following ischemic preconditioning. Hoshida and colleagues (1993) described the temporal dynamics of manganese-SOD activity following preconditioning in canine myocardium and described a biphasic pattern of enzyme activity over a 24-hour period similar to the pattern of ischemic tolerance observed in a related study (Kuzuya et al., 1993). Following four 5-minute coronary occlusions in the dog, manganese-SOD *activity* was found to increase in the epicardial risk zone within 1 hour, and returned to normal within 3 hours, and was then elevated again 24 hours later. Myocardial manganese-SOD *content* increased gradually in the ischemic and nonischemic zones over 72 hours following ischemic preconditioning. Twenty-four hours following ischemic preconditioning, manganese-SOD activity had increased significantly in the subepicardial and subendocardial regions of the ischemic and nonischemic zones, but the increase was greatest in the subendocardial region of the ischemic zone. Interestingly, at no point were there any differences in either activity or content of the cytosolic copper-zinc-SOD between the ischemic and nonischemic zones. In a recent preliminary study, we have found that the activities of both manganese-SOD and copper-zinc-SOD are increased 24 hours after preconditioning of rabbit myocardium (Heads et al., 1995a). In elegant studies with isolated rat cardiac myocytes, Yamashita and coworkers (1994) reported that hypoxic preconditioning of these cells resulted in increased activity of manganese-SOD 24 hours later, at which time marked protection was observed against a prolonged hypoxic insult. Both the rise in enzyme activity after preconditioning and the acquisition of cellular tolerance to hypoxia were abolished when myocytes were treated with staurosporine, a protein kinase inhibitor, or with antisense oligonucleotide directed against manganese-SOD during preconditioning. The involvement of a protein kinase mediator in this regulation of SOD activity is particularly interesting to us in view of our finding that both adenosine and PKC are involved in the second window of protection in vivo.

Inducible nitric oxide synthase

Parratt and coworkers have suggested that endothelial-derived nitric oxide is an endogenous antiarrhythmic substance and that classic ischemic preconditioning against arrhythmias in the dog is mediated by release of nitric oxide (Vegh et al., 1992). More recently, they demonstrated that the second window of protection against arrhythmias in this species, induced by rapid ventricular pacing, was abolished by administration of dexamethasone (Vegh et al., 1994). This corticosteroid is appreciated to have many actions, including inhibition of cyclo-oxygenase and inducible nitric oxide synthase activities. It is interesting to note that bacterial endotoxins induce nitric oxide synthase activity and treatment of animals with low doses of endotoxin induces delayed myocardial protection. For example, Parratt's group has shown that enhanced tolerance to ischemia/reperfusion arrhythmias is seen several hours after endotoxin treatment in rats, an effect that is abolished by dexamethasone pretreatment (Song et al., 1994). So far, however, there is no direct evidence that nitric oxide synthase activity is increased in myocardium 24 hours after ischemic or other preconditioning stimuli.

Induction of collateralization

In considering the mechanisms through which protection is manifested in the second window, a further possibility that must be considered is that preconditioning might open coronary collateral vessels or stimulate angiogenesis, providing collateral support in the ischemic region. However, this is unlikely to account for the protection observed in experimental studies to date. In the dog, Kuzuya and associates (1993) observed no differences in regional myocardial blood flow (determined by radiolabeled microspheres) 24 hours after four 5-minute coronary occlusions, obviating the possibility that opening of preformed collaterals could account for delayed protection in this species. The rabbit is deficient in preformed collateral vessels (Maxwell et al., 1987). Moreover, this species has a very limited capacity to develop collaterals in response to ischemia. For example, Cohen and associates (1994) demonstrated that even after 3 to 4 days of repetitive coronary artery occlusion in the conscious rabbit, the ratio of collateral to normal tissue blood flow remained at a constant low level of around 5%.

ADENOSINE AND THE SECOND WINDOW OF PROTECTION

As with classic preconditioning, it seems likely that our understanding of the second window of protection may profit from attention to intracellular signal transduction pathways (Fig 5-3). In the rabbit, there is a wealth of evidence that the early protection against infarction associated with preconditioning is initiated by adenosine, generated as a consequence of ATP catabolism during the preconditioning ischemic stimulus (see Chapter 4). With regard to the delayed protection in the rabbit we have shown that adenosine receptor blockade with 8-sulphophenyltheophylline (SPT) during preconditioning abolished the protection against infarction 24 hours later (Baxter et al., 1994a). We also demonstrated in the same study that a single bolus of a selective adenosine A_1 receptor agonist CCPA (25, 50, or 100 μg kg^{-1}) led to enhanced resistance to infarction 24 hours later in a rabbit model of coronary occlusion in vivo. These observations suggested that adenosine receptor activation during preconditioning in the rabbit might be an important trigger of not only early protection, but of the delayed protection as well. Interestingly, we have observed a prolonged period of delayed protection following CCPA treatment: An approximately 50% reduction in I/R was observed over a period between 24 and 72 hours after CCPA treatment, but no protection was observed 96 hours after treatment (Baxter & Yellon, 1994). Thus the temporal profile of delayed protection following CCPA closely parallels the time course of delayed protection following ischemic preconditioning in the rabbit. The similarity of time course and magnitude of protection evoked by ischemic preconditioning and CCPA pretreatment provide further indirect evidence that in the rabbit adenosine is an important trigger of the second window of protection. We cannot exclude the possibility, however, that other locally released mediators may be involved as triggers of delayed protection in the rabbit. For example

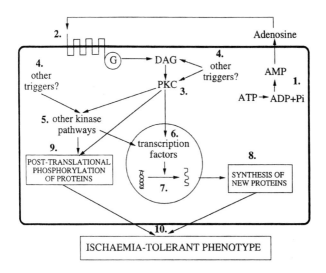

Figure 5-3. The sequence of cellular events that results in delayed protection following a sublethal ischemic stress is at present largely speculative. The scheme shown here is a proposal based on our knowledge of the physiology of the second window of protection in rabbit myocardium, which is known to involve adenosine, PKC, and the altered activity of various putative cytoprotective proteins (see text for a complete account). During ischemia, catabolism of ATP results in production of adenosine, which diffuses into the extracellular space [1]. Adenosine binds to specific receptors on the plasma membrane [2]. There are various subtypes of adenosine receptor, the A1 and A3 receptor subtypes are found on cardiac myocytes. A1 receptors are coupled to a guanylate triphosphate regulatory protein (G-protein), activation of which causes the liberation of diacylglycerol (DAG) from phosphoinositol bisphosphate. DAG, in the presence of Ca2+, causes the activation of a family of cytosolic enzymes called protein kinase C (PKC) [3]. Which PKC isoenzymes are activated depends on the nature and intensity of the triggering stimulus. In addition to DAG, PKC isoenzymes may be activated by other triggers such as free radicals and a variety of hormones and cytokines [4]. In addition, other triggers may activate other kinases such as protein tyrosine kinase and mitogen-activated protein kinase [5]. Also, there may be interactions ("cross talk") between PKC and certain other kinase pathways. The activation of multiple kinase cascades results in a complex signaling pattern. Kinases effect diverse chemical reactions including phosphorylation of proteins. Certain kinases, including some PKC isoenzymes, translocate to the nucleus where they could phosphorylate and activate transcription factors [6]. When activated by PKC or other kinases, transcription factors will interact with DNA and promote the production of mRNA, encoding the gene sequence for particular proteins [7]. The mRNA for these proteins may appear very rapidly (within 1 or 2 hours). Translation of the message may follow with ribosomal synthesis of the proteins [8]. In addition to this genomic control of protein synthesis de novo, kinases may cause the modification of newly synthesized or existing proteins. An example of such modification would be the posttranslational phosphorylation of proteins [9]. The presence of newly synthesized cytoprotective proteins [8] and posttranslationally modified cytoprotective proteins [9] could confer the ischemia-tolerant phenotype on the adapted cell [10]. The identity of these proteins is unknown. At present we suggest that HSPs and antioxidants are likely candidate proteins.

it is known that noradrenaline may be an important trigger for early preconditioning in the rat (Banerjee et al., 1993), and treatment with noradrenaline in the rat can induce a delayed phase of protection in this species that extends to 72 hours (Meng et al., 1993).

There is some indirect evidence for the involvement of PKC in the second window of protection. Delayed protection was abolished when preconditioning occurred in the presence of chelerythrine, a PKC inhibitor (Baxter et al., 1995b). More recently we have observed that pretreatment of rabbits in vivo with dioctanoyl-sn-glycerol, a synthetic diacylglycerol analog that reversibly activates PKC, resulted in an approximately 50% reduction in infarct size 24 hours later (unpublished results). PKC could influence many nuclear transcription events either directly by phosphorylation of transcription factors or indirectly through activation of other kinase signal cascades (e.g., raf kinase and MAP kinase families) (Hug & Sarre, 1993). Certainly, there is some evidence that activation of PKC is associated with new protein synthesis or posttranslational phosphorylation (Issandou & Darbon, 1991). Faucher and associates (1993) have shown that a low-molecular weight protein in the HSP27 family is phosphorylated by PKC in an adenocarcinoma cell line, and in our laboratory we have observed that hyperthermia-induced HSP expression is PKC dependent in myogenic cells (unpublished results). As mentioned earlier, we found that 24 hours following CCPA pretreatment, activities of both mitochondrial and cytosolic fractions of SOD are increased in rabbit myocardium (Heads et al., 1995a) although changes in myocardial HSP70i content were not observed. Maggirwar and coworkers (1994) proposed a link between adenosine receptor activation and increased SOD activity, possibly by both transcriptional and posttranslational mechanisms. This association between adenosine, an obviously important paracrine substance in myocardial ischemia, and SOD would appear to be very relevant to further exploration of the second window of protection. However, the complex relationships between protein activity and the protected state following preconditioning and A_1 agonist treatment remain to be more fully investigated.

POSSIBLE PATHOPHYSIOLOGICAL CONSIDERATIONS AND RELEVANCE TO CLINICIANS

At the time of this writing, there have been no studies examining subacute adaptive responses to ischemia in human myocardium and so any extrapolation of our knowledge of the second window of protection to humans is speculative. However, it is almost certain that, like classic preconditioning, late preconditioning is a universal phenomenon, not limited to laboratory animal species. It has been suggested that preconditioning in general may occur as a natural feature of some ischemic syndromes in humans (see Chapter 6). In this context, the relationship between angina (a marker of sublethal myocardial ischemia) and myocardial infarction has been highlighted in some reports. Although the prognostic significance of angina before acute myocardial infarction is by no means certain, three recent studies of patients with a history of *unstable* angina before myocardial infarction suggest a beneficial effect in terms of reduced infarct size and short-term mortality (Kloner et al., 1995; Nakagawa et al., 1995; Ottani et al., 1995). In all three studies, these beneficial effects appeared to be poorly correlated with the extent of coronary collateralization and previous antianginal drug therapies. The studies suggested that episodes of angina within a critical period before infarction might protect the myocardium in the absence of collateralization. One possible explanation of this protective effect of angina is that a state of enhanced tolerance to ischemia is elicited in myocardium by antecedent angina. Interestingly, the kinetics of this preconditioning effect of angina occur over many hours or days rather than the 1 or 2 hours associated with the classic preconditioning phenomenon and would suggest a form of adaptation temporally related to the second window of protection rather than to classic preconditioning. For example, in a carefully conducted study by Ottani and colleagues (1995) patients were selected with a history of angina within the 24-hour period prior to infarction and compared to those who had no such history. The mean time between the last episode of angina and onset of infarction was around 11 hours, a time that clearly falls outside the time frame of experimentally defined classic preconditioning and yet the patients with antecedent angina experienced smaller infarcts (see Marber et al., 1995a for further commentary). Adenosine A_1 receptors in human myocardium are located principally on myocytes and perivascular sympathetic nerves (Bohm et al., 1993; Burnstock, 1989). The pain associated with myocardial ischemia, angina pectoris, is thought to be mediated by adenosine acting on A_1 receptors and stimulating afferent sensory pathways (Gaspardone et al., 1995). This raises the intriguing possibility that, in human myocardium, adenosine released during episodes of angina and acting via A_1 receptors could trigger an adaptive cytoprotective response analagous to that seen in experimental studies of the second window of protection.

Ultimately, the aim of this research is to understand the mechanisms of myocardial adaptation to transient ischemia. With this knowledge we may be in a position to stimulate adaptation therapeutically and thereby enhance endogenous cytoprotective mechanisms by a pharmacological means or other form of treatment. One can envisage such a treatment being a valuable method of myocardial preservation in situations of scheduled ischemia such as coronary bypass grafting and the storage of hearts removed from donors prior to transplantation. As we learn more about its characteristics and mechanisms we may find that the second window of protection, because of its longevity, has greater potential for therapeutic exploitation than classic preconditioning. Furthermore, adaptive cytoprotection may be relevant to other tissues and organs, particularly the brain.

SUMMARY

Myocardium may be preconditioned by ischemic stress in two ways: The first form of adaptation immediately confers a brief period of protection against subsequent ischemia (classic preconditioning); the other form of adaptation confers a second window of protection against ischemia many hours or days later. Investigation of this delayed form of preconditioning is still at an early stage. We know that during the second window of protection, myocardium shows enhanced resistance to ischemic necrosis, ischemia- and reperfusion-induced arrhythmias, and postischemic stunning. The mechanisms of protection are unknown; they are likely to be different for each end point of protection, but may share some common features. We believe that increased resistance to ischemia is the result of altered activity of cytoprotective proteins in the preconditioned myocardium. Some of these cytoprotective proteins may be regulated at the level of gene transcription. We hope that an understanding of the physiology and mechanisms of the second window of protection will shed light on the associations between antecedent angina pectoris and myocardial infarction, and promote the rational development of new therapeutic approaches to cardioprotection based on manipulation of this innate adaptive capacity of myocardium.

REFERENCES

Banerjee A, Locke-Winter C, Rogers KB, et al. Preconditioning against myocardial dysfunction after ischemia and reperfusion by an alpha-adrenergic mechanism. *Circ Res* 1993; 73: 656–670.

Baxter GF, Goma FM, Yellon DM. Involvement of protein kinase C in the delayed cytoprotection following sublethal ischemia in rabbit myocardium. *Br J Pharmacol* 1995a; 115: 222–224.

Baxter GF, Goma FM, Yellon DM. Duration of the "second window of protection" following ischemic preconditioning in the rabbit [abstract]. *J Mol Cell Cardiol* 1995b; 27: A162.

Baxter GF, Marber MS, Patel VC, Yellon DM. Adenosine receptor involvement in a delayed phase of protection 24 hours following ischemic preconditioning. *Circulation* 1994a; 90: 2993–3000.

Baxter GF, Yellon DM. Temporal characterization of the "second window of protection:" prolonged anti-infarct effect after adenosine A1 receptor activation [abstract]. *Circulation* 1994b; 90(Suppl I): I-475.

Bohm M, Ungerer M, Erdmann E. Adenosine receptors in the human heart pharmacological characterization in nondiseased and cardiomyopathic tissue. *Drug Dev Res* 1993; 28: 268–276.

Burnstock G. Vascular control by purines with emphasis on the coronary system. *Eur Heart J* 1989; 10: 15–21.

Cohen MV, Yang X-M, Downey JM. Conscious rabbits become tolerant to multiple episodes of ischemic preconditioning. *Circ Res* 1994; 74: 998–1004.

Cumming DVE, Heads RJ, Brand NJ, et al. The ability of heat stress and metabolic preconditioning to protect primary rat cardiac myocytes. *Basic Res Cardiol* 1996a; (in press).

Cumming DVE, Heads RJ, Watson A, et al. Differential protection of primary rat cardiocytes by transfection of specific heat stress proteins. *J Mol Cell Cardiol* 1996b; (in press).

Currie RW, Karmazyn M, Kloc M, Mailer K. Heat shock response is associated with enhanced post-ischemic ventricular recovery. *Circ Res* 1988; 63: 543–549.

Currie RW, Tanguay RM, Kingma JG. Heat shock response and limitation of tissue necrosis during occlusion-reperfusion in rabbit hearts. *Circulation* 1993; 87: 963–971.

Dillmann WH, Mehta HB, Barrieux A, et al. Ischemia of the dog heart induces the appearance of a cardiac mRNA coding for a protein with migration characteristics similar to the heat shock/stress protein 71. *Circ Res* 1986; 59: 110–114.

Faucher C, Capdevielle J, Canal I, et al. The 28-kDa protein whose phosphorylation is induced by protein kinase C activators in MCF-7 cells belongs to the family of low molecular mass heat shock proteins and is the estrogen-regulated 24-kDa protein. *J Biol Chem* 1993; 268: 15168–15173.

Gaspardone A, Crea F, Tomai F, et al. Muscular and cardiac adenosine-induced pain is mediated by A_1 receptors. *J Am Coll Cardiol* 1995; 25: 251–257.

Heads RJ, Baxter GF, Latchman DS, Yellon DM. Delayed protection in rabbit heart following ischemic preconditioning is associated with modulation of HSP27 and superoxide dismutase at 24 hours [abstract]. *J Mol Cell Cardiol* 1995a; 27: A163.

Heads RJ, Yellon DM, Latchman DS. Differential cytoprotection against heat stress or hypoxia following expression of specific stress protein genes in myogenic cells. *J Mol Cell Cardiol* 1995b; 27: 1669–1678.

Hoshida S, Kuzuya T, Fuji H, et al. Sublethal ischemia alters myocardial antioxidant activity in canine heart. *Am J Physiol* 1993; 264: H33–H39.

Hug H, Sarre TF. Protein kinase C isoenzymes: divergence in signal transduction. *Biochem J* 1993; 291: 329–343.

Issandou M, Darbon J-M. Activation of protein kinase C by phorbol esters induces DNA synthesis and protein phosphorylation in glomerular mesangial cells. *Febs Lett* 1991; 281: 196–206.

Kaszala K, Vegh A, Parratt JR, Papp JG. Time course of pacing induced preconditioning in dogs [abstract]. *J Mol Cell Cardiol* 1995; 27: A145.

Kloner RA, Shook T, Przyklenk K, et al. Previous angina alters in-hospital outcome in TIMI 4: a clinical correlate to preconditioning? *Circulation* 1995; 91: 37–47.

Knowlton AA, Brecher P, Apstein CS. Rapid expression of heat shock protein in the rabbit after brief cardiac ischemia. *J Clin Invest* 1991; 87: 139–147.

Kuzuya T, Hoshida S, Yamashita N, et al. Delayed effects of sublethal ischemia on the acquisition of tolerance to ischemia. *Circ Res* 1993; 72: 1293–1299.

Lindquist SC. The heat shock response. *Annu Rev Biochem* 1986; 55: 1151–1191.

Maggirwar SB, Dhanraj DN, Somani SM, Ramukumar V. Adenosine acts as an endogenous activator of the cellular antioxidant defense mechanism. *Biochem Biophys Res Commun* 1994; 201: 508–515.

Marber MS, Baxter GF, Yellon DM. Prodromal angina limits infarct size: a role for ischemic preconditioning [letter with authors' reply]. *Circulation* 1995a; 92: 1061–1062.

Marber MS, Latchman DS, Walker JM, Yellon DM. Cardiac stress protein elevation 24 hours after brief ischemia or heat stress is associated with resistance to myocardial infarction. *Circulation* 1993; 88: 1264–1272.

Marber MS, Mestril R, Chi S-H, et al. Overexpression of the rat inducible 70-kD heat stress protein in a transgenic mouse increases the resistance of the heart to ischemic injury. *J Clin Invest* 1995b; 95: 1446–1456.

Maxwell MP, Hearse DJ, Yellon DM. Species variation in the coronary collateral circulation during regional myocardial ischemia: a critical determinant of the rate of evolution and extent of myocardial infarction. *Cardiovasc Res* 1987; 21: 737–746.

Mehta HB, Popovich BK, Dillmann WH. Ischemia induces changes in the level of mRNAs coding for stress protein 71 and creatine kinase M. *Circ Res* 1988; 63: 512–517.

Meng X, Brown JM, Ao L, et al. Norepinephrine induces late cardiac protection preceded by oncogene and heat shock protein overexpression [abstract]. *Circulation* 1993; 88(Suppl I): I-633.

Mestril R, Chi S-H, Sayen MR, et al. Expression of inducible stress protein 70 in rat heart myogenic cells confers protection against simulated ischemia induced injury. J Clin Invest 1994; 93: 759-767.

Minowada G, Welch WJ (1995). Clinical implications of the stress response. *J Clin Invest* 1995; 95: 3–12.

Nakagawa Y, Ito H, Kitakaze M, et al. Effect of angina pectoris on myocardial protection in patients with reperfused anterior wall myocardial infarction: retrospective clinical evidence of "preconditioning." *J Am Coll Cardiol* 1995; 25: 1076–1083.

Ottani F, Galvani M, Ferrini D, et al. Prodromal angina limits infarct size: a role for ischemic preconditioning. *Circulation* 1995; 91: 291–297.

Plumier J-CL, Ross BM, Currie RW, et al. Transgenic mice expressing the human heat shock protein 70 have improved postischemic myocardial recovery. *J Clin Invest* 1995; 95: 1854–1860.

Qiu Y, Tang X-L, Sun J-Z, et al. Does the late phase of ischemic preconditioning protect against infarction and reperfusion arrhythmias in conscious pigs? [abstract]. *Circulation* 1995; 92(Suppl I): I-389.

Shiki K, Hearse DJ. Preconditioning of ischemic myocardium: reperfusion-induced arrhythmias. *Am J Physiol* 1987; 253: H1470–H1476.

Song W, Furman BL, Parratt JR. Attenuation by dexamethasone of endotoxin protection against ischemia-induced ventricular arrhythmias. *Br J Pharmacol* 1994; 113: 1083–1084.

Strasser R, Arras M, Vogt A, et al. Preconditioning of porcine myocardium: how much ischemia is required for induction? What is its duration? Is a renewal of effect possible? [abstract]. *Circulation* 1994; 90(Suppl): I-109.

Sun J-Z, Tang X-L, Knowlton AA, et al. Late preconditioning against myocardial stunning: an endogenous protective mechanism that confers resistance to postischemic dysfunction 24 h after brief ischemia in conscious pigs. *J Clin Invest* 1995; 95: 388–403.

Tanaka M, Fujiwara H, Yamasaki K, et al. Ischemic preconditioning elevates cardiac stress protein but does not limit infarct size 24 or 48 h later in rabbits. *Am J Physiol* 1994; 267: H1476–H1482.

Tang X-L, Qiu Y, Sun J-Z, et al. Time-course of late preconditioning against myocardial stunning in conscious pigs [abstract]. *Circulation* 1995; 92(Suppl I): I-388.

Vegh A, Papp JG, Parratt JR. Prevention by dexamethasone of the marked antiarrhythmic effects of preconditioning induced 20 h after rapid cardiac pacing. *Br J Pharmacol* 1994; 113: 1081–1082.

Vegh A, Szekeres L, Parratt JR. Preconditioning of ischemic myocardium: involvement of L-arginine nitric oxide pathway. *Br J Pharmacol* 1992; 107: 648–652.

Yamashita N, Kuzuya T, Hoshida S, et al. A "second window of protection" occurs 24 hours after ischemic preconditioning in rat heart [abstract]. *J Mol Cell Cardiol* 1995; 27: A517.

Yamashita N, Nishida M, Hoshida S, et al. Induction of manganese superoxide dismutase in rat cardiac myocytes increases tolerance to hypoxia 24 hours after preconditioning. *J Clin Invest* 1994; 94: 2193–2199.

Yang X-M, Baxter GF, Heads RJ, et al. Infarct limitation in the second window of protection in conscious rabbits. *Cardiovasc Res* 1996; 31: 777–783.

Yellon DM, Baxter GF. A second window of protection or delayed preconditioning phenomenon: future horizons for myocardial protection? *J Mol Cell Cardiol* 1995; 27: 1023–1034.

Yellon DM, Latchman DS, Marber MS. Stress proteins—an endogenous route to myocardial protection: fact or fiction? *Cardiovasc Res* 1993; 27: 158–161.

Yellon DM, Pasini E, Cargnoni A, et al. The protective role of heat stress in the ischemic and reperfused rabbit myocardium. *J Mol Cell Cardiol* 1992; 24: 895–907.

CHAPTER 6

Cardiac Preconditioning in Humans

Robert A. Kloner
Derek M. Yellon

The concept of ischemic preconditioning is universal in all species tested to date. Brief episodes of ischemia precondition the heart so that it is more resistant to subsequent periods of prolonged and severe ischemia. It is easy to demonstrate this phenomenon in experimental animals using standardized techniques of coronary artery occlusion, measurement of ischemic risk zone, and zone of necrosis. It is much more difficult to demonstrate that this phenomenon occurs in human patients. However, recent data suggests that the human heart probably can be preconditioned (Kloner & Yellon, 1994). The good news regarding these observations is the possibility that if preconditioning exists in humans, then pharmacological agents that mimic preconditioning without causing ischemia might be developed for a host of cardiovascular entities, as we describe later. This review describes studies that support the concept that the human heart can be preconditioned. We begin with data on isolated human heart cells, then move to human heart tissue and trabeculae, and finally discuss the clinical evidence for preconditioning in the whole patient, including evidence from the angioplasty, angina, and myocardial infarction literature.

PRECONDITIONING HUMAN MYOCYTES AND MUSCLE

Ikonomidis and associates (1994a; 1994b) studied human ventricular cardiomyocytes in culture. They simulated ischemia by placing the cells into a chamber that exposed them to 100% nitrogen and anoxic buffer. Cells underwent 90 minutes of sustained ischemia with or without reoxygenation. Cells were either sustained in buffer prior to the 90 minutes of ischemia or were exposed to brief periods of preconditioning ischemia and reperfusion (10–30 minutes) prior to longer duration of ischemia. The investigators observed that those human cells that were exposed to preconditioning were more likely to re-

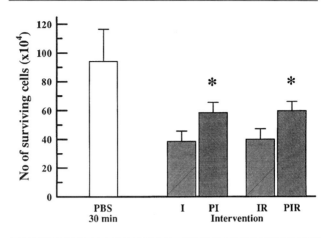

Figure 6-1. *Surviving human myocytes in culture exposed to phosphate-buffered saline (PBS) (stabilization in perfusion PBS). I = 90 minutes of ischemia; PI = preconditioning plus ischemia; IR = 90 minutes of ischemia plus 30 minutes of reperfusion; PIR = preconditioning plus ischemia plus reperfusion. (From Ikonomidis and colleagues [1994b].)*

tain viability (assessed by trypan blue exclusion) than those cells not preconditioned (Fig 6-1). In addition, preconditioned cells produced less hydrogen ion and had less lactate dehydrogenase (LDH) release. This was an important study for several reasons: First, it showed that myocytes could be preconditioned and, second, it showed that the preconditioning could occur independent of other cell types. A second study by Ikonomidis and colleagues (1994a) showed that preconditioning of human cardiomyocytes was dependent on adenosine A_1 receptors. In this clever study the authors removed the supernatant from plates of human ventricular myocytes following preconditioning ischemia and gave it to nonpreconditioned myocytes prior to a 90-minute period of sustained ischemia followed by 30 minutes of reperfusion. They also assayed the supernatant for adenosine. Administration of the supernatant (which was shown to contain nM ranges of adenosine) reduced cell injury to those cells subjected to prolonged ischemia and reperfusion. Addition of an adenosine receptor blocker (SPT) negated the protective effect, while preincubating the ventricular myocytes in adenosine or the adenosine agonist R-PIA protected the myocytes from subsequent ischemia plus reperfusion. The authors concluded that, "for the first time, human ventricular myocyte protection is demonstrated using supernatant from preconditioned cells and that a preconditioning effect in human cardiomyocytes is achieved via endogenously released adenosine acting on cardiac A_1 receptors" (Ikonomidis et al., 1994b).

Besides studies that suggest that preconditioning protects ventricular myocytes in culture, studies have suggested that preconditioning can protect myocardial trabeculae studied in in vitro preparations. Yellon's group (Walker et al., 1995) exposed one group of human right atrial trabeculae in a muscle bath to simulated ischemia consisting of rapid pacing and hypoxic, substrate-free perfusion for 90 minutes followed by 120 minutes of reoxygenation. Another group received preconditioning with 3 minutes of rapid pacing plus hypoxic, substrate-free perfusion followed by 10 minutes of reoxygenation prior to the 90-minute period of simulated ischemia. The preconditioned group of muscles demonstrated greater recovery of developed tension at 120 minutes of reoxygenation compared to the nonpreconditioned group. Similar to Ikonomidis's study in isolated myocytes, Yellon and colleagues showed that the human right atrial trabeculae could be preconditioned pharmacologically by exposure to the adenosine A_1 agonist R-PIA. Further studies by this group (Speechly-Dick et al., 1996) have recently shown that activation of PKC also protected atrial trabeculae exposed to simulated ischemia and that blocking the K_{ATP} channel prevented protection induced by either preconditioning or PKC activation. This study is important, as it suggests that in humans the K_{ATP} channel may be the end effector of the preconditioning phenomenon.

Wollmering and associates (1994) studied diseased human ventricular myocardial trabeculae in a tissue bath in which the muscles were subjected to 30 minutes of global ischemia followed by 60 minutes of reoxygenation. Pharmacological preconditioning with adenosine or phenylephrine was shown to improve the recovery of contractile function and preserve tissue creatine kinase MB isoenzyme (CK-MB) levels. The authors concluded that either transient "α 1-adrenoreceptor or adenosine (P1 purinergic receptor) stimulated preconditioning in human ventricular myocardium and that diseased human ventricles retain the ability to be preconditioned" (Wollmering et al., 1994).

PRECONDITIONING THE HUMAN HEART DURING CARDIOPULMONARY BYPASS

That human ventricular myocardium can be preconditioned was demonstrated directly in a study by Yellon and associates that analyzed human myocardial biopsies obtained for ATP levels during cardiopulmonary bypass (Yellon et al., 1993). Previous studies by Murry and colleagues (1990) in the canine myocardium demonstrated a biochemical signature of preconditioned tissue—that tissue demonstrated a much slower rate of ATP depletion during prolonged ischemia compared to nonpreconditioned tissue. In this surgical study (Yellon et al., 1993), one group of patients received a direct preconditioning protocol consisting of two 3-minute episodes of aortic cross-clamping with 2 minutes of reperfusion interspersed between each episode. This was followed by 10 minutes of sustained ischemia with aortic cross-clamping while the heart was electrically fibrillated and distal aortocoronary anastomoses were attached. The control patients did not receive the brief episodes of intermittent aortic cross-clamping prior to the 10-minute period of test ischemia. The rate of fall of ATP during the 10-minute test ischemia was much greater in nonpreconditioned hearts compared to the preconditioned hearts. In fact, in the control group ATP levels fell by 13 μmol/g/dry weight, during the 10-minute phase of ischemia;

in the preconditioned group, ATP levels actually increased slightly during this time. The importance of this study is two-fold. It suggests that in the in vivo setting (in contrast to the in vitro setting of the previous studies the human heart can demonstrate the biological signature of preconditioning—that is, slow depletion of ATP during sustained ischemia. In addition, there is a practical implication to this study: Brief periods of intermittent, aortic, cross-clamp ischemia may be an effective way of protecting the hearts of some patients undergoing coronary artery bypass procedures.

ANGIOPLASTY AND PRECONDITIONING

Another clinical situation in which preconditioning is likely to occur in vivo is that of repetitive balloon inflations during percutaneous transluminal coronary angioplasty. Deutsch and coworkers (1990) performed two sequential 90-second balloon inflations in 12 patients. They observed that the second balloon-induced coronary artery occlusion was associated with less chest pain, less ST-segment elevation, less lactate production, and a lower mean pulmonary artery pressure (Fig 6-2). Cribier and associates (1992) subjected 17 patients with left anterior descending coronary stenosis to five successive balloon inflations. With each successive balloon inflation, patients reported less chest pain, there was less ST-segment elevation, and less deterioration in left ventricular function (Figs 6-3 and 6-4). Similar results were reported by Taggart and colleagues (1993) as well as other investigators (Kerensky et al., 1995). Whether this phenomenon represents true preconditioning or not has been debated. In Deutsch's study (1990), measurement of great cardiac vein flow did not show an increase during the second inflation, suggesting that the beneficial effects observed during the second inflation were not due to recruitment of

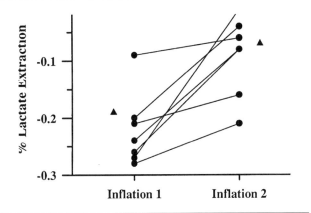

Figure 6-2. Transmyocardial lactate extraction during segmental percutaneous coronary angioplasty. There is more lactate extraction (less production) during a second compared to first balloon inflation. (From Deutsch and coworkers [1990], with permission from the American Heart Association.)

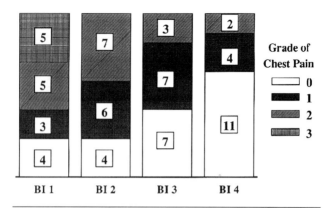

Figure 6-3. *Decrease in chest pain with four segmental percutaneous coronary angioplasty balloon inflations (BIs). The decrease in pain that occurs may be related to ischemic preconditioning. (From Cribier and associates [1992].)*

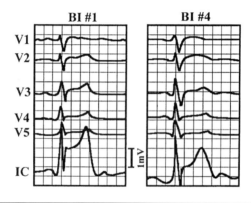

Figure 6-4. *Decrease in ST-segment elevation on surface leads and intracoronary lead on the fourth compared to the first balloon inflation. (From Cribier and associates [1992].)*

substantial coronary collateral flow. However, in Cribier's study (1992), coronary collateral grade assessed by angiography increased in 10 out of 17 patients. Therefore, some of the improvement observed in some of the patients may have been due to acute recruitment of collateral vessels rather than the intrinsic myocardial cell adaptive process of preconditioning. The other 7 patients, who did not acutely recruit collaterals, still demonstrated less chest pain and ECG change. It is likely that these patients demonstrated a true preconditioning phenomena. Birnbaum and associates (unpublished observations) observed in Kloner's laboratory, using a rabbit model of repetitive brief coronary artery occlusion, that there is a progressive decrease in ST-segment elevation with sequential 5-minute occlusions. This decrease in ST-segment elevation was not associated with acute recruitment of collaterals, determined by measurement of collateral flow with radioactive microspheres. This study suggests that the progressive decrease in ST elevation seen with repetitive coronary artery occlusion/reperfusion is not a recruitment of collateral flow-mediated phenomena. Another study that supports the concept that the protective effect of repetitive balloon inflation stimulates preconditioning was suggested by Tomai and coworkers (194a). These investigators blocked the K_{ATP} channel (thought to be important in the mechanism of preconditioning in several species) with glibenclamide, in patients undergoing angioplasty. Glibenclamide blocked benefits of repetitive balloon inflation compared to control patients just as it blocks the protective effect of preconditioning on infarct size in some models (Gross et al., 1994). In another clinical study (Kerensky et al., 1995), a first balloon inflation was again shown to decrease ischemia-induced injury during later inflation, and intracoronary adenosine appeared to modify the preconditioning effect—although in this study adenosine surprisingly tended to abolish the protective effect of the first inflation. The authors concluded, "adenosine plays a role in ischemic preconditioning in humans" (Kerensky et al., 1995), although it would appear that exactly what role adenosine plays is not clear. However in two recent reports, aminophylline (Claeys et al., 1994) and bamiphylline (Tomai et al., 1994b), both adenosine receptor antagonists, were shown to block the beneficial ischemic preconditioning effect of repetitive angioplasty.

In summary, most studies of repetitive coronary angioplasty have suggested that a first brief balloon inflation (usually on the order of 90–120 seconds) is capable of preconditioning the heart (or at least putting it in a preconditioned state) to subsequent balloon inflations. This phenomenon does not appear to depend on gross recruitment of collaterals in some patients, and in these patients probably does represent a manifestation of ischemic preconditioning. Glibenclamide, a K_{ATP} blocker that can block the beneficial effects of preconditioning in large-animal models, and adenosine receptor antagonists block the protective effect of repetitive balloon inflations in humans.

WARM-UP ANGINA AND PRECONDITIONING

Another facet of potential preconditioning in humans is acute tolerance to angina. It is not uncommon for a patient to develop angina during a walk, rest for a few minutes, and then continue walking without further symptoms. This so-called *warm-up phenomenon* has also been described in several clinical studies in which patients undergo two consecutive exercise tests with a brief rest period in between (MacAlpin & Kattus, 1966; (Marber et al., 1996); Okazaki et al., 1993; Williams et al., 1985). Typically patients exercise longer before developing angina on the second test and also develop less ECG evidence of ischemia on the second compared to the first test (Okazaki et al., 1993). Some of these trials have measured parameters such as great cardiac vein flow, showing that there was no increase in this flow during the second test, implying that acute recruitment of collateral flow was not the explanation for less ischemia (Okazaki et

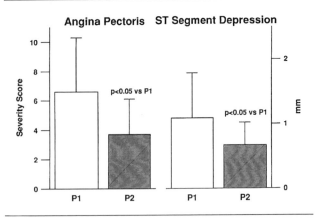

Figure 6-5. *Effect of sequential pacing-induced tachycardia on angina and ST-segment change. P1 = first pacing episode; P2 = second pacing episode. (Adapted from Williams and colleagues [1985], with permission from the American Heart Association.)*

al., 1993). Williams and colleagues (1985) observed a similar phenomenon in the catheterization laboratory when ischemia was induced by pacing-induced tachycardia. They showed that the severity of angina, degree of ST-segment depression, and lactate production decreased during a second compared to a first period of pacing (Fig 6-5). This benefit was associated with no change in peak coronary artery blood blow during the second period of ischemia, but a decrease in regional myocardial oxygen consumption in this area. Maybaum and coworkers (1995) reported one of the most recent studies investigating the preconditioning effect of repeated exercise. Patients with coronary artery disease had three exercise treadmill tests at 30-minute intervals. The authors investigated several ECG parameters: time to 1 mm of ST depression, time to ECG recovery, total ischemic time, and double product at 1 mm of ST depression. They also measured exercise duration. An improvement of 10% or more was observed in two or more of these measurements in 76% of the patients. The authors concluded that preconditioning occurs during repeated exercise ischemia. Thus it is likely that the warm-up phenomenon represents preconditioning; however, it is also conceivable that small collaterals, which cannot be visualized by coronary angiography or which do not reflect a change in great cardiac vein flow, might "open up" between the two exercise periods and this, rather than true preconditioning, might explain the benefit.

PRECONDITIONING, ANGINA PECTORIS, AND INFARCT SIZE LIMITATION?

The initial descriptions of ischemic preconditioning centered on the concept that brief periods of ischemia prior to coronary artery occlusion could reduce myocardial infarct size in animals (Murry et al., 1986). Is there evidence that angina pectoris (a form of brief ischemia), prior to an acute myocardial infarction in humans, can limit infarct size? The recent data from studies published just in the last year suggest that prior angina does limit infarct size. In the thrombolysis in myocardial infarction (TIMI-4) trial (Kloner et al., 1995c), Kloner and colleagues observed that patients with any history of angina prior to myocardial infarction had a smaller infarct size (Fig 6-6) determined by creatine kinase (CK) (119 CK integrated units) compared to patients with no history of angina (154 CK integrated units; $p = .01$). Patients who experienced angina within 48 hours before infarction also had smaller infarct size (115 CK units) versus those who did not (151 CK units; $p = .03$). Patients with histories of prior angina also had less heart failure and shock, and less in-hospital mortality compared to patients without prior angina (Fig 6-7). While there was no difference in appearance of large epicardial coronary arteries between patients with prior angina and those without prior angina (Fig 6-8), we cannot rule out the possibility that collaterals, too small for detection on an-

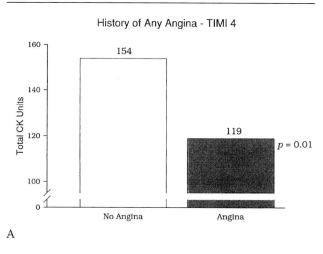

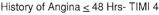

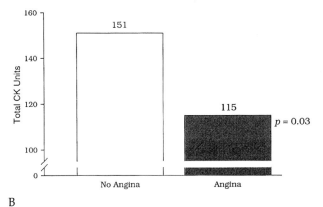

Figure 6-6. *In the TIMI 4 study, patients with any history of angina (A) or a history of angina within 48 hours of the infarct (B) had a smaller infarct size determined by creatine kinase curves compared to patients without a history of angina. (Adapted from Kloner and colleagues [1995c], with permission from the American Heart Association.)*

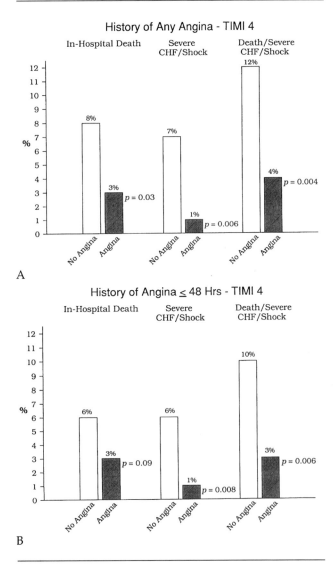

Figure 6-7. *In the TIMI 4 study, patients with any history of angina (A) or a history of angina within 48 hours of infarct (B) were less likely to die and develop severe congestive heart failure (CHF) or shock in hospital. (Adapted from Kloner and colleagues [1995c].)*

giography, might have "opened up" with repetitive episodes of angina. Since patients may have derived benefit even when the angina did not occur within hours of the myocardial infarction, it is conceivable that the second window of protection as described by Yellon and Baxter (1995) was playing a role in this preconditioning phenomena. An example of this second window effect could be argued to be part of the protection seen, for example, in the study by Ottani and associates (1995). In this study patients were selected with a 24-hour history of angina prior to infarction. The mean time between the last episode of angina was around 11 hours, a time that clearly falls outside the onset of the time frame of experimentally defined classic preconditioning. In another study by Nakagawa and coworkers (1995), patients in the

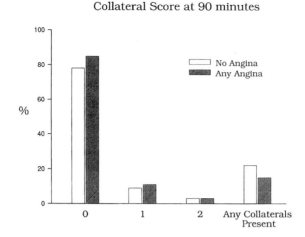

Figure 6-8. *In the TIMI 4 study there was no difference in angiographic collateral score between patients with versus patients without angina, suggesting that at least large epicardial collaterals were not responsible for the beneficial effects associated with a history of previous angina. (Adapted from Kloner and colleagues [1995c], with permission from the American Heart Association.)*

group that showed benefit had their last episode of angina a mean 25 hours before the onset of infarction and, although the greatest benefit was seen in patients who had experienced angina near to infarction, none of these patients experienced their last episode of angina within the time frame of classic preconditioning (60–90 minutes). Including those just mentioned, there have now been at least a half dozen other clinical reports besides the TIMI 4 study showing that angina prior to myocardial infarction has beneficial effects including reduction of infarct size, reduction in mortality, improvement in left ventricular function, and reduction in arrhythmias (Ottani et al., 1995; Nakagawa et al., 1995; Anzai et al., 1994; Pasceri et al., 1995; Marber et al., 1996; Andreotti et al., 1996; Iwasaka et al., 1994; Anzai et al., 1995). These studies are reviewed in detail elsewhere (Kloner & Yellon, 1994; Kloner et al., 1995a). We even found evidence for this phenomenon in patients who demonstrated spontaneous thrombolysis in a nonthrombolytic trial (the MILIS study). In this study (Kloner et al., 1995b), some patients exhibited early CK peaking and were thus likely to have experienced spontaneous reperfusion. Within this subgroup of patients, those with histories of previous myocardial infarction were more likely to develop smaller infarct sizes compared to those without previous angina.

Thus previous angina confers a beneficial effect on the early stages of acute myocardial infarction. This phenomenon has been observed by several different investigators throughout the world. One likely mechanism is ischemic preconditioning—either classic preconditioning and/or delayed preconditioning related to the second window of protection. Again, however, the studies published to date have not measured regional myocardial blood flow or myocardial perfusion within the ischemic zone prior to thrombolysis. Thus it is not entirely possible to rule out microcollateralization in the infarct region of those patients with histories of previous angina. Unfortunately, we may never have the answer to the question of whether prior to thrombolysis, myocardial collateral perfusion was better in previous angina patients. Since the rule of thumb in most hospitals is to induce thrombolysis as soon as possible after chest pain, to minimize the size of the infarct, it is unlikely that investigators currently would be willing to take the time to perform a myocardial perfusion study prior to inducing thrombolysis.

Is It Time to Reevaluate the Pathophysiology of Angina?

An intriguing but unanswered question is whether suppression of angina by antianginal agents could prevent preconditioning as might occur with warm-up angina or angina prior to myocardial infarction. Certainly, many of the patients in myocardial infarct studies who had experienced previous angina were taking some antianginal medicines, which do not always fully suppress all anginal episodes. Had full suppression of angina prior to infarction been achieved with medications, it is conceivable that the infarct-reducing effect of prior angina might have been lost, but we have no way of proving this concept. Another unanswered question is whether silent ischemia prior to infarction could precondition the heart. Medicines, including antianginal agents can suppress silent ischemia, but could they suppress the preconditioning stimulus? These questions await further research in order to be answered. Certainly, at the present time, clinicians should not "not treat" angina for fear that they might be preventing preconditioning.

Practical Implications for Preconditioning in the Human

What are the practical implications of the findings that support the concept that ischemic preconditioning probably occurs in humans? It might be possible to develop preconditioning mimetic agents that stimulate the same biochemical pathways that are "turned on" during ischemic preconditioning, but without inducing ischemia. Likely candidates are adenosine, adenosine receptor agonists, and ATP-dependent potassium channel openers such as nicorandil, which is currently used to treat angina in some countries. These agents could be used to treat a number of cardiovascular events. For example, they might be administered prior to cardiopulmonary bypass procedures to better preserve the heart during surgery. Perhaps they could be administered to high-risk patients undergoing general surgery, such as patients scheduled for vascular surgery, who often have coexisting coronary artery disease. Perhaps they could be administered to harvested hearts prior to transplantation. They might be given to high-risk patients with angina or to patients with acute coronary syndromes such as unstable angina and threatened myocardial infarction. Finally, they might be administered to patients with coronary artery disease prior to an exercise activity or an activity known to exacerbate ischemia.

SUMMARY

In summary, there are a number of clinical phenomena that support the concept t hat preconditioning occurs in humans: less chest pain, ST change, and lactate production with sequential compared to a first coronary angioplasty balloon inflation; less ischemia during a second compared to a first exercise test; and smaller infarct size and other beneficial effects of angina prior to a myocardial infarction. In vitro studies using isolated human myocytes and isolated atrial and ventricular trabeculae also support the concept that the human heart can be preconditioned. Finally, brief episodes of intermittent aortic cross-clamping slow the loss of ATP during a subsequent period of more prolonged ischemia in the human heart. All of these observations, taken together, suggest that the endogenous protective mechanism of ischemic preconditioning may be operative in humans. What we believe is important, however, is not to demonstrate that preconditioning occurs in specific clinical settings such as angina, bypass surgery, or angioplasty (those patients who may be undergoing preconditioning in these settings are indeed fortunate), but more importantly to find the mechanisms associated with the profound protection observed and then develop the pharmacology and use it to protect the unstable patient directly in those specific clinical settings mentioned here.

REFERENCES

Andreotti F, Pasceri V, Maseri A, et al. Is the benefit of preinfarction angina on infarct size due to faster coronary recanalization? [letter]. *Circulation* 1996; (in press).

Anzai T, Yoshikawa T, Asakura Y, et al. Effect on short-term prognosis and left ventricular function of angina pectoris prior to first Q-wave anterior wall acute myocardial infarction. *Am J Cardiol* 1994; 74: 755–759.

Anzai T, Yoshikawa T, Asakura Y, et al. Preinfarction angina as a major predictor of left ventricular function and long-term prognosis after a first Q-wave myocardial infarction. *J Am Coll Cardiol* 1995; 26: 319–327.

Claeys MJ, Vrints CJ, Bosmans JM, et al. Aminophylline abolishes ischemic preconditioning during angioplasty. *Circulation* 1994; (Suppl I, Part 2): I-477 [abstract].

Cribier A, Korsatz L, Koning R, et al. Improved myocardial ischemic response and enhanced collateral circulation with long repetitive coronary occlusion during angioplasty: a prospective study. *J Am Coll Cardiol* 1992; 20: 578–586.

Deutsch E, Berger M, Kussmaul WG, et al. Adaption to ischemia during percutaneous transluminal coronary angioplasty. Clinical, hemodynamic, and metabolic features. *Circulation* 1990; 82: 2044–2051.

Gross GJ, Yao Z, Auchampach JA. Role of ATP-sensitive potassium channels in ischemic preconditioning. In: Przyklenk K, Kloner RA, Yellon DM, eds. *Ischemic preconditioning: the concept of endogenous cardioprotection.* Norwell, MA: Kluwer Academic Publishers, 1994.

Ikonomidis JS, Shirai T, Weisel RD, Mickle DAG. Human cardiomyocyte preconditioning is adenosine A1 receptor dependent [abstract]. *Circulation* 1994a; 90(Suppl I, Part 2): I-477.

Ikonomidis JS, Tumiati LC, Weisel RD, et al. Preconditioning human ventricular cardiomyocytes with brief periods of simulated ischemia. *Cardiovasc Res* 1994b; 28: 1285–1291.

Iwasaka T, Nakamura S, Karakawa M, et al. Cardioprotective effect of unstable angina prior to acute anterior myocardial infarction. Chest 1994; 105: 57–61.

Kerensky RA, Kutcher MA, Braden GA, et al. The effects of intracoronary adenosine on preconditioning during coronary angioplasty. Clin Cardiol 1995; 18: 91–96.

Kloner RA, Muller J, Davis V. Effects of previous angina pectoris in patients with first acute myocardial infarction not receiving thrombolytics. *Am J Cardiol* 1995a; 75: 615–617.

Kloner RA, Przyklenk K, Shook T, et al. Clinical aspects of preconditioning and implication for the cardiac surgeon. *J Card Surg* 1995b; 10: 369–375.

Kloner RA, Shook T, Przyklenk K, et al. Previous angina alters inhospital outcome in TIMI 4: a clinical correlate to preconditioning? Circulation 1995c; 91: 37–45.

Kloner RA, Yellon DM. Does ischemic preconditioning occur in patients? *J Am Coll Cardiol* 1994; 24: 1133–1142.

MacAlpin RN, Kattus AA. Adaptation to exercise in angina pectoris: the electrocardiogram during treadmill walking and coronary angiographic findings. *Circulation* 1966; 33: 183–201.

Marber MS, Baxter GF, Yellon DM. Prodromal angina limits infarct size. A role for ischemic preconditioning [letter]. *Circulation* 1996: 1061.

Marber MS, Joy MD, Yellon DM. Warm-up in angina: is it ischemic preconditioning? *Br Heart J* 1994; 72(3): 213–215.

Maybaum S, Ilan M, Mogilevski J, Tzivoni D. Repeated exercise induced ischemia causes myocardial preconditioning. *J Am Coll Cardiol* 1995; (Suppl): 22A.

Murry CE, Jennings RB, Reimer KA. Preconditioning with ischemia: a delay of lethal cell injury in ischemic myocardium. *Circulation* 1986; 75: 1124–1136.

Murry CE, Richard VJ, Reimer KA, Jennings RB. Ischemic preconditioning slows energy metabolism and delays ultrastructural damage during a sustained ischemic episode. *Circ Res* 1990; 66: 913–931.

Nakagawa Y, Ito H, Kitakaze M, et al. Effects of angina pectoris on myocardial protection in patients with reperfused anterior wall myocardial infarction: retrospective clinical evidence of "preconditioning." *J Am Coll Cardiol* 1995; 25: 1076–1083.

Okazaki Y, Kodama K, Sato H, et al. Attenuation of increased regional myocardial oxygen consumption during exercise as a major cause of warm-up phenomenon. *J Am Coll Cardiol* 1993; 21: 1597–1604.

Ottani F, Galvani M, Ferrini D, et al. Prodromal angina limits infarct size. A role for ischemic preconditioning. *Circulation* 1995; 91: 291–297.

Pasceri V, Cianflore D, Finocchiaro ML, et al. Relation between myocardial infarction site and pain location in Q-wave acute myocardial infarction. *Am J Cardiol* 1995; 75: 224–227.

Speechly-Dick ME, Grover GJ, Yellon DM. Does ischemic preconditioning in the human involve protein kinase C and the ATP-dependent K+ channel? Studies of contractile function following simulated ischemia in an atrial in-vivo model. *Circ Res* 1995; 77: 1030–1035.

Taggart PI, Sutton PMI, Oliver RM, Swanton RH. Ischemic preconditioning may activate potassium ATP channels in humans? [abstract]. *Circulation* 1993; 88(Suppl I, Part 2): I-569.

Tomai F, Crea F, Gaspardone A, et al. Ischemic preconditioning during coronary angioplasty is prevented by glibenclamide, a selective ATP-sensitive K+ channel blocker. Circulation 1994a; 90: 700–705.

Tomai F, Crea F, Gaspardone A, et al. Blockade of A1-adenosine receptors prevents myocardial preconditioning in man [abstract]. *Eur Heart J* 1994b; 15(Suppl): 553.

Walker DM, Walker JM, Pugsley WB, et al. Preconditioning in isolated superfused human muscle. *J Mol Cell Cardiol* 1995; 27: 1349–1357.

Williams DO, Bass TA, Gerwitz H, et al. Adaptation to the stress of tachycardia in patients with coronary artery disease: insight into the mechanism of the warm-up phenomenon. *Circulation* 1985; 71: 687–692.

Wollmering MM, Fullerton DA, Walther JM, et al. Preconditioning protects function and viability in human ventricle. *Circulation* 1994; 90(Suppl I, Part 2): I-477.

Yellon DM, Alkhulaif AM, Pugsley WB. Preconditioning the human myocardium. *Lancet* 1993; 342: 276–277.

Yellon DM, Baxter GF. A "second window of protection" or delayed preconditioning phenomenon: future horizons for myocardial protection? *J Mol Cell Cardiol* 1995; 27: 1023–1034.

CHAPTER 7

Stunning in Ischemic Left Ventricular Dysfunction: Proposed Role for Calcium and Calcium Antagonists

Lionel H. Opie

Ischemic left ventricular (LV) dysfunction conventionally includes a number of established clinical entities, such as the transient acute LV failure of effort or unstable angina, the more sustained pattern of LV dysfunction in acute myocardial infarction (AMI), and ischemic cardiomyopathy, one of the end results of severe chronic coronary artery disease. Recently, new ischemic syndromes have been identified that expand the overall spectrum of conditions linked directly or indirectly to ischemia. The first of these was silent ischemia, followed by stunning, hibernation, and postinfarct LV dysfunction. A further dimension has been added by the description of preconditioning whereby one period of ischemia can lessen the adverse response to subsequent severe ischemia. As clinical ischemia is so often repetitive, preconditioning must be considered among the new ischemic syndromes, even if its full clinical relevance is not yet established. To add to the current complexity, there is the tantalizing possibility that several of these states can coexist. In patients with prior infarction or established coronary artery disease, there are at least nine or possibly ten clinical conditions that may occur singly or together:

I. *Conventional clinical ischemic syndromes*
   A. Angina pectoris of effort
   B. Unstable angina pectoris
   C. Acute myocardial infarction
   D. Ischemic cardiomyopathy

II. *"New" ischemic syndromes recently recognized*
   A. Silent ischemia
   B. Stunning, acute and chronic (including maimed myocardium)
   C. Maimed myocardium (Boden et al., 1995)
   D. Hibernation
   E. Mixed postinfarct ischemic syndrome including LV dysfunction and LV remodeling
   F. Preconditioning

Bearing in mind the heterogeneity of coronary artery disease and the unpredictability of collateral development, it is clear that no 2 patients with symptomatic coronary artery disease will have the same pathophysiology or identical clinical features. This chapter examines the contribution of the new ischemic syndromes to ischemic LV dysfunction, with the emphasis on stunning.

ACUTE ISCHEMIA AND LV DYSFUNCTION

It is well established that acute ischemia can cause contractile dysfunction. A common clinical example is effort angina, in which transient ischemia is sufficiently severe to cause pain and to precipitate LV systolic failure. The mechanism of this failure is still disputed, but one of the prime candidates is a rise of inorganic phosphate following breakdown of ATP and creatine phosphate (see Chapter 1). Similarly, a rise of adenosine, also from breakdown of ATP, or ATP itself may stimulate the pain fibers (Kennedy & Leff, 1995; Sylven, 1993).

Silent ischemia

Silent ischemia, the first of the new ischemic syndromes, has now attained maturity, being over 21 years old (Stern & Tzivoni, 1974). Of importance is that silent ischemia can cause temporary heart failure, presenting as increased LV systolic and diastolic volumes during mental stress (Legault et al., 1995). Why the ischemia is silent is still not well understood. Possible explanations include an increased threshold for pain, a milder rather than more severe form of ischemia, and increased release of pain modifiers such as beta-endorphins (Sheps et al., 1995). Of note is the finding that episodes of silent ischemia are accompanied by defective perfusion of the myocardium, thereby proving their ischemic etiology (Deanfield et al., 1983). Silent ischemia is, therefore, a cause of LV dysfunction.

Postischemic diastolic failure

While the recovery from angina by cessation of exertion has been known from the early descriptions centuries ago, more recent work has shown that myocardial mechanical recovery is also delayed. For example, after the induction of pacing-induced angina, there was a rise in LV end diastolic pressure and a stiffening of the myocardium with a decreased rate of LV wall thinning (Bourdillon et al., 1983). Similarly, regional wall-motion abnormalities persist for at least 30 minutes after treadmill exercise testing (Kloner et al., 1991). In another postischemic clinical situation, bypass surgery seems to promote diastolic dysfunction with an increase in LV diastolic chamber stiffness (McKenney et al., 1994). These clinical observations tie in well with the now established concept that "ischemia does something" that impairs mechanical activity even after the actual ischemic event is over.

The evolution of the concept of stunning

In 1975 Heyndrickx and coworkers made the seminal discovery that regional ischemia in the dog heart when induced for only 5 minutes was followed by depressed mechanical function lasting for more than 3 hours. Furthermore, 15 minutes of coronary occlusion resulted in more than 6 hours of LV dysfunction. Of considerable importance was the point that the short periods of ischemia did not result in any residual necrosis. The impaired postischemic function could not be accounted for by any impairment of blood flow in the previously occluded vessel (Heyndrickx et al., 1978). There was a small decrease in blood flow in the endocardium relative to the epicardium, probably accounted for by the decreased mechanical function. Later, Braunwald and Kloner (1982) described the delayed myocardial contractile recovery as the *stunned myocardium*.

Myocardial stunning occurs in the following experimental conditions: (1) in the zones adjacent to necrotic tissue, (2) after myocardial oxygen demands have been transiently elevated in the presence of partial arterial stenosis, (3) after subendocardial ischemia in exercising dogs with LV hypertrophy, even without coronary occlusion, and (4) in isolated hearts when reperfused after global ischemia or reoxygenated after anoxia (Braunwald, 1991). Braunwald also noted that diastolic dysfunction is an important aspect of stunning.

For how long might stunning continue? If the absence of necrosis is an essential part of the definition, as required by Bolli (1990, 1992), then it becomes clear that the longer and more severe the period of ischemia, the less the contribution of true stunning and the more the contribution of permanent damage to postinfarct dysfunction. Even with 1 hour of complete coronary artery occlusion in the dog followed by 4 weeks of reperfusion, recovery was not complete (Lavallee et al., 1983). This type of gradual but incomplete recovery over several days and even weeks seems very different from the rapid reversible stunning found after short-lived periods of ischemia. To emphasize these differences, such very delayed recovery has been called either *chronic stunning* (Opie, 1995) or the closely related entity called *the maimed myocardium* (Boden et al., 1995; see also Chapter 9). In contrast, the typical duration of total ischemia that is followed by completely reversible stunning is 15 to 20 minutes (Du Toit & Opie, 1992).

Mechanism of incomplete recovery from prolonged acute ischemia

Experimentally, during prolonged (30 minutes) of severe hypoxia in the guinea pig papillary muscle, there is a slow, steady increase in the diastolic tension (i.e., hypoxic contracture) that decreases only slightly on reoxygenation when there is also automaticity (Opie, 1989). Because the automaticity is thought to be calcium based (Brooks et al., 1995; Gao et al., 1995; Opie & Coetzee, 1988; Saman et al., 1988), it is reasonable to suppose that there is a posthypoxic rise in calcium. Additional evidence is that reoxygenation of the hypoxic interventricular septum of the rabbit leads to an increased uptake of radiocalcium (Poole-Wilson et al., 1984). Likewise, measurements of cytosolic calcium during early postischemic reperfusion show increased calcium levels and oscillations (Brooks et al., 1995; Gao et al., 1995) that soon revert to normal.

By now, considerable data have accumulated to show that in certain circumstances there can be calcium uptake during early reperfusion or reoxygenation, resulting from sodium-calcium exchange (Du Toit & Opie, 1994; Myers et al., 1995) or from calcium ion entry via the L-channels (Du Toit & Opie, 1992). These data suggest that cytosolic calcium overload is an important component of reperfusion stunning and of the failure to recover from ischemia (Fig 7-1). In addition, there is likely to an important contribution from the formation of free radicals as reviewed elsewhere (Bolli, 1992; Hearse, 1991). A reasonable concept is that formation of free radicals increases cytosolic calcium by a variety of mechanisms: an effect on membrane phospholipids with an increase in cytosolic calcium, mitochondrial production of free radicals with mitochondrial injury, additive or parallel effects to calcium overload on ATP depletion, and an effect on the calcium release channel of the sarcoplasmic reticulum (SR) with enhanced release of calcium (Du Toit & Opie, 1994). Free radicals may also (1) inhibit the uptake of calcium by the SR, (2) inhibit the sodium pump, (3) stimulate sodium/calcium (Na/Ca) exchange, and (4) decrease the rate of inactivation of the calcium current (Du Toit & Opie, 1994). The "Cape Town hypothesis" is that free radicals constitute one of several causes of the early rise of cytosolic calcium on reperfusion (Fig 7-2) and it is these changes in calcium that are crucial.

Despite these important observations, therapy by neither calcium antagonists nor by free radical scavengers has yet been established as a means of diminishing stunning in patients, although one study with the calcium antagonist nisoldipine is promising (Sheiban et al., 1997). Furthermore, because stunning is transient by definition, it may be argued that there is no necessity to treat a self-healing condition. This argument becomes less viable when it is considered that repetitive stunning may be a cause of hibernation (Shen & Vatner, 1995) and may therefore contribute to critically impaired LV failure.

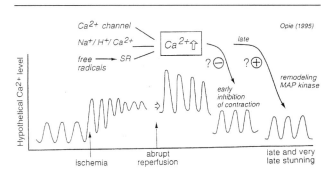

Figure 7-1. Proposed role of increased cytosolic calcium in causing early stunning after reperfusion and in hypothetically playing a role in late remodeling by stimulation of protein synthesis, possibly at the level of mitogen-activated protein (MAP) kinase. $Na^+/H^+/Ca^{2+}$ = sodium/proton and sodium/calcium exchange mechanisms; SR = sarcoplasmic reticulum. For data on cytosolic calcium measurements, see Gao and colleagues (1995) and Brooks and associates (1995). (Figure copyright L. H. Opie, 1995.)

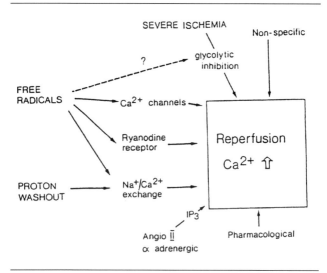

Figure 7-2. *Proposed mechanisms whereby the cytosolic calcium rises in the early reperfusion period. (Figure copyright by L. H. Opie, 1995.)*

Early versus late phases of short-term stunning

The effects of excess cytosolic calcium can be separated into two phases: It is proposed that in the first the damage is being done and in the second the myocardium is hypocontractile as a result of the damage already done. This is the so-called two-stage model (Du Toit & Opie, 1994). The origin of the hypocontractile state differs according to the stage and so does the proposed therapy. In the first stage, it can be hypothesized that all procedures leading to excess cytosolic calcium should be harmful and that the use of calcium antagonists as well as Na+/H+ exchange inhibitors should be beneficial (Table 7-1). In the second stage, calcium agonists such as beta-adrenergic stimulants may be useful to stimulate the hypocontractile left ventricle (Ito et al., 1987). Cardiac surgeons have acknowledged this distinction by using low-calcium reperfusion solutions following cardiac arrest and coronary bypass surgery, and then later when LV failure is manifest in the early postoperative phase, experience shows that calcium or calcium agonists are beneficial in sustaining the cardiac output.

Repetitive stunning

Repetitive ischemia frequently occurs in patients with coronary disease. Hypothetically, each ischemic episode could be followed by stunning. Each ischemic episode would also precondition against subsequent ischemia (Bolli et al., 1996). To model this situation, Park and associates (1995) gave ten rapidly repetitive coronary occlusions to conscious pigs. After the tenth occlusion, reperfusion was followed by delayed recovery that was still suboptimal at 5 hours. The calcium channel blocker nisoldipine given before, during, and after the ischemic episodes greatly enhanced the rate of recovery. These data show how ischemia that is cumulative (even though short lived) can cause prolonged stunning. Other evidence, also on conscious animal models, support the con-

TABLE 7-1. PROPOSED ROLE OF CALCIUM IN TWO PHASES OF
REPERFUSION STUNNING*

Parameter	Established calcium overload (phase 1)	Early stunning with hypocontractile myocardium (phase 2)
Cytosolic calcium (proposed patterns)	Increased (for a few minutes)	Initially increased, then normal or possibly decreased
Myocardial performance	Transiently normal	Depressed
Calcium antagonists	Benefit	Harm
Inorganic blockers	Benefit	Not tested
Ryanodine	Benefit	Harm?
Low-medium calcium	Benefit	Harm
Na^+/H^+ blockers	Benefit	No effect
High-medium calcium	Worsen	Benefit
Calcium agonists	Worsen	Benefit
Catecholamines	Worsen	Benefit

* Modified from Opie (1991) and Opie and Du Toit (1992), with permission.

cept that repetitive ischemia can give rise to stunning so severe and prolonged that it approximates hibernation (Shen
& Vatner, 1995).

HIBERNATION AND ISCHEMIC DYSFUNCTION

Hibernation was first described as a clinical condition in
which part of the myocardium does not contract normally
(systolic dysfunction) in the presence of coronary artery disease but without another obvious cause such as concurrent
angina or myocardial infarction. The original description of
Rahimtoola was: "a state of persistently impaired myocardial
and left ventricular function at rest due to reduced coronary
blood flow that can be partially or completely restored to normal if the myocardial oxygen supply/demand relationship is
favorably altered, either by improving blood flow and/or by
reducing demand" (Rahimtoola, 1985, 1989). It is now known,
however, that the resting blood flow may only be modestly or
marginally reduced despite coronary artery disease, and that
the flow reduction when present is not so low that it causes
anginal pain or permanently damages the myocardium.

Hibernation therefore poses an interesting challenge to
the definition of ischemia already given. Experimentally, the
blood flow is "too little" for normal contractility especially
during tachycardia (Shen & Vatner, 1995) and it could therefore be said that there is chronic ischemia. On the other
hand, when the ischemia does occur, it is mild enough to be
"compensated" by the decreased contractility, so that any
metabolic impairment is arrested and in fact there is no true
ischemia, at least not in a model of acute hibernation described by Schulz and coworkers (Schulz et al., 1993). An
important recent proposal is that the myocardial blood flow

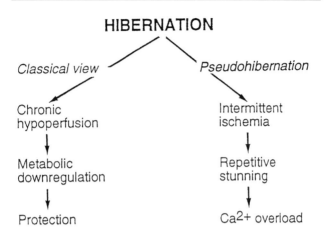

Figure 7-3. *Two current views on the genesis of hibernation.*

at rest may be normal, or nearly normal, with superimposed episodes of ischemia causing repetitive episodes of stunning that when summated translate into chronic impairment of LV function (Shen & Vatner, 1995). Clinically, there remains an impressive link between chronic ischemia and hibernation (see Chapter 13). Thus there are at present two main hypotheses for hibernation (Fig 7-3). Whatever the mechanism, when revascularization occurs, the hibernating segments "wake up" either rapidly (Ferrari et al., 1994) or sometimes only after many months (Rahimtoola, 1989; Vanoverschelde et al., 1993). Detection of the hibernating myocardium by PET is now used for preoperative detection of hibernation (Brunken & Armbrecht, 1990; Uren & Camici, 1992; Vanoverschelde et al., 1993), although the exact criteria are still open to dispute. A problem with this technique is that subendocardial flow cannot be measured separately and that very low flows are not accurate.

Hibernation without prior infarction

The extreme difficulty of deriving a simple hypothesis for hibernation is highlighted by the complex situation in patients as revealed by the study of Vanoverschelde and colleagues (1993). Their 26 patients with hibernation were carefully selected and did not have any prior myocardial infarction, but rather had repetitive attacks of angina pectoris. There were highly specific angiographic findings, consisting of an occluded proximal coronary artery filled by collaterals. Seventeen of the patients had resting mechanical dysfunction of myocardial segments as shown at contrast ventriculography. In these segments, myocardial blood flow was modestly depressed, oxidative metabolism was less than normal, yet glucose extraction had increased ("mismatch" pattern on PET). Collateral flow reserve was severely blunted. Despite marked histological changes shown by biopsy, wall motion had improved 5 to 8 months after revascularization.

These patients had the major criterion for hibernation in that recovery of poorly functioning segments took place after revascularization. The blood flow in those segments recovering best was only modestly reduced. Yet the severe histological changes found in the hibernating segments raised the possibility that the segments supplied by the collaterals were in fact intermittently severely ischemic, compatible with the history of angina pectoris.

Disuse atrophy versus phenotype change

Ventricular unloading can cause shrinkage of myocardial cells, and accumulation of collagen and fibroblasts (Kent et al., 1985). Certain changes, such as the loss of myofibrils, are common to the histology of the hibernating segments of patients studied by Vanoverschelde and colleagues (1993) or Schwarz and associates (1996), and also to disuse atrophy. A simple hypothesis would therefore be that during sustained hibernation, disuse atrophy may eventually occur. Additionally, in response to an unknown signal, there can be reversion to a fetal "downgraded" phenotype with delayed recovery to the normal pattern (Vanoverschelde et al., 1993). This phenotype has less well-differentiated myofibrils with small mitochondria, severely reduced contractile filaments, a reduced content of SR, and increased glycogen—a combination suggesting an adaptation whereby increased energy reserves (glycogen) are combined with decreased myocardial contraction (downgraded myofibrils).

Hibernation: another spectrum of changes?

It is thus evident that hibernation stretches all the way from the condition recognized by Ferrari and colleagues (1994), where regional function returns promptly at the operation table on revascularization, to another condition recognized by a much delayed mechanical recovery and overt histological changes (Schwarz et al., 1996; Vanoverschelde et al., 1993). The important point is that different observers are likely to be describing different entities under the same title of hibernation, which is not, however, a uniform condition but rather another spectrum of conditions. Hibernation stretches from acute to chronic hibernation, and from rapid to slow recovery of the contractile elements.

PRECONDITIONING—AN INEVITABLE PARTICIPANT IN THE NEW ISCHEMIC SYNDROMES?

Whereas many repetitive episodes of ischemia should produce cumulative damage, relatively few episodes or even one burst of short-lived, severe ischemia followed by complete reperfusion causes preconditioning (see Chapters 4–6). Although preconditioning is classically initiated by one or more periods of total ischemia each followed by reperfusion, nonetheless there are important variants. First, ischemic preconditioning can be achieved by a *partial coronary occlusion* (rather than total) and without intermittent reperfusion (Koning et al., 1994), explaining why in the Harris model, when coronary ligation is applied in two stages, there are less fatal arrhythmias than with one single occlusion of equal anatomic size. This finding raises the possibility that myocardial infarction of a "stuttering" pattern of onset may be less severe than expected. Another deviation from the classic pattern of preconditioning is *intraischemic preconditioning*, whereby an initial brief period of no-flow ischemia increases myocardial tolerance to subsequent low-flow ischemia without any intervening reperfusion period (Schulz et al., 1995). A third variation is that preconditioning can follow transient *vigorous beta-adrenergic stimulation* (Asimakis et al., 1994). Preconditioning may follow rapid pacing (Szilvassy et al., 1994). Protection may not be limited to the ischemic zone but may extend to remote "virgin" myocardial territory (Przyklenk et al., 1993). Thus, preconditioning may be invoked by more stimuli than previously appreciated, the common factor being a temporary energy imbalance between myocardial oxygen supply and demand (Headrick, 1996).

Is preconditioning related to some of the less common clinical aspects of effort angina? These may include warm-up angina (effort provokes pain, rest relieves pain, but renewed exertion is pain free) and angina of second wind (walk-through angina, in which continued exertion appears to overcome the angina). If these phenomena are related to preconditioning (Marber et al., 1994) then, logically, silent ischemia could also cause preconditioning. As silent ischemia is so common in patients with coronary disease, it is at least possible that preconditioning is an integral part of the clinical picture of repetitive ischemia, whether symptomatic or silent.

As already emphasized, first principles suggest that in the postinfarct period there is a mixture of stunned, necrotic, hibernating, and normal myocardium:

I. *Variations in myocardial response to ischemia*
   A. Transient anaerobic metabolism
   B. Anaerobic metabolism plus serious ionic imbalance ($Na/Ca/H$) with threatened necrosis
   C. Tissue necrosis and eventual fibrosis, including inflammatory response and cytokine production
   D. Tissue repair including activation of protein synthesis and remodeling/hypertrophy

II. *Variations in coronary blood supply*
   A. Coronary artery disease with one or more of the following
      1. Endothelial damage with impaired production of nitric oxide
      2. Increased vascular smooth muscle (vasoconstriction) or if severe and localized vasospasm
      3. Platelet thrombi
      4. Plaque rupture
      5. Occluding thrombus with or without recanalization
      6. Inadequate supply as a result of increased oxygen demand (exercise, emotion, acute hypertension)

III. *Response to ischemia/reperfusion*
   A. Repetitive stunning including maiming
   B. Hibernation (may include above)
   C. Repetitive preconditioning

A significant percentage of postinfarct patients, almost 40% in one study, may have exercise-induced ischemia, and in almost three quarters of such individuals the ischemia will be silent (Jespersen et al., 1985). Such repetitive ischemia may hypothetically result in postischemic stunning and/or hibernation, and hypothetically could even be limited by concurrent preconditioning (discussed later).

An additional complexity is the late recovery, from 5 weeks to 7 months postinfarct, of hypocontractile myocardium and the delayed improvement in ejection fraction (Galli et al., 1994). Because of the spontaneous lessening of the perfusion defect in the apparently infarcted area, this defect may represent hibernation, at least in part. It is perhaps a question of semantics whether chronic stunning (Opie, 1995) can really be dissociated from true hibernation. In either case, the crucial observation is the prolonged postinfarct improvement in mechanical function. Of interest is the recent observation that the calcium antagonist nisoldipine can hasten the delayed return of LV function after primary coronary angioplasty for AMI (Sheiban, 1997). These reports may only apply to a highly selected group of patients with recent myocardial infarction, but nonetheless support the concept of reversible postinfarct LV dysfunction that, when prolonged, may be a form of chronic stunning (Opie, 1995).

CALCIUM IONS—A CRUCIAL ROLE IN THE NEW ISCHEMIC SYNDROMES?

Because calcium ion regulation is crucial for normal cardiac contraction and relaxation, it would not be surprising if the altered myocardial function of the new ischemic syndromes could be explained at least in part in terms of altered calcium ion regulation (Table 7-1). The following hypothetical proposals are an attempt at a unitary explanation, while recognizing the complexity of each condition and the likelihood that other multiple mechanisms are also at work.

Starting with *stunning*, an important hypothesis is that cytosolic calcium overload during the reperfusion period is the crucial abnormality (Brooks et al., 1995; Du Toit & Opie, 1992; Du Toit & Opie, 1994; Gao et al., 1995; Myers et al., 1995; Opie, 1989). The proposed mechanism is that calcium-dependent proteins are activated and the thin filaments damaged, thereby impairing systolic force generations, while the increased cytosolic calcium augments diastolic tone and predisposes to diastolic dysfunction and after-contractions (Gao et al., 1995). The prominent role ascribed to free radicals by several groups (Bolli, 1990, 1992; Hearse, 1990, 1991) could be incorporated into the "calcium hypothesis" because free radicals by damaging membranes may enhance cytosolic calcium (Hearse, 1991; Opie, 1989, 1991).

Next, considering *hibernation*, if viewed as a series of repetitive attacks of stunning, then likewise there are repetitive episodic rises of cytosolic calcium that immobilize the myocardium. If viewed as persistent, chronic, mild ischemia, with a down-regulated energy demand following contractile arrest, then the proposal would be that energy production from enhanced glycolysis is sufficient to prevent ischemic contracture, but insufficient to allow for normal contractile activity. There is some evidence for enhanced glycolysis in the hibernating myocardium in that the extraction of F18-fluorodeoxyglucose is enhanced relative to the modestly decreased coronary flow so that there is a mismatch pattern (Uren & Camici, 1992; Vanoverschelde et al., 1993).

In the case of *preconditioning*, the mechanism may be exceedingly complex. The preconditioned myocardium could be protected from the normally adverse effects of ischemic calcium overload by a series of mechanisms including (1) activation, possibly by adenosine, of the inhibitory G-protein, G_i (Niroomand, 1995; Thornton et al., 1993); (2) decreased release of calcium from the SR (Zucchi et al., 1995); and (3) decreased tissue levels of cyclic AMP (Sandhu et al., 1996; Szilvassy et al., 1994). These specific changes could explain the decreased cytosolic calcium ion levels found in preconditioned cells (Okumura et al., 1995). In view of the complex mechanisms proposed for preconditioning, it would be simplistic to suppose that there is a simple role for calcium ions. For example, activation of PKC, often invoked as crucial to preconditioning, is more likely to be accompanied by a rise than a fall of cytosolic calcium (because of the simultaneous release of the calcium-mobilizing compound inositol trisphosphate). Nonetheless, possibly an increased subsarcolemmal calcium level may facilitate the link between phospholipase C, PKC, and the ATP-dependent potassium channel. The link between calcium and adenosine and PKC may also depend on the isoform of PKC. For example the delta-isoform may be linked to adenosine A_1 stimulation in the rat (Henry et al., 1996). In the neonatal rat cardiomyocytes the epsilon-isoform decreases contraction (Johnson & Mochly-Rosen, 1995). Hypothetically, phosphorylation of a contractile protein may be involved. Thus, it is likely that the role of calcium ions in preconditioning is, like the phenomenon itself, unlikely to be simple.

Rather, the present evidence is that calcium ions play an important and possibly dominant role in stunning and hence, possibly, indirectly in some types of hibernation and therefore in the new ischemic syndromes.

In *stunning* in the isolated rat heart, provision of nisoldipine at the time of reperfusion diminishes reperfusion stunning (Du Toit & Opie, 1992), yet it is sometimes argued that calcium ions entering at the time of reperfusion do not play a role because Ehring and colleagues (1992) found a protective effect of nisoldipine only when it was given before reperfusion and not at the time of reperfusion. This argument neglects the fact that nisoldipine was in fact given 4 to 6 minutes after the onset of reperfusion in the study of Ehring and colleagues (1992), whereas increased cytosolic levels on reperfusion returned to normal within a few minutes of the onset of reperfusion, as also acknowledged by Park and associates (1996). The clinical analogy, similar in design and concept to the rat heart experiments of Du Toit and Opie (1992), is the benefit obtained by intracoronary nisoldipine given at the time of primary angioplasty for AMI (Sheiban et al., 1997). Possibly the "window of opportunity" for protection against stunning by the acute use of calcium antagonists at the time of reperfusion is rather brief.

In patients with postinfarct hypokinetic myocardium, Pouler and coworkers (1992) gave nisoldipine, which improved systolic and diastolic dysfunction, possibly due to afterload reduction or else by better control of cytosolic calcium. The left ventricles returned to a more ellipsoid, less spherical shape. Of note, these patients had a mean ejection fraction of 37 to 39% and no clinical features of heart failure.

In early postinfarct diastolic dysfunction in patients studied 2 days after thrombolytic reperfusion, intravenous gallopamil improved diastolic dysfunction (Natale et al., 1992). There are several noteworthy points: (1) the study did not comment on systolic function, which might have been impaired; (2) the calcium antagonist was more able than the beta-blocker atenolol to improve indices of diastolic function; and (3) gallopamil changed the peak filling time from late to early diastole (i.e., the early filling improved). Two possible mechanisms were proposed, one being reduced stunning and the other the existence of viable, underperfused ischemic myocardium that responded to the antiischemic effect of gallopamil.

In postinfarct diastolic dysfunction in patients entered within 5 weeks of AMI, the DEFIANT study (1992) showed the benefits of the calcium antagonist nisoldipine. The patients had a low mean ejection fraction of 42%. The latter value is just above that required for allocation to angiotensin-converting enzyme (ACE) inhibitor therapy (Pfeffer et al., 1992). The striking changes after 4 weeks were those in isovolumic relaxation, which prolonged during placebo treatment and decreased with nisoldipine. It is important to note that the patients were not in overt heart failure, almost all being in New York Heart Association classes I and II. Recently, the data in a similar but separate and larger study (DEFIANT II) over a longer period of 6 months also supported the improvement of diastolic function found in the first study (Poole-Wilson, 1995). These observations, taken together, provide further indirect support for the potential role of calcium in stunning.

SUMMARY

Ischemic heart disease was once the province of the bedside clinician who could specifically diagnose entities such as angina of effort, unstable angina, and myocardial infarction. Ischemia must now be regarded as much more complex and elusive because of the discovery of the new ischemic syndromes, including stunning, hibernation, and preconditioning. In stunning, there is postreperfusion mechanical dysfunction that recovers spontaneously. In hibernation, there is prominent contractile dysfunction, apparently out of proportion to any reduction in coronary flow, and recovery after revascularization is good. In preconditioning, severe ischemia followed by reperfusion protects against subsequent ischemia so that precondition variably alters the severity of ischemic damage in the other new ischemic syndromes. It is proposed that cytosolic calcium overload at the time of reperfusion plays a major role in the causation of stunning. In ischemic LV diastolic dysfunction without major systolic dysfunction, calcium antagonists may be appropriate therapy, which could point to a role for abnormal regulation of cytosolic calcium.

REFERENCES

Asimakis GK, Inners-McBride K, Conti VR, Yang C. Transient beta-adrenergic stimulation can precondition the rat heart against postischemic contractile dysfunction. *Cardiovasc Res* 1994; 28: 1726–1734.

Boden WE, Brooks WW, Conrad CH, et al. Incomplete, delayed functional recovery late after reperfusion following acute myocardial infarction: "maimed myocardium." *Am Heart J* 1995; 130: 922–932.

Bolli R. Mechanism of myocardial "stunning." *Circulation* 1990; 82: 723–738.

Bolli R. Myocardial "stunning" in man. *Circulation* 1992; 86: 1671–1692.

Bolli R, Zughaib M, Li X-Y, et al. Recurrent ischemia in the canine heart causes recurrent bursts of free radical production that have a cumulative effect on contractile function: a pathophysiological basis for chronic myocardial "stunning." *J Clin Invest* 1995; 96: 1066–1084.

Bourdillon PD, Lorell BH, Mirsky I, et al. Increased regional myocardial stiffness of the left ventricle during pacing-induced angina in man. *Circulation* 1983; 67: 316–323.

Braunwald E. Stunning of the myocardium: an update. *Cardiovasc Drugs Ther* 1991; 5: 849–852.

Braunwald E, Kloner RA. The stunned myocardium: prolonged, postischemic ventricular dysfunction. *Circulation* 1982; 66: 1146–1149.

Brooks WW, Conrad CH, Morgan JP. Reperfusion induced arrhythmias following ischemia in intact rat heart: role of intracellular calcium. *Cardiovasc Res* 1995; 29: 536–542.

Brunken RC, Armbrecht JJ. Detection of hibernating myocardium with positron emission tomography. In: Zipes DP, Rowlands DJ, eds. *Progress in cardiology*. Philadelphia: Lea & Febiger, 1990: 161–179.

Deanfield JE, Maseri A, Selwyn AP, et al. Myocardial ischemia during daily life in patients with stable angina: its relation to symptoms and heart rate changes. *Lancet* 1983; 2: 753–758.

DEFIANT (Doppler Flow and Echocardiography in Functional Cardiac Insufficiency: Assessment of Nisoldipine Treatment) Research Group. Improved diastolic function with the calcium antagonist nisoldipine (coat-core) in patients post myocardial infarction: results of the DEFIANT study. *Eur Heart J* 1992; 13: 1496–1505.

Du Toit EF, Opie LH. Inhibitors of Ca^{2+}-ATPase pump of sarcoplasmic reticulum attenuate reperfusion stunning in isolated rat heart. *J Cardiovasc Pharmacol* 1994; 24: 678–684.

Du Toit J, Opie LH. Modulation of severity of reperfusion stunning in the isolated rat heart by agents altering calcium flux at onset of reperfusion. *Circ Res* 1992; 70: 960–967.

Ehring T, Boehm M, Heusch G. The calcium antagonist nisoldipine improves the functional recovery of reperfused myocardium only when given before ischemia. *J Cardiovasc Pharmacol* 1992; 20: 63–74.

Ferrari R, La Canna G, Giubbini R, et al. Left ventricular dysfunction due to stunning and hibernation in patients. *Cardiovasc Drugs Ther* 1994; 8: 371–380.

Galli M, Marcassa C, Imparato A, et al. Effects of nitroglycerin by technetium-99m sestamibi tomoscintigraphy on resting regional myocardial hypoperfusion in stable patients with healed myocardial infarction. *Am J Cardiol* 1994; 74: 843–848.

Gao WD, Atar D, Backx PH, Marban E. Relationship between intracellular calcium and contractile force in stunned myocardium. Direct evidence for decreased myofilament Ca^{2+} responsiveness and altered diastolic function in intact ventricular muscle. *Circ Res* 1995; 76: 1036–1048.

Headrick JP. Ischemic preconditioning: bioenergetic and metabolic changes and the role of endogenous adenosine. *J Mol Cell Cardiol* 1996; 28: 1227–1240.

Hearse DJ. Ischemia, reperfusion and the determinants of tissue injury. *Cardiovasc Drugs Ther* 1990; 4: 767–776.

Hearse DJ. Stunning: a radical review. *Cardiovasc Drugs Ther* 1991; 5: 853–876.

Henry P, Demolombe S, Pucèat, Escande D. Adenosine A_1 stimulation activates δ-protein kinase C in rat ventricular myocytes. *Circ Res* 1996; 78: 161–165.

Heyndrickx GR, Baig H, Nellens P, et al. Depression of regional blood flow and wall thickening after brief coronary occlusions. *Am J Physiol* 1978; 234: H653–H659.

Heyndrickx GR, Millard RW, McRitchie RJ, et al. Regional myocardial function and electrophysiological alterations after brief coronary occlusion in conscious dogs. *J Clin Invest* 1975; 56: 978–985.

Ito BR, Tate H, Kobayashi M, Schaper W. Reversibly injured, postischemic canine myocardium retains normal contractile reserve. *Circ Res* 1987; 61: 834–846.

Jespersen CM, Kassis E, Edeling CJ, Madsen JK. The prognostic value of maximal exercise testing soon after first myocardial infarction. *Eur Heart J* 1985; 6: 769–772.

Johnson JA, Mochly-Rosen D. Inhibition of the spontaneous rate of contraction of neonatal cardiac myocytes by protein kinase C isozymes. A putative role for the epsilon isozyme. *Circ Res* 1995; 76: 654–663.

Kennedy C, Leff P. Painful connection for ATP. *Nature* 1995; 377: 385–386.

Kent RL, Uboh CE, Thompson EW, et al. Biochemical and structural correlates in unloaded and reloaded cat myocardium. *J Mol Cell Cardiol* 1985; 17: 153–165.

Kloner RA, Allen J, Cox TA, et al. Stunned left ventricular myocardium after exercise treadmill testing in coronary artery disease. *Am J Cardiol* 1991; 68: 329–334.

Koning MMG, Simonis LAJ, de Zeeuw S, et al. Ischemic preconditioning by partial occlusion without intermittent reperfusion. *Cardiovasc Res* 1994; 28: 1146–1151.

Lavallee M, Cox D, Patrick TA, Vatner SF. Salvage of myocardial function by coronary artery reperfusion 1, 2 and 3 hours after occlusion in conscious dogs. *Circ Res* 1983; 53: 235–247.

Legault SE, Freeman MR, Langer A, Armstrong PW. Pathophysiology and time course of silent myocardial ischemia during mental stress: clinical, anatomical, and physiological correlates. *Br Heart J* 1995; 73: 242–249.

Marber MS, Joy MD, Yellon DM. Is warm-up in angina ischemic preconditioning? *Br Heart J* 1994; 72: 213–215.

McKenney PA, Apstein CS, Mendes LA, et al. Increased left ventricular diastolic chamber stiffness immediately after coronary artery bypass surgery. *J Am Coll Cardiol* 1994; 24: 1189–1194.

Mitchell MB, Meng X, Ao L, et al. Preconditioning of isolated rat heart is mediated by protein kinase C. *Circ Res* 1995; 76: 73–81.

Moolman J, Genade S, Tromp E, Lochner A. Ischemic preconditioning: interaction with antiadrenergic interventions [abstract]. *J Mol Cell Cardiol* 1995; 27: A161.

Murry CE, Jennings RB, Reimer KA. Preconditioning with ischemia: a delay of lethal cell injury in ischemic myocardium. *Circulation* 1986; 74: 1124–1136.

Myers ML, Mathur S, Li G-H, Karmazyn M. Sodium-hydrogen exchange inhibitors improve postischemic recovery of function in the perfused rabbit heart. *Cardiovasc Res* 1995; 29: 209–214.

Natale E, Ricci R, Tubaro M, Milazzotto F. Diastolic ventricular dysfunction in noncomplicated acute myocardial infarction: the influence of gallopamil. *J Cardiovasc Pharmacol* 1992; 20(Suppl 7): S48–S56.

Niroomand F, Weinbrenner C, Weis A, et al. Impaired function of inhibitory G proteins during acute myocardial ischemia of canine hearts and its reversal during reperfusion and a second period of ischemia. Possible implications for the protective mechanism of ischemic preconditioning. *Cir Res* 1995; 76: 861–870.

Okumura H, Takeda S, Tamura K, et al. Ischemic preconditioning attenuates increases in $[H^+]_i$ and $[Ca^{2+}]_i$ during prolonged ischemia in isolated rat hearts [abstract]. *J Mol Cell Cardiol* 1995; 27: A145.

Opie LH. Reperfusion injury and its pharmacologic modification. *Circulation* 1989; 80: 1049–1062.

Opie LH. Postischemic stunning—the case for calcium as the ultimate culprit. *Cardiovasc Drugs Ther* 1991; 5: 895–900.

Opie LH. Cardiac metabolism—emergence, decline, and resurgence. Part I. *Cardiovasc Res* 1992; 26: 721–733.

Opie LH. Chronic stunning: the new switch in thought. *Basic Res Cardiol* 1995; 90: 303–304.

Opie LH, Coetzee WA. Role of calcium ions in reperfusion arrhythmias. Relevance to pharmacological intervention. *Cardiovasc Drugs Ther* 1988; 2: 623–636.

Opie LH, Du Toit EF. Post-ischemic stunning: the two-phase model for the role of calcium as pathogen. *J Cardiovasc Pharmacol* 1992; 20(Suppl 5): S1–S4.

Park SW, Tang X-L, Qiu Y, et al. Nisoldipine attenuates myocardial stunning induced by multiple coronary occlusions in conscious pigs and this effect is independent of changes in hemodynamics or coronary blood flow. *J Mol Cell Cardiol* 1996; 28: 655–666.

Pfeffer MA, Braunwald E, Moye LA, et al. Effect of captopril on mortality and morbidity in patients with left ventricular dysfunction after myocardial infarction. Results of the survival and ventricular enlargement trial. *N Engl J Med* 1992; 327: 669–677.

Poole-Wilson PA. DEFIANT-II: the effect of nisoldipine vs placebo on ventricular function and exercise capacity [abstract]. Presented at the XVIIth Congress of the European Society of Cardiology. Amsterdam, The Netherlands. August 1995.

Poole-Wilson PA, Harding DP, Bourdillon PDV, Tones MA. Calcium out of control. *J Mol Cell Cardiol* 1984; 16: 175–187.

Pouler H, van Eyll C, Gurnè O, Rousseau MF. Effects of prolonged nisoldipine administration on the "hibernating" myocardium. *J Cardiovasc Pharmacol* 1992; 20(Suppl 5): S73–S78.

Przyklenk K, Bauer B, Ovize M, et al. Regional ischemic "preconditioning" protects remote virgin myocardium from subsequent sustained coronary occlusion. *Circulation* 1993; 87: 893–899.

Rahimtoola SH. A perspective on three large multicenter randomized clinical trials of coronary bypass surgery for chronic stable angina. *Circulation* 1985; 72(Suppl V): 123–125.

Rahimtoola SH. The hibernating myocardium. *Am Heart J* 1989; 117: 211–221.

Saman S, Coetzee WA, Opie LH. Inhibition by simulated ischemia or hypoxia of delayed afterdepolarizations provoked by cyclic AMP: significance for ischemic and reperfusion arrhythmias. *J Mol Cell Cardiol* 1988; 20: 91–95.

Sandhu R, Thomas U, Diaz RJ, Wilson GJ. Effect of ischemic preconditioning of the myocardium on cAMP. *Circ Res* 1996; 78: 137–147.

Schulz R, Post H, Sakka S, et al. Intraischemic preconditioning. Increased tolerance to sustained low-flow ischemia by a brief episode of no-flow ischemia without intermittent reperfusion. *Circ Res* 1995; 76: 942–950.

Schulz R, Rose J, Martin C, et al. Development of short-term myocardial hibernation. Its limitation by the severity of ischemia and inotropic stimulation. *Circulation* 1993; 88: 684–695.

Schwarz ER, Schaper J, vom Dahl J, et al. Myocyte degeneration and cell death in hibernating human myocardium. *J Am Coll Cardiol* 1996; 27: 1577–1585.

Sheiban I, Tonni S, Chizzoni A, et al. Recovery of left ventricular function following early reperfusion in acute myocardial infarction: a potential role for the calcium antagonist nisoldipine. *Cardiovasc Drugs Ther* 1997; (in press).

Shen Y-T, Vatner SF. Mechanism of impaired myocardial function during progressive coronary stenosis in conscious pigs. Hibernation versus stunning? *Circ Res* 1995; 76: 479–488.

Sheps DS, Ballenger MN, De Gent GE, et al. Psychological responses to a speech stressor: correlation of plasma beta-endorphin levels at rest and after psychological stress with thermally measured pain threshold in patients with coronary artery disease. *J Am Coll Cardiol* 1995; 25: 1499–1503.

Stern S, Tzivoni D. Early detection of silent ischemic heart disease by 24-hour electrocardiographic monitoring of active subjects. *Br Heart J* 1974; 36: 481–486.

Sylven C. Mechanisms of pain in angina pectoris—a critical review of the adenosine hypothesis. *Cardiovasc Drugs Ther* 1993; 7: 745–759.

Szilvassy Z, Ferdinandy P, Bor P, et al. Ventricular overdrive pacing-induced anti-ischemic effect: a conscious rabbit model of preconditioning. *Am J Physiol* 1994; 266: H2033–H2041.

Thornton JD, Liu GS, Downey JM. Pretreatment with pertussis toxin blocks the protective effects of preconditioning: evidence for a G-protein mechanism. *J Mol Cell Cardiol* 1993; 25: 311–320.

Uren NG, Camici PG. Hibernation and myocardial ischemia: clinical detection by positron emission tomography. In: Opie LH, ed. *Stunning, hibernation, and calcium in myocardial ischemia and reperfusion.* Boston: Kluwer Academic Publishers, 1992: 202–215.

Vanoverschelde J-L, Wijns W, Depre C, et al. Mechanisms of chronic regional post-ischemic dysfunction in humans. New insights from the study of noninfarcted collateral-dependent myocardium. *Circulation* 1993; 87: 1513–1523.

Wang YG, Lipsius SL. β-adrenergic stimulation induces acetylcholine to activate ATP-sensitive K^+ current in cat atrial myocytes. *Circ Res* 1995; 77: 565–574.

Zucchi R, Ronca-Testoni S, Yu G, et al. Postischemic changes in cardiac sarcoplasmic reticulum Ca^{2+} channels. A possible mechanism of ischemic preconditioning. *Circ Res* 1995; 76: 1049–1056.

CHAPTER 8

Ischemic Diastolic Dysfunction and Postischemic Diastolic Stunning

Carl S. Apstein
Niraj Varma
Franz R. Eberli

Cardiac failure is the result of either systolic or diastolic dysfunction, or both. Systolic dysfunction can be defined as a decreased ejection from one or both ventricles. Diastolic dysfunction can be defined as an impaired filling of one or both ventricles. Systolic dysfunction is easily assessed by measuring ejection fraction and regional wall-motion abnormalities. Clinical manifestations of pure LV systolic dysfunction include a decreased cardiac output, increased heart rate, and peripheral vasoconstriction. However, patients hospitalized for congestive heart failure almost always present with the additional symptom of shortness of breath, at rest, or with exertion, due to pulmonary congestion as a result of LV diastolic dysfunction (Grossman, 1991; Packer, 1990). Clinical manifestations of diastolic dysfunction include:

1. Exertional dyspnea
2. Congestive heart failure
3. Acute ischemic pulmonary edema
4. Respiratory symptoms of angina pectoris
5. Postcardiac surgery dysfunction

In fact, approximately one third of all cases of congestive heart failure are due primarily to diastolic dysfunction. Classical examples of isolated diastolic dysfunction are hypertrophic cardiomyopathy, the hypertensive hypertrophic cardiomyopathy of the elderly, and aortic stenosis with a normal ejection fraction (Fifer et al., 1986; Hess et al., 1986; Topol et al., 1985). Such patients have normal systolic function despite clinical signs and symptoms of left-sided heart failure (i.e., dyspnea on exertion or pulmonary congestion). The fraction of patients with congestive heart failure due primarily to diastolic dysfunction is higher in elderly patients than in the general population (Gaasch, 1994).

Understanding the pathophysiology of diastolic dysfunction is important, because it affects therapy and prognosis. Diastolic properties are determined by a complex

TABLE 8-1 DIASTOLIC DYSFUNCTION: PARAMETERS AND ETIOLOGY

Physiological abnormality	Alteration in parameter of assessment	Common etiology
Delayed or incomplete relaxation	↑Tau ↑IVRT ↓E/A ratio	LV hypertrophy Myocardial ischemia LV asynchrony Abnormal loading
Early diastolic filling abnormalities	↓Peak filling rate ↑Time to peak filling ↓E/A ratio	Delayed relaxation LV asynchrony
Late diastolic filling abnormalities	↑Diastolic P/V relationship Normal or ↑E/A ratio	LV chamber dilation Restrictive/constrictive filling pattern
Increased LV passive chamber stiffness	↑Diastolic P/V relationship ↑Stiffness constant	↑Collagen and fibrosis Myocardial infiltration (e.g., amyloid) ↑Vascular turgor Concentric LVH Postmyocardial infarction hypertrophy and fibrosis LV chamber dilation

Tau = time constant of isovolumic pressure decay; IVRT = isovolumic relaxation time; E/A ratio = ratio of early and late LV inflow as detected by Doppler echocardiography; peak filling rate = dV/dt max; time to peak filling = time to dV/dt max; ↑ diastolic P/V relationship = upward shift and/or increased slope of LV diastolic pressure/volume relationship; stiffness constant = K_p constant of chamber stiffness calculated from simple exponential of pressure-volume relationship ($\ln P = K_p V + \ln c$).

interplay of functional and structural components. The major components contributing to diastolic dysfunction are (1) slowed and incomplete myocardial relaxation, (2) impaired LV filling, and (3) altered passive elastic properties of the ventricle, resulting in increased passive stiffness. Table 8-1 lists the most common etiologies leading to these forms of diastolic dysfunction and some of the parameters used to measure diastolic dysfunction. Measurements of diastolic properties are more complicated than those of systolic function. Usually high-fidelity pressure measurements and/or simultaneous LV pressure-volume measurements are required. Changes in the isovolumic relaxation are most often assessed by changes in the time constant of the isovolumic LV pressure decay (Tau), filling abnormalities by changes in the filling rate and the time to peak filling, and changes in passive elastic properties by changes in the diastolic pressure-volume relationship. In a given patient, impairment of one or more of these parameters will result in decreased LV chamber distensibility as manifested by an increase in diastolic pressure at any given LV volume.

Widespread use of noninvasive methods of cardiac imaging has led to the recognition that LV diastolic dysfunction commonly occurs as a result of myocardial hypertrophy and/or ischemia. Myocardial resistance to diastolic filling is usually the result of common structural abnormalities such as hypertrophy and interstitial fibrosis and/or impaired myocyte relaxation as a result of ischemia. The increased mass of the hypertrophied myocardium, and the increased collagen content that frequently accompanies hypertrophy, both represent structural abnormalities that reduce diastolic distensibility. Ischemia also causes a functional impairment of myocyte relaxation. Important interactions connect hypertrophy and ischemia. The left ventricle with concentric hypertrophy is more susceptible to ischemia, especially subendocardial ischemia, and such myocardium generally exhibits exaggerated ischemic diastolic dysfunction (for reviews see Gaasch, 1994; Grossman, 1991; Lorell, 1994). For a given degree of ischemia the functional impairment of relaxation is more severe in the hypertrophied heart than occurs in the absence of hypertrophy (Eberli et al., 1992a; Lorell, 1994). Thus, patients with concentric left ventricular hypertrophy (LVH) secondary to chronic hypertension or aortic stenosis are particularly susceptible to ischemic diastolic dysfunction.

Ischemic diastolic dysfunction is a reversible impairment of myocyte relaxation caused by ischemia. The slowing or failure of myocyte relaxation means that a fraction of actin-myosin cross-bridges persist and continue to generate tension throughout diastole, especially in early diastole, creating a state of *partial persistent systole*. As a result, LV pressure decay, as assessed by Tau, is impaired and the left ventricle is functionally stiffer than normal during diastole. Such ischemic diastolic dysfunction can continue during and after reperfusion, resulting in a phase of postischemic diastolic stunning, analogous to postischemic stunning of contractile function. For example, diastolic dysfunction is usually present early after cardiac surgery, after the myocardium has been exposed to cardioplegic arrest (i.e., to ischemia and reperfusion) (McKenney et al., 1994a, 1994b).

This chapter considers the clinical syndromes of diastolic dysfunction listed earlier by reviewing the physiology of ischemic diastolic dysfunction, the subcellular mechanisms responsible for it, and current therapy.

NORMAL LV DIASTOLIC FUNCTION: MATCHING INPUT TO OUTPUT

Cardiac function, especially during exercise, is critically dependent on diastolic physiological mechanisms to increase LV filling (cardiac input) in parallel with LV ejection (cardiac output). Furthermore, adequate pulmonary function is also dependent on LV diastolic function because LV diastolic pressure directly affects pulmonary capillary pressure. Figure 8-1 presents this relationship by illustrating the heart and lungs during diastole (the mitral valve is open). During diastole the left ventricle, left atrium, and pulmonary veins form a "common chamber" that is continuous with the pulmonary capillary bed. Therefore, an increase in LV diastolic pressure will increase pulmonary capillary pressure, and, if high enough, will cause pulmonary congestion and edema.

LV diastolic pressure is determined by the volume of blood in the LV during diastole and by LV diastolic distensibility or compliance. At the onset of diastole, relaxation of the contracted myocardium occurs. This is a dynamic process that takes place during isovolumic relaxation (between aortic valve closure and mitral valve opening) and during early rapid filling of the ventricle. The rapid pressure decay,

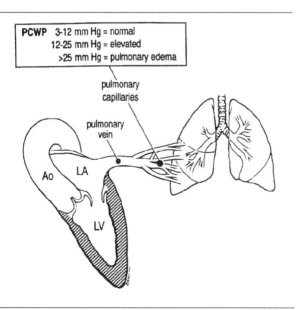

Figure 8-1. *Left ventricular diastolic pressure and pulmonary congestion. The heart is drawn in diastole with the mitral valve open to illustrate that during diastole the left ventricle (LV), the left atrium (LA), and the pulmonary veins form a common chamber continuous with the pulmonary capillary bed. Thus, left ventricular diastolic pressure determines pulmonary capillary pressure and the presence or absence of pulmonary congestion or edema. Ao = aorta.*

and the concomitant "untwisting" and elastic recoil of the left ventricle, produce a ventricular suction that augments the left atrial-ventricular pressure gradient and thus enhances diastolic filling. During the later phases of diastole the normal left ventricle is composed of completely relaxed myocytes and is very compliant and easily distensible, offering minimal resistance to LV filling over a normal volume range. Therefore, LV filling can normally be accomplished by very low "filling" pressures in the left atrium and pulmonary veins, preserving a low pulmonary capillary pressure (normal pulmonary capillary pressure is <12 mmHg) and a high degree of lung distensibility. A loss of normal LV diastolic relaxation and distensibility, due to either structural or functional causes, impairs LV filling, resulting in increases in LV diastolic, left atrial, and pulmonary venous pressures, which directly increase pulmonary capillary pressure.

Measurement of LV diastolic distensibility

LV diastolic distensibility is quantified by the position and slope of the LV filling curve, or diastolic pressure-volume (P-V) curve, which plots LV diastolic pressure as a function of LV diastolic volume throughout diastole. A relatively stiff, nondistensible ventricle will require higher pressures to achieve filling of a given volume. Therefore an increase in LV diastolic chamber stiffness (or decrease in distensibility or compliance) shifts the LV diastolic P-V curve upward and often also increases its slope. Definition of LV filling curves in humans requires the simultaneous measurement of LV diastolic pressure and volume. Such LV volume measurements have been achieved by angiography, echocardiography, or radionuclide imaging techniques simultaneous with measurements of LV diastolic pressure. Figure 8-2 illustrates LV filling curves in a patient at rest and during myo-

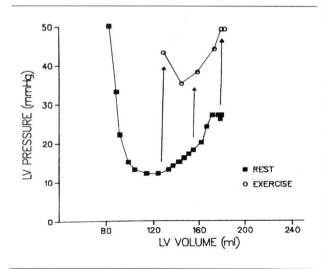

Figure 8-2. *The classical LV diastolic pressure-volume shift of ischemia is illustrated by this patient. At all diastolic volumes pressure is clearly elevated compared to the resting coordinates. (Reprinted with permission from Carroll and Carroll [1991].)*

cardial ischemia caused by exercise. During exercise the diastolic P-V curve is shifted upward, indicating decreased LV diastolic distensibility.

LV-filling dynamics

The normal left ventricle has a characteristic pattern of inflow velocities that are altered with the development of diastolic dysfunction. Because inflow velocities are readily measured by Doppler echocardiography, a characteristic abnormal inflow pattern provides diagnostic evidence for the presence of diastolic dysfunction. The altered inflow pattern also has important physiological consequences.

Figure 8-3 depicts an idealized change of LV volume versus time during systole and diastole. Normally, LV in-

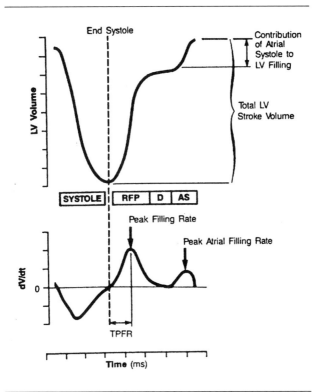

Figure 8-3. Idealized plot of LV volume versus time (top) and the rate of change of volume (dV/dt) versus time (bottom) as might be obtained from contrast or radionuclide ventriculography. The representative cardiac cycle begins at end diastole. Subsequent events as depicted by the bars in the center of the figure are (1) systole, during which LV volume decreases to a minimum, and (2) diastole, the beginning of which is signaled by the opening of the mitral valve and the onset of LV filling. Diastole has three distinct phases in normal individuals: (1) the rapid filling phase (RFP), during which the left ventricle fills rapidly, dV/dt reaches its maximum, and the peak filling rate occurs; (2) diastasis (D), during which relatively little LV volume change occurs; and (3) atrial systole (AS), in which active atrial contraction fills the left ventricle to its end diastolic volume. The diastolic parameters that have been derived from such analysis are the peak filling rate, the time to peak filling rate (TPFR), the percent contribution of atrial systole, and the first third filling fraction. (Reprinted with permission from Labovitz and Pearson [1987].)

flow velocity and the volume rate of LV filling is greatest early in diastole, immediately after mitral valve opening, and is responsible for the normally tall E-wave of the Doppler echocardiogram. Relatively little LV filling occurs in late diastole because most atrial-to-ventricular transfer of blood has occurred in early and mid-diastole. The amount of blood transported by atrial contraction is relatively small, the velocity imparted by the atrial contraction (the A-wave of the Doppler echocardiogram) is relatively low, and the normal E/A wave ratio is greater than 1 and approaches a value of 2 in younger individuals (Cohen et al., 1996; Hatle, 1993; Labovitz & Pearson, 1987).

With the diastolic dysfunction that accompanies ischemia and/or hypertrophy, myocardial relaxation is characteristically impaired and the rate and amount of early diastolic LV filling is reduced with a resultant shift of LV filling to the later part of diastole. The Doppler E-wave is decreased. The hemodynamic load on the atrium is increased and atrial contraction makes a more important contribution to ventricular filling than in normals. This is reflected by an increase in the Doppler A-wave and a decrease in the E/A ratio. A typical example of changes in the mitral flow velocities during short periods of ischemia (i.e., balloon angioplasty) is given in Figure 8-4. The chronic atrial overload often eventually results in atrial fibrillation, and the loss of atrial contraction can dramatically reduce LV filling, left atrial emptying, and LV stroke volume. The redistribution of filling from early to late diastole also means that LV filling and left atrial emptying are compromised more in patients with diastolic dysfunction than in normals by the occurrence of tachycardia; an increased heart rate shortens the duration of diastole and truncates the important late phase of diastolic filling.

Doppler echocardiographic assessment of LV filling has its limitations, since diastolic filling parameters are a func-

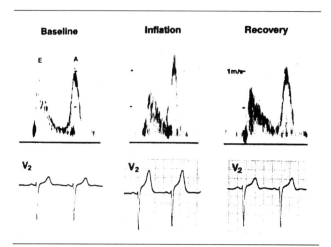

Figure 8-4. *Pulsed Doppler ultrasound recording of LV inflow velocities with accompanying electrocardiographic lead V_2 during left anterior descending coronary artery occlusion (inflation of angioplasty balloon). Note the marked reversal of early (E) and atrial (A) peak velocities and ST-segment elevation with coronary occlusion. (Reprinted with permission from Labovitz and colleagues [1987].)*

tion of multiple determinants. The typical but nonspecific mitral filling patterns, such as the pattern of increased isovolumic relaxation time and the decreased E/A ratio can be altered (i.e., pseudonormalized) by changes in atrial pressure. When severe LV systolic dysfunction and a restrictive pattern exists, the isovolumic relaxation time might even be decreased and the E/A ratio increased (Hatle, 1993). A detailed discussion of Doppler echocardiography is beyond the scope of this chapter and the interested reader is referred to recent reviews of Doppler echocardiographic assessment of diastolic dysfunction (Cohen et al., 1996; Hatle, 1993).

IMPORTANCE OF LV DIASTOLIC FUNCTION DURING EXERCISE

During exercise the cardiac output can increase severalfold. The increase in LV output must be matched by an increase in LV input. The increase in LV output during exercise is accomplished by an increase in heart rate, a modest increase in stroke volume, a decrease in peripheral vascular resistance, and an increase in contractile force that increases LV systolic pressure and the force of ejection. However, the left ventricle cannot accomplish an increase in input by those mechanisms that increase output during exercise. Tachycardia shortens the duration of diastole (i.e., the time in which LV filling must occur), thereby mandating that the diastolic filling rate during exercise be increased out of proportion to cardiac output. Nor can an increase in left atrial pressure be utilized as a mechanism to increase LV filling without sacrificing a low pulmonary capillary pressure.

How can this requirement for a marked increase in LV input (i.e., diastolic filling rate) during exercise be accomplished? An increase in flow rate across the mitral valve requires that the transmitral diastolic pressure gradient increase. However, this increase in the transmitral gradient cannot be achieved by increasing the pressure in the left atrium for that would increase pulmonary capillary pressure, cause pulmonary congestion, and precipitate dyspnea and respiratory compromise during exercise. Rather, the normal left ventricle accomplishes a remarkable increase in diastolic filling rate during exercise by rapidly and markedly decreasing intra-LV pressure during early diastole. This early diastolic LV pressure decrease creates a relative LV "suction" effect, which increases the transmitral pressure gradient without increasing left atrial pressure (Cheng et al., 1992, 1993; Little & Cheng, 1994; Yellin & Nikolic, 1994) (Fig 8-5). In other words, during exercise the LV increases its force of ejection during systole to "push" the LV output more forcefully, but it also "pulls" blood in during diastole more forcefully to increase input in parallel with output. This LV diastolic "suction" occurs as a result of several mechanisms. During exercise, the increased force of contraction during systole (observed clinically as an increase in systolic LV and arterial pressure) increases early diastolic myocardial elastic recoil due to the greater systolic shortening forces and extent of systolic fiber shortening, manifested as a smaller end systolic volume, which occurs during exer-

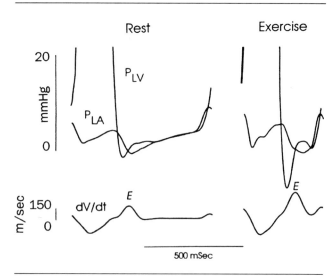

Figure 8-5. *Recording of LV pressure (P_{LV}) and left atrial pressure (P_{LA}), and the rate of change of LV volume (dV/dt) at rest and during exercise. During exercise, minimal LV pressure decreases without any increase in left atrial pressure. This leads to an increase in the peak mitral valve gradient and produces a larger peak filling rate (E). (Reprinted with permission from Cheng and colleagues [1992].)*

cise (Little & Cheng, 1994). Also, an acceleration of myocyte relaxation occurs during exercise due to an increased rate of calcium uptake by the SR. Increased cyclic AMP, generated by the beta adrenergic response to exercise, phosphorylates the regulatory SR membrane protein, phospholamban, to increase the rate of calcium uptake by the SR during diastole (Katz, 1992).

Thus during exercise the normal heart has an elegant balance and symmetry of physiological mechanisms to ensure that cardiac input keeps pace with cardiac output, with preservation of a low pulmonary capillary pressure. The beta adrenergic system increases cyclic AMP levels to increase systolic calcium entry and SR calcium release, with a consequent increase in contractility and systolic fiber shortening. But the rate of diastolic SR calcium reuptake is also accelerated by the cyclic AMP increase, and the greater extent of systolic fiber shortening results in the early diastolic recoil mechanism, decreasing intra-LV pressure in early diastole to "pull" blood into the left ventricle and facilitate LV filling. These mechanisms result in an increase in measured LV distensibility during exercise in normal patients, as manifested by a downward shift of the LV diastolic P-V curve (Carroll et al., 1983a, 1983b) (Fig 8-6, left panel).

EFFECTS OF ISCHEMIA

If ischemia occurs during exercise, not only is the normal increase in LV distensibility lost, but even worse, a rapid and marked increase in LV diastolic chamber stiffness occurs and LV diastolic pressures quickly increase, resulting in acute pulmonary congestion (see Fig 8-2). The responses of LV diastolic

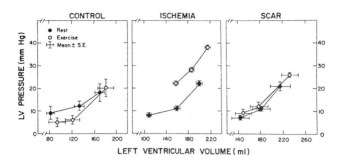

Figure 8-6. *The LV diastolic pressure-volume relation in controls, patients with exercise-induced ischemia, and in patients with scar from prior infarction but no exercise-induced ischemia. The coordinates of pressure and volume are averages at three diastolic points: the early diastolic pressure nadir, mid-diastole, and end diastole. For details see text. (Reprinted with permission from Carroll and colleagues [1983b].)*

distensibility during exercise in normal patients, in patients with coronary artery disease and exercise-induced ischemia, and in patients with healed myocardial infarction but without ischemia during exercise are illustrated in Figure 8-6.

Figure 8-6 reports LV diastolic P-V curves in the three patient groups at rest and during exercise (Carroll et al., 1983a). The simultaneous measures of LV diastolic pressure and volume define LV distensibility or compliance. In normal patients (control, left panel Fig 8-6), during the resting state LV pressure was approximately 9 mmHg in early diastole and increased to about 15 mmHg at end diastole. Exercise caused a marked downward shift of the LV diastolic P-V curve in early diastole and a lesser decrease of mean LV diastolic pressure relative to the resting state. During exercise, these control patients increased their cardiac output three- to fourfold. Because of this physiological increase in LV diastolic distensibility, the increase in cardiac output was accomplished without an increase of LV diastolic pressure and pulmonary capillary pressure.

By contrast, the middle panel of Figure 8-6 reports the LV diastolic P-V curves in patients with coronary artery disease who developed angina and ischemia with exercise. The P-V curve at rest was similar to that of the control patients, but with exercise a marked upward shift occurred, such that LV end diastolic pressure was 40 mmHg and LV mean diastolic pressure was approximately 30 mmHg. As discussed earlier (see Fig 8-1), such an increase in LV diastolic pressure would cause significant pulmonary congestion.

This upward shift of the LV diastolic P-V curve, and the consequent pulmonary congestion during exercise-induced ischemia, explains why many patients with coronary disease have respiratory symptoms together with their anginal pain, often complaining of wheezing, chest tightness, inability to take a deep breath, or shortness of breath. Such respiratory symptoms may occur in the absence of anginal pain and are often referred to as *anginal equivalents*. Often these "anginal" symptoms are quite similar to symptoms of heart failure, which is not surprising since the responsible mechanism is an increase of pulmonary capillary pressure in both cases. The acute decrease in LV distensibility during angina and its consequences on pulmonary mechanics have been documented by Pepine and Wiener (1972). They showed that airway resistance and lung compliance decreased during an anginal episode concomitant with the increase in LV diastolic chamber stiffness and LV diastolic pressure. Thus, during angina, acute left-sided "diastolic" heart failure often occurs as the result of an acute increase in LV diastolic chamber stiffness as illustrated in Figure 8-2 and the middle panel of Figure 8-6. This upward shift of the LV diastolic P-V curve was completely reversible with recovery after exercise.

The right panel of Figure 8-6 reports the LV diastolic P-V curves in patients with a healed myocardial infarction but without exercise-induced ischemia. Such patients lost the early diastolic increase in distensibility during exercise that was seen in the control patients, so that LV diastolic filling was not facilitated by an increase in distensibility. Because exercise-induced ischemia did not occur, there was no upward shift of the LV diastolic P-V curve.

Ischemic diastolic stunning after cardiac surgery

A sequence of ischemia and reperfusion occurs during most types of cardiac surgery. Contractile dysfunction after cardiopulmonary bypass is characterized by decreased function despite normal flow, with slow recovery to normal levels, and is considered a classical example of myocardial stunning (Bolli, 1992). Postischemic mechanical dysfunction results not only in systolic dysfunction, but also in diastolic dysfunction. In fact, diastolic dysfunction might be a more sensitive parameter of ischemic injury than systolic dysfunction (Apstein & Grossman, 1987). During reperfusion LV chamber stiffness is increased. Thus, it is not surprising that LV diastolic chamber stiffness is commonly increased after coronary artery bypass surgery and after aortic valve replacement (McKenney et al., 1994a, 1994b). Over time diastolic dysfunction will resolve and it is therefore reasonable to refer to reversible postischemic diastolic dysfunction as postischemic diastolic stunning (McKenney et al., 1994a, 1994b) (Fig 8-7). Recognition of this phenomenon is important for physicians dealing with postoperative patients because a reduced cardiac output or elevated pulmonary capillary pressure in the early postoperative setting may reflect an increase in LV diastolic chamber stiffness rather than a decrease in contractile function. This distinction can be made readily by echocardiography.

Hypertrophy/ischemia interactions and their effects on LV diastolic dysfunction

The conditions of LVH and ischemia have important interactions. Hearts with concentric LVH (e.g., secondary to chronic hypertension or aortic stenosis) are highly susceptible to subendocardial ischemia for several reasons (adapted from Isoyama [1992]).

1. There is some evidence that an inadequate coronary growth relative to muscle mass, with a resulting de-

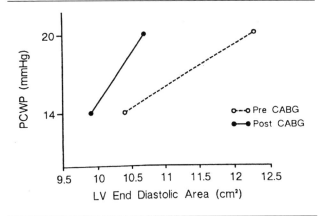

Figure 8-7. *LV pressure-area relation of a patient before (Pre) and immediately after (Post) coronary artery bypass graft (CABG) surgery. LV diastolic area was measured by two-dimensional cross-sectional echocardiography. Volume loading (1–2 liters of saline) resulted in an increase of the baseline pulmonary capillary wedge pressure (PCWP) and the LV diastolic area. After bypass surgery, the LV diastolic area was smaller at each pressure level, as reflected by a leftward shift of the area-pressure relationship, indicating an increase in LV diastolic chamber stiffness. (Reprinted with permission from McKenney and colleagues [1994a].)*

crease in capillary density and increased capillary-to-myocyte oxygen diffusion distance, renders the hypertrophied myocyte more susceptible to ischemia (Tomanek et al., 1991).

2. The increase in ventricular wall thickness results in an increased epicardial-endocardial distance. The coronary arterial circulation consists of epicardial vessels that penetrate transmurally, giving rise to midmyocardial branches that perfuse the thickened LV wall before serving the subendocardium. Thus coronary perfusion pressure is dissipated in proportion to LV wall thickness, leaving the subendocardium as the region most vulnerable to ischemia (Isoyama, 1992).

3. Coronary arterial remodeling accompanies concentric hypertrophy and is manifested by an increase in coronary arterial medial thickness and perivascular fibrosis, which can restrict the extent of coronary arterial vasodilatation.

4. Coronary vasodilator reserve is usually diminished with concentric LVH, because vascular tone at rest is usually abnormally reduced and coronary flow at rest is increased (Eberli et al., 1991b; Marcus et al., 1983; Tomanek et al., 1991). The increased coronary flow is required in the resting state to supply the increased muscle mass. Since maximal achievable coronary flow is similar to that of normal ventricles, coronary flow reserve is decreased. When metabolic demand and the need for oxygen increases, coronary reserve is often inadequate to meet the increased oxygen requirements, and ischemia occurs (Marcus et al., 1983).

5. Increased LV diastolic pressures can cause vascular compression, thereby reducing coronary flow and

perfusion of the subendocardial layer (Isoyama, 1992). Furthermore, a decrease in coronary flow reserve is partly due to an endothelial dysfunction in the vasculature of hearts with LVH secondary to pressure overload hypertrophy (Ishihara et al., 1992).

6. Coronary artherosclerosis incidence and severity is increased in the presence of systemic arterial hypertension, which is often the cause of concentric LVH. Thus patients with concentric LVH on a hypertensive basis often have significant concomitant coronary artery disease.

Taken together, these factors make the heart with concentric LVH exquisitely sensitive to subendocardial ischemia. Such hearts also have a structural basis for diastolic dysfunction because of their increased mass and increased interstitial and subendocardial fibrosis, which commonly accompanies concentric LVH, particularly when it results from hypertension (Lorell, 1994). The combination of structural abnormality, susceptibility to subendocardial ischemia, and exaggerated impairment of myocyte relaxation in response to ischemia make the heart with concentric LVH highly vulnerable to frequent and severe ischemic diastolic dysfunction.

The exaggerated ischemic diastolic dysfunction of concentric LVH has been demonstrated in several clinical settings and experimental models (Lorell, 1994). For example, during pacing-induced ischemia, patients with aortic stenosis and concentric LVH developed marked increases in LV end diastolic pressure and a substantial upward shift of the LV diastolic P-V curve (Fifer et al., 1986). In experimental studies, rat hearts with concentric LVH due to sodium overload hypertension developed greater diastolic dysfunction during hypoxia than control rat hearts (Cunningham et al., 1990; Lorell et al., 1986; Wexler et al., 1988). Hearts from rabbits with LVH secondary to renal vascular hypertension exhibited exaggerated diastolic dysfunction during demand ischemia (Lorell et al., 1989). Rat hearts with concentric LVH due to aortic banding had exaggerated ischemic LV diastolic dysfunction when subjected to low-flow ischemia (Eberli et al., 1992a).

The increased susceptibility of LVH hearts to ischemia/reperfusion injury is also evident during cardiac surgery. In the early days, open heart surgery was sometimes complicated by the development of extreme contracture of the heart after the ischemia/reperfusion injury induced by cardiopulmonary arrest. This extreme form of ischemic diastolic dysfunction was called the *stone heart* (Katz & Tada, 1972) and occurred more often in hearts with LVH than in nonhypertrophied hearts. This phenomenon has almost disappeared with the introduction of cardioplegic solutions, but postischemic diastolic dysfunction remains a clinical problem in particular in patients with LVH. For example, patients with concentric LVH who had aortic valve replacement for aortic stenosis manifested exaggerated diastolic dysfunction in the immediate postoperative period (McKenney et al., 1994b). The extent of early postoperative diastolic dysfunction was significantly greater in these patients than it was in patients without LVH after coronary artery bypass graft surgery.

SUBCELLULAR MECHANISMS POTENTIALLY RESPONSIBLE FOR ISCHEMIC DIASTOLIC DYSFUNCTION IN NORMAL AND HYPERTROPHIED HEARTS

Myocyte relaxation occurs by reversal of those processes that cause contraction. The sodium and calcium movements that comprise excitation-contraction coupling are reversed to effect repolarization-relaxation coupling, the tension-generating actin-myosin interaction abates, and myofilament tension is dissipated. Hypertrophy and ischemia can alter myocyte sodium and calcium movements, high-energy phosphate metabolism (levels of ATP, ADP, creatine phosphate, and inorganic (phosphate [P_i]), and intracellular pH, all of which can affect the rate and extent of myocyte relaxation. Furthermore, both pH and P_i alter myofilament sensitivity to calcium and can thereby influence both systolic and diastolic myofilament tension at any calcium level. (For a recent review, see Apstein & Morgan [1994].) Diastolic dysfunction at the myofilament level can result from either the persistence of excessive cytosolic calcium or the persistence of actin-myosin rigor complexes throughout diastole (Fig 8-8).

Role of calcium

Contraction is initiated during myocyte activation. An inward calcium current occurs during the action potential

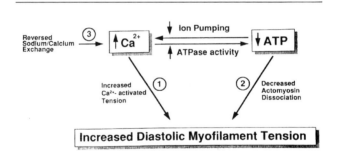

Figure 8-8. *Synergistic interaction between an increase in cytosolic calcium and a decrease in ATP availability to increase diastolic myofilament tension. This figure illustrates how an increased cytosolic calcium level or a decrease in ATP availability can directly increase diastolic myofilament tension and cause or exacerbate ischemic diastolic dysfunction. (1) An increase in diastolic calcium can directly increase diastolic myofilament tension by binding to troponin-C and/or can accelerate a decrease in ATP levels by activating a number of myocyte calcium ATPases. (2) A decrease in ATP availability can directly increase diastolic tension by decreasing the rate or amount of actomyosin dissociation from the rigor complex state. A decrease in ATP availability can also impair the calcium removal from the cytosol by the sarcolemmal and sarcoplasmic reticular calcium ATPases. (3) A decrease in ATP availability can also decrease the sarcolemmal sodium-potassium ATPase (sodium pump) activity resulting in an increase in intracellular sodium, which increases intracellular calcium by means of sodium-calcium exchange. Thus either cytosolic calcium overload or a decrease in ATP availability can initiate a "vicious cycle" of calcium-ATP interactions that are synergistic in causing or exacerbating diastolic dysfunction.*

when the sarcolemmal (SL) voltage-dependent calcium channel opens and calcium diffuses into the cell driven by its 10,000-fold transmembrane concentration gradient. This calcium influx triggers a much greater amount of calcium release from the SR. Cytosolic calcium levels rise rapidly, calcium binds to its myofilament receptor on troponin-C, activating contractile protein tension generation via the actin-myosin cross-bridge cycle. For complete myocyte relaxation to occur, the cytosol must be cleared of calcium so that calcium dissociates from troponin-C, and all tension-generating actin-myosin bonds must be lysed. The diastolic clearance of cytosolic calcium requires ATP to fuel the SR and SL calcium ATPases that transport calcium into the SR or across the sarcolemma, respectively. Calcium removal may also occur via Na^+/Ca^{++} exchange, and ATP is required to fuel the Na^+ pump, which maintains a low intracellular Na^+ level, which is favorable to Ca^{++} extrusion by this mechanism.

During ischemia and hypoxia an intracellular accumulation of calcium occurs. This increase in cytosolic calcium could potentially result from excessive calcium entry into the cytosol, a decrease in calcium efflux, or from inadequate calcium reuptake by the SR during diastole, but seems not to be due to an excessive calcium influx via slow "L"-type calcium channels (Applegate et al., 1987). The reversible increase in diastolic chamber stiffness observed in patients with angina (Bronzwaer et al., 1991; Carroll et al., 1983a; Fifer et al., 1986), as well as the similar reversible increase in diastolic chamber stiffness in experimental models of ischemia have been explained by an increase in intracellular calcium $[Ca^{2+}]_i$ and a consequent increase in calcium-activated cross-bridge cycling and tension development (Apstein & Grossman, 1987; Eberli et al., 1991b, 1991c; Kihara et al., 1989; Mochizuki et al., 1992; Paulus et al., 1982; Serizawa et al., 1981; Wexler et al., 1986). $[Ca^{2+}]_i$ measurements by ^{19}F NMR spectroscopy, and bioluminescent and fluorescent calcium indicators that showed an increase of $[Ca^{2+}]_i$ both during hypoxia and zero-flow ischemia in the whole heart have supported this notion (Camacho et al., 1993; Kihara et al., 1989; Lee et al., 1988; Marban et al., 1987; Mohabir et al., 1991; Steenbergen et al., 1987). More recently, Camacho and colleagues (1994) also reported an increase in $[Ca^{2+}]_i$ during low-flow ischemia in the rabbit heart and they found a correlation between the impaired relaxation of the left ventricle, as assessed by the constant of the pressure decay, Tau, and the intracellular calcium reuptake.

In addition to its potential for persistently activating the actin-myosin cross-bridge interaction, excessive calcium levels can decrease phosphocreatine and ATP levels, and increase ADP levels by increasing the activities of Ca^{++}-activated ATPases such as the SR and SL calcium pumps, as well as other ATPases (Cross et al., 1995). Thus an increase in cell calcium can also impair relaxation indirectly by decreasing phosphocreatine and/or the ATP/ADP ratio, because such changes in the levels of high-energy phosphate metabolites affect the actin-myosin cross-bridge cycle (see Fig 8-8).

Much recent research has been devoted to determining the relative roles of disordered calcium regulation and/or abnormalities of high-energy phosphate metabolism as primary mechanisms for diastolic dysfunction during demand and supply ischemia, and during postischemic reperfusion. For example, in some studies the increases in diastolic calcium level preceded and did not occur simultaneously with the onset of contracture (Kihara et al., 1989; Lee et al., 1988). Conversely others have reported an increase in intracellular calcium before the onset of increased diastolic force in isolated hearts (Koretsune & Marban, 1990), or contracture occurring before any increase in intracellular calcium in isolated myocytes (Allshire et al., 1987; Miyata et al., 1992). Furthermore, in recent studies from our laboratory, interventions that altered intracellular calcium after the onset of ischemic diastolic dysfunction in isolated heart models of both supply and demand ischemia did not affect the degree of ischemic diastolic dysfunction. However, during postischemic reperfusion, after both demand and supply ischemia, an experimentally imposed calcium load immediately worsened the degree of diastolic dysfunction, suggesting that it was calcium driven during reperfusion (Eberli et al., 1990, 1991a, 1992b; Varma et al., 1994, 1995a, 1995b).

Role of decreased ATP and increased ADP in increased ischemic diastolic chamber stiffness

As discussed earlier, ATP and ADP play a critical role in myocyte relaxation. ATP is required to fuel the ion pumps that regulate diastolic levels of cytosolic calcium, and ATP and ADP have a complex number of interactions with the contractile proteins.

It was recognized early that the beginning of ischemic or hypoxic contracture was associated with a fall of ATP below a critical level. Therefore a decrease in tissue ATP levels causing actin-myosin cross-bridges to "lock" in a noncycling rigor state was proposed as the mechanism for the initiation of increased diastolic chamber stiffness (Hearse et al., 1977; Lowe et al., 1979). In support of an ATP-based, rather than a calcium-based, mechanism of contracture, Koretsune and Marban (1990), using NMR spectroscopy in ferret hearts showed that $[Ca^{2+}]_i$ began to rise after about 10 minutes of zero-flow ischemia and peaked in a steady-state level of about twofold systolic concentration after 30 to 35 minutes. By contrast, contracture began only after 40 minutes in this model. This dissociation of $[Ca^{2+}]_i$ and contracture has also been observed in ferret papillary muscle (Allen & Orchard, 1983) and in isolated myocytes during anoxia or metabolic inhibition (Allshire et al., 1987; Cobbold & Bourne, 1984; Haigney et al., 1992). These studies supported the concept that contracture occurs when cytosolic ATP decreases below a critical level. The critical decrease in ATP level in whole heart preparations for contracture to develop has been found to be 10 to 50% depending on metabolic parameters such as glycolytic activity (Hearse et al., 1977; Kingsley et al., 1991; Koretsune & Marban, 1990; Lowe et al., 1979). However, these decreases of 10 to 50% result in ATP levels that are higher than ATP levels associated with contracture in skinned muscle fiber preparations or isolated myocytes. In skinned muscle fibers ATP had to fall below 0.1 mM before rigor developed; alternatively it could be prevented by adding 30 μM ATP (Allen & Orchard, 1987; Ventura-Clapier et al., 1987). In metabolically inhibited isolated myocytes contracture occurred when ATP had dropped to about 0.2 mM (Bowers et al., 1991).

There are several possible, hypothetical explanations for this discrepancy i.e., how increased diastolic chamber stiffness could arise at ATP levels in the millimolar range, as measured in whole heart preparations. Firstly, it is conceivable that the increase in diastolic chamber stiffness observed in a whole heart at ATP levels in the millimolar range simply represents a number of myocytes that have depleted their ATP and have gone in contracture, and a number of myocytes that have preserved ATP and preserved contractile function. This explanation of loss of ATP substrate and classic rigor formation in a subset of myocytes is supported by the observation that after ATP depletion isolated myocytes go into contracture within a short period of time (Allshire et al., 1987; Bowers et al., 1991; Cobbold & Bourne, 1984; Haigney et al., 1992). Secondly, during ischemia increased diastolic chamber stiffness could result from a loss of the plasticizing effect of ATP (Katz, 1992). The plasticizing effect of ATP describes the role of ATP in the relaxation of myofilaments, as opposed to its role in the contraction. For relaxation to occur, ATP has to bind to the myosin head to initiate actomyosin dissociation. This plasticizing effect is facilitated by ATP concentrations in the millimolar range (i.e., by much higher concentrations than are needed to saturate the substrate site of myosin), which requires only micromolar concentrations of ATP. A third explanation is a classic product inhibition of the myofibrillar ATPase (i.e., on the myosin head), whereby ADP competes for the binding of ATP to the actomyosin complex or for an allosteric regulatory site on the actomyosin complex (Ventura-Clapier & Veksler, 1994; Yamashita et al., 1994). As ADP increases during ischemia, the decreased binding of ATP to the rigor complex would decrease dissociation of the rigor complex and result in an increased tension of diastolic chamber stiffness (Ventura-Clapier & Veksler, 1994; Yamashita et al., 1994). Fourthly, there could be a compartmentation of ATP within the myocyte (mitochondrial vs. cytosolic ATP pool) (Illingworth et al., 1975). Localization of glycolytic enzymes and the creatine kinase system have both been proposed to contribute to a compartmentation of ATP pools (Bessman et al., 1980; Han et al., 1992; Kurganov et al., 1985; Weiss & Hiltbrand, 1985).

In addition to these effects at the level of the actin-myosin cross-bridge cycle, ATP is necessary to fuel the ion pumps that maintain normal intracellular calcium movements (i.e., the SR Ca-ATPase and the sarcolemmal Ca^{++} and Na^{+} pumps), as discussed earlier. Thus a decrease in ATP can result in cytosolic calcium overload and impaired relaxation because of a failure to maintain normal ionic homeostasis.

Demand and supply ischemia

The term *ischemic diastolic dysfunction* implies a single pathophysiological process, but recent studies suggest that diastolic function may be affected somewhat differently by supply and demand ischemia. Demand ischemia typically occurs during exercise or pacing-induced angina, resulting from an increase in oxygen demand in the setting of limited coronary flow (e.g., due to a coronary stenosis), which reduces or eliminates coronary vasodilator reserve. By contrast, supply ischemia results from a marked reduction of coronary flow (e.g., a coronary occlusion), resulting in inadequate coronary perfusion even for the resting state, such that ischemia occurs without any increase in myocardial oxygen demand.

The initial effects of acute ischemia on diastolic compliance differ, depending on whether it is of the supply or demand type. Experimental coronary ligation, resulting in acute supply ischemia, resulted in an initial downward and rightward shift of the diastolic P-V curve such that end diastolic volume increased relative to end diastolic pressure, indicating an increase in diastolic compliance. Conversely, during demand ischemia diastolic compliance acutely decreased in patients with coronary artery disease during pacing or exercise-induced angina, in dogs with coronary arterial stenoses and pacing tachycardia, and in isolated hearts with low coronary flow and tachycardia (Apstein & Grossman, 1987; Isoyama et al., 1987; Varma et al., 1994, 1995a, 1995b).

These opposite initial compliance changes with demand and supply ischemia may be explained by differences in the pressure and volume within the coronary vasculature; the mechanical effects of the normal, non-ischemic myocardium that is adjacent to the ischemic region; and tissue metabolic factors. An acute coronary occlusion (supply ischemia) increases diastolic compliance initially because (1) the coronary vasculature distal to the occlusion is collapsed, causing a loss of coronary turgor; (2) the marked decrease in ischemic segmental force development permits repetitive systolic stretching, resulting in ischemic segment lengthening; and (3) tissue acidosis and increased inorganic phosphate levels decrease any calcium-mediated diastolic fiber tension. By contrast, with demand ischemia there is less acidosis and less of an increase in inorganic phosphate. The coronary vascular space is not collapsed and the ischemic segment is not stretched by the surrounding non-ischemic myocardium. The sum of these processes results in an acute decrease in diastolic compliance during demand ischemia (Apstein & Grossman, 1987). After more sustained ischemia (e.g., 30–60 minutes or longer), both demand and supply ischemia result in decreased diastolic compliance.

Importance of glycolysis in ischemic diastolic dysfunction

Additional evidence for a critical role of altered ATP levels in causing ischemic diastolic dysfunction comes from studies of ischemic glycolysis. During conditions of oxygen supply limitation such as ischemia, the glycolytic pathway becomes a relatively more important source of ATP synthesis because of this pathway's ability to achieve ATP synthesis anaerobically. In general, the rate of development of ischemic contracture or diastolic dysfunction is inversely related to the activity of the glycolytic pathway. Metabolic interventions that inhibited glycolysis accelerated the development of is-chemic contracture, and provision of additional exogenous glycolytic substrate (a high level of glucose with or without insulin) increased levels of ATP and partially or completely prevented ischemic contracture (Apstein et al., 1978, 1983; Eberli et al., 1991c; Schaefer et al., 1995; Vanoverschelde et al., 1994). In studies comparing the sources and rates of ATP pro-duction during low-flow ischemia, the rate of glycolytic flux from glucose was the metabolic parameter that best corre-lated with the prevention or delay of ischemic contracture (Owen et al., 1990). Glycolysis also plays a very important role in the diastolic function of certain forms of pressure overload hypertrophy. Inhibition of glycolysis in hypertro-phied hearts resulted in a much greater impairment of dias-tolic relaxation than in controls (Kagaya et al., 1995). Furthermore, the exaggerated ischemic diastolic chamber stiffness in hypertrophied hearts could be attenuated by pro-vision of an abundance of glycolytic substrate (Cunningham et al., 1990). In dogs with decompensated hypertrophy after chronic aortic stenosis, exaggerated ischemic diastolic dys-function was associated with a loss of glycolytic flux (Gaasch et al., 1990).

These results were consistent with the hypothesis that the glycolytic pathway may provide a small but critically localized pool of ATP, which may have a high turnover rate relative to its pool size (Weiss & Hiltbrand, 1985). In support of this hypothesis it has been shown in skeletal muscle that certain glycolytic enzymes are bound to the contractile ap-paratus (Kurganov et al., 1985) and that membrane frag-ments consisting of transverse tubules connected to adjacent terminal cisternae of the SR contain a compartmentalized glycolytic reaction that is not in equilibrium with the bulk cell ATP stores (Han et al., 1992).

However, although these studies demonstrate the im-portance of an active glycolytic pathway in protecting against ischemic diastolic dysfunction, they do not define the mechanism of protection or distinguish between an ef-fect on high-energy phosphate metabolites at the level of the myofilaments versus an improvement in sodium and/or calcium homeostasis secondary to increased glycolytic en-ergy supply. Evidence that the protective effect of glycolysis during low-flow ischemia is mediated, at least in part, by improving cation homeostasis comes from recent NMR studies (Cross et al., 1995). Provision of glucose to rat hearts during low-flow ischemia protected against ischemic dia-stolic dysfunction, and this protection was associated with a more active sarcolemmal Na^+/K^+ ATPase activity (i.e., so-dium pump activity), which prevented an increase in intra-cellular Na^+ during ischemia. Since intracellular Na^+ excess can lead to cell Ca^{++} uptake via Na^+/Ca^{++} exchange, the glu-cose probably also protected against calcium overload.

From this discussion it is clear that calcium homeostasis, high-energy phosphate metabolism, and myocardial relax-ation are intimately related and interdependent. During is-chemia, either or both processes may become primarily or secondarily abnormal with resultant diastolic dysfunction. The relative importance of primary disturbances of calcium regulation in comparison with high-energy phosphate metabolism, under different circumstances of ischemia and hypertrophy, remains an area of active research. Despite lack of complete understanding of all of the subcellular mechanisms responsible for ischemic diastolic dysfunction, the current level of knowledge supports certain clinical principles.

CLINICAL CONSIDERATIONS: THE DIAGNOSIS AND MANAGEMENT OF ISCHEMIC DIASTOLIC DYSFUNCTION

In 1923, Henderson observed, "If an old man's heart relaxes slowly, his capacity for physical exertion is thus limited . . . even though the systolic contractions were still like those of youth" (Henderson, 1923, p. 166), thus recognizing that dyspnea with exertion (also occurring at rest in severe cases) is the most characteristic symptom of LV diastolic dysfunction. The shortness of breath results from pulmonary congestion due to elevated pressures in the pulmonary capillaries, pulmonary veins, and left atrium and ventricle because of the impairment of LV diastolic filling as illustrated in Figures 8-1 and 8-2. Clinical management requires recognition of this condition and therapeutic measures that improve the diastolic physiology and relieve the pulmonary congestion. A general approach to the treatment of diastolic dysfunction is outlined in Table 8-2 and is adapted from the recommendations of Levine and Gaasch (1994).

Diagnosis

The patient with symptomatic LV diastolic dysfunction usually presents with dyspnea on exertion, or at rest in severe cases. The signs and symptoms are those of left-sided congestive heart failure with pulmonary congestion ranging

TABLE 8-2 A GENERAL APPROACH TO THE TREATMENT OF DIASTOLIC DYSFUNCTION*

Treatment goals	Treatment methods
Reduce central vascular volume to decrease pulmonary capillary pressure	Venodilators (nitrates, ACE inhibitors, diuretics, morphine, tourniquets, salt restriction
Maintain atrial contraction	Cardioversion of atrial fibrillation, avoid atrial distension
Enhance ventricular systolic emptying	Antihypertensive therapy
Regression of hypertrophy	Antihypertensive therapy
Control heart rate	Exercise limitation, beta adrenergic blocker, cardioversion of atrial fibrillation
Prevent/treat ischemia	Antihypertensive therapy, control heart rate, lipid-lowering therapy, beta adrenergic blockers, calcium channel blockers, nitrates, revascularization
Improve myocardial relaxation	Calcium channel blockers (?), ACE inhibitors (?)

*Adapted from Levine and Gaasch (1994).

from mild to severe, and are typically worse with exertion. The diagnosis of diastolic dysfunction is made when further evaluation, usually by echocardiography, reveals normal systolic function (i.e., a normal ejection fraction) and the absence of valvular disease. In most cases, LVH is present on the echocardiogram and/or electrocardiogram, but occasionally it is not. Doppler echocardiography of mitral valve inflow may demonstrate diminished early diastolic filling velocities (an abnormally low E-wave) and increased late diastolic filling as manifest by an increased A-wave if the patient is in normal sinus rhythm. Evidence of ischemia is often present in the form of typical electrocardiographic abnormalities (ST-segment and T-wave changes), by myocardial perfusion scan defects, and by symptoms of angina pectoris. In patients with marked LVH, subendocardial ischemia is often a contributing or precipitating factor.

Chronic management of patients with exertional dyspnea due to LV diastolic dysfunction

During exercise the aging or hypertensive heart characteristically has preserved systolic function (ejection fraction, cardiac output), but diastolic function is usually impaired (Kitzman et al., 1991; Nixon & Burns, 1994). Therefore it is not surprising that patients presenting with exertional dyspnea and a normal ejection fraction are more often elderly and/or have LVH. Characteristically these patients show no signs of pulmonary congestion at rest. However, they may show cardiomegaly by chest radiograph, falsely suggesting LV systolic pump failure. Direct objective assessment of systolic function is very important, since treatment of dyspnea on exertion secondary to pure diastolic dysfunction differs from treatment of dyspnea due to systolic pump failure.

The most important principle is the prevention of recurrent episodes of pulmonary congestion by decreasing or reversing those factors that predispose to diastolic dysfunction. The goals of chronic management of the patient with LV diastolic dysfunction are outlined in Table 8-2.

In patients with hypertensive LVH, antihypertensive therapy is the mainstay of treatment. The choice of a specific antihypertensive agent must be individualized, as each has specific characteristics relevant to the management of diastolic dysfunction. Regression of LVH is an important therapeutic goal and can be accomplished by effective antihypertensive treatment with diuretics, calcium channel blockers, beta adrenergic blockers, or ACE inhibitors (Dahloef et al., 1992).

Angiotensin converting enzyme (ACE) inhibitors possess some features that make them particularly attractive for treating patients with diastolic dysfunction due to hypertensive LVH. Some experimental evidence suggests that ACE inhibitors may reduce the myocardial fibrosis that accompanies hypertensive LVH (Weber & Brilla, 1991). This action, if verified clinically, could be a theoretical advantage. Recently, ACE inhibitors have been shown to improve LV diastolic dysfunction in patients with ischemic heart disease (Rousseau et al., 1990), in patients with LVH due to aortic stenosis (Friedrich et al., 1994), and during experimental low-flow ischemia in hypertrophied hearts with ischemic diastolic dysfunction (Eberli et al., 1992a). Furthermore, unlike beta adrenergic and calcium channel blockers, the use of ACE inhibitors is not proscribed by the presence of concomitant systolic dysfunction.

Ischemia often precipitates and/or contributes to diastolic dysfunction. Ischemia can result from the presence of coronary atherosclerosis, LVH with subendocardial ischemia as described earlier, or both. Therefore, drugs with anti-ischemic effects such as the beta adrenergic blockers, calcium antagonists, and nitrates are useful agents.

Beta adrenergic blockers provide salutary bradycardic and negatively inotropic actions, reducing myocardial oxygen demand by these mechanisms in addition to their antihypertensive action. Slowing of the heart rate is particularly important in the treatment of pulmonary congestion due to ischemic diastolic dysfunction. In addition to decreasing myocardial oxygen demand, a relative bradycardia increases the duration of diastole, thereby increasing the time available for both coronary flow and LV filling, both of which are usually compromised, especially in patients with LVH and ischemic diastolic dysfunction. Furthermore, the amount of myocyte calcium and sodium entry is directly proportional to the frequency of depolarization or heart rate, and tachycardia can contribute to cellular calcium overload by this mechanism. Thus beta-blockers and calcium channel blockers with strong bradycardic actions are particularly useful.

Calcium channel blockers, especially verapamil, have been reported to be useful in the treatment of pure diastolic dysfunction. In a randomized, placebo-controlled, prospective, crossover trial in patients with primary diastolic dysfunction, verapamil significantly reduced the signs and symptoms of heart failure, and increased LV diastolic filling rate and treadmill exercise time, providing objective evidence of this drug's efficacy in this syndrome (Setaro et al., 1990). In hypertrophic cardiomyopathy, verapamil acutely improved LV diastolic function and prolonged long-term survival (Hess & Krayenbuehl, 1994). Calcium antagonists have been purported to have a direct "lusitropic" (relaxation-enhancing) effect, but it is difficult to distinguish between such an action and benefit that is secondary to reduction or prevention of ischemia.

Both short- and long-acting nitrates may be useful in the management of ischemic diastolic dysfunction because of multiple effects. Their venodilating action reduces central blood volume and pulmonary capillary pressure concomitant with relief of ischemia. Relief of ischemia results from both a decrease in myocardial oxygen demand and improved myocardial perfusion. Oxygen demand is decreased because the venodilating effect reduces LV volume and wall stress. Myocardial perfusion can be increased by virtue of coronary arterial dilation, relief of coronary vasospasm, and improved collateral flow. The nitrate-induced reduction of LV diastolic pressure also relieves subendocardial vascular compression and improves subendocardial perfusion by this mechanism.

Relief of ischemia by means of coronary artery bypass graft surgery or angioplasty may be required for management of severe "drug-resistant" ischemic diastolic dysfunction.

An important caveat is that the patient with LV diastolic dysfunction with a small, stiff LV chamber is particularly susceptible to excessive preload reduction with resultant underfilling of the left ventricle, a consequent decrease in stroke volume and cardiac output, and subsequent hypotension. In patients with severe LVH, excessive preload reduction can also create a sub-aortic outflow obstruction. Thus treatment with diuretics or venodilators such as the nitrates, calcium antagonists, and ACE inhibitors must be done cautiously with careful attention to symptoms of ventricular underfilling such as weakness, dizziness, near-syncope, and syncope.

In patients with chronic atrial fibrillation, where sinus rhythm cannot be restored and maintained, heart rate control is particularly important because the loss of atrial contraction is cumulative with the myocardial resistance to LV filling in contributing to diastolic dysfunction. Digitalis, beta adrenergic blockers, and verapamil are useful in blocking atrio-ventricular nodal conduction and controlling ventricular rate. It is important to measure heart rate during moderate exercise and not to assume heart rate control is adequate based on the resting state. Often a combination of these drugs is required to achieve adequate heart rate control.

Management of patients with acute pulmonary edema

Despite the best management strategy, patients with LV diastolic dysfunction often present with severe pulmonary congestion or pulmonary edema requiring emergent treatment. The treatment goal of acute pulmonary edema for such patients is identical to that for all forms of cardiogenic pulmonary edema: reduction of pulmonary capillary pressure by means of diuretics and vasodilators. Commonly such patients have chronic, inadequately controlled hypertension with secondary LVH. The acute episode of pulmonary edema frequently occurs with concomitant exacerbation of hypertension, and aggressive antihypertensive therapy may be required as part of the treatment of pulmonary edema.

However, as discussed earlier, patients with a small, stiff LV chamber are particularly susceptible to excessive preload reduction with resultant underfilling of the left ventricle. Such patients should have frequent monitoring of arterial blood pressure. If hypotension occurs it can usually be promptly reversed by decreasing the dosage of preload reducing agents and by intravenous volume replacement with saline. Often such patients are hemodynamically unstable and small changes in intravascular volume can have profound effects on the arterial blood pressure and/or on the pulmonary capillary pressure. In such cases continuous monitoring of the pulmonary capillary pressure and intra-arterial pressure is useful in guiding the administration of vasodilators and intravenous volume replacement.

When a patient presents with acute pulmonary edema it is often unclear as to whether systolic or diastolic dysfunction (or both) is primarily responsible, and the presence and significance of any concomitant myocardial ischemia may also be uncertain. The relative roles of systolic versus diastolic dysfunction can be rapidly clarified by echocardiography. Until such clarification, treatment with diuretics and vasodilators should proceed to relieve the pulmonary congestion. Intravenous nitroglycerin is particularly useful because it also treats any concomitant ischemia, and its vasodilatory effects can be rapidly and readily titrated in response to hemodynamic changes. The use of ACE inhibitors is not proscribed by the presence of concomitant systolic dysfunction; thus these agents are theoretically attractive, but their efficacy in the setting of acute pulmonary edema due to diastolic dysfunction has not been definitively established. Similarly, calcium channel blockers without negative inotropic effects (e.g., felodipine and amlodipine) have been shown to reduce experimental ischemic diastolic dysfunction without worsening residual ischemic contractile function (Bernstein et al., 1996). Such agents are also theoretically attractive, but need to be tested in this specific clinical setting. Both ACE inhibitors and these calcium channel blockers may be useful when antihypertensive therapy is required.

Other drugs useful in the treatment of acute pulmonary edema due to diastolic dysfunction are those discussed earlier in chronic management. In the absence of significant systolic dysfunction, beta adrenergic blockers and calcium channel blockers with negative inotropic effects, such as diltiazem and verapamil, are potentially useful. These drugs are antihypertensive, anti-ischemic, and antitachycardic, thus reversing the triad of factors often responsible for decompensation in patients with diastolic dysfunction.

The occurrence of atrial fibrillation can precipitate acute pulmonary edema in patients with LVH and diastolic dysfunction as a result of the associated tachycardia, and also because of the loss of atrial contraction. Atrial contraction is particularly important for atrial emptying in such patients because early LV filling is impaired. A disproportionate amount of LV filling and left atrial emptying occurs in late diastole and is dependent on atrial contraction. A decrease in atrial emptying due to atrial fibrillation can result in both increased pulmonary capillary pressure and relative LV underfilling, with a resultant sympathetic drive to increased heart rate. Therefore, rapid restoration of normal sinus rhythm is an important treatment goal.

From this discussion it should be apparent that no simple or single therapeutic plan exists for the management of this condition. Because the major symptom of chronic diastolic dysfunction is dyspnea with exertion, a practical clinical approach is to use the patient's exercise tolerance as a guide to the efficacy of drug therapy, adjusting dosage and adding combination therapy accordingly.

SUMMARY

Ischemic diastolic dysfunction is a major cause of dyspnea on exertion and left-sided congestive heart failure. Ischemia, resulting from coronary atherosclerosis and/or the relative subendocardial hypoperfusion common with LVH, impairs myocyte relaxation. A malefic synergism exists between ischemia and LVH. Hearts with LVH are particularly susceptible to subendocardial ischemia. With pressure overload

LVH, ischemic relaxation abnormalities are themselves ex-aggerated, and also add to the structural abnormalities of LVH (increased LV muscle mass and fibrosis) in impairing LV filling and increasing the pulmonary capillary pressure. Exercise often precipitates symptomatic diastolic dysfunction, not only by causing ischemia, but also because the cardiac output response to exercise must be accompanied by a disproportionate increase in cardiac input (i.e., diastolic filling rate), since the tachycardia of exercise shortens the diastolic filling period. By a mechanism of early diastolic elastic recoil and LV "suction," the normal ventricle can markedly augment diastolic filling during exercise without increasing left atrial and pulmonary capillary pressures. This mechanism is absent with ischemic diastolic dysfunction and, as a result, pulmonary capillary pressures increase markedly during exercise, causing dyspnea on exertion as well as the dyspnea that frequently accompanies angina. Diastolic dysfunction also occurs after the ischemia-reperfusion that accompanies cardiac surgery. The ischemic relaxation impairment appears to result from reduced myocyte ATP availability and/or excessive cytosolic calcium levels, both of which can interfere with normal actin-myosin cross-bridge cycling. Treatment goals include reduction of the pulmonary capillary pressure, maintenance of atrial contraction, regression of LVH, prevention of ischemia, and improvement of myocyte relaxation. Useful drugs include ACE inhibitors, calcium antagonists, beta adrenergic blockers, nitrates, and diuretics. Treatment should be individualized with the goal of improving exercise tolerance.

REFERENCES

Allen DG, Orchard CH. Intracellular calcium concentration during hypoxia and metabolic inhibition in mammalian ventricular muscle. *J Physiol (Lond)* 1983; 339: 107–122.

Allen DG, Orchard CH. Myocardial contractile function during ischemia and hypoxia. *Circ Res* 1987; 60: 153–168.

Allshire A, Piper HM, Cuthbertson KSR, Cobbold PH. Cytosolic free Ca^{2+} in single rat heart cells during anoxia and reoxygenation. *Biochem J* 1987; 244: 381–385.

Applegate RJ, Walsh RA, O'Rourke RA. Effects of nifedipine on diastolic function during brief periods of flow-limiting ischemia in the conscious dog. *Circulation* 1987; 76: 1409–1421.

Apstein CS, Deckelbaum L, Hagopian L, Hood Jr WB. Acute cardiac ischemia and reperfusion. Contractility, relaxation and glycolysis. *Am J Physiol* 1978; 235: H637–H648.

Apstein CS, Gravino FN, Haudenschild CC. Determinants of protective effect of glucose and insulin on the ischemic myocardium: effects on contractile function, diastolic compliance, metabolism and ultrastructure during ischemia and reperfusion. *Circ Res* 1983; 52: 515–526.

Apstein CS, Grossman W. Opposite initial effects of supply and demand ischemia on left ventricular diastolic compliance: the ischemia-diastolic paradox. *J Mol Cell Cardiol* 1987; 19: 119–128.

Apstein CS, Morgan JP. Cellular mechanisms underlying left ventricular diastolic dysfunction. In: Gaasch WH, LeWinter MM, eds. *Left ventricular diastolic dysfunction and heart failure.* Philadelphia: Lea & Febiger, 1994: 3–24.

Bernstein EA, Eberli FR, Silverman AM, et al. The calcium channel blocker felodipine protects against ischemia-reperfusion injury by a mechanism other than reducing O_2 demand. *Cardiovasc Drugs Ther* 1996; 10: 167–178.

Bessman SP, Yang WCT, Geiger PJ, Erickson-Viitanen S. Intimate coupling of creatine phosphokinase and myofibrillar adenosinetriphosphatase. *Biochem Biophys Res Commun* 1980; 96: 1414–1420.

Bolli R. Myocardial "stunning" in man. *Circulation* 1992; 86: 1671–1691.

Bowers KC, Allshire AP, Cobbold PH. Bioluminescent measurement in single cardiomyocytes of sudden cytosolic ATP depletion coincident with rigor. *J Mol Cell Cardiol* 1991; 24: 213–218.

Bronzwaer JGF, de Bruyne B, Ascoop CAPL, Paulus WJ. Comparative effects of pacing-induced and balloon coronary occlusion ischemia on left ventricular diastolic function in man. *Circulation* 1991; 84: 211–222.

Camacho SA, Brandes R, Figueredo VM, Weiner MW. Ca^{2+} transient decline and myocardial relaxation are slowed during low flow ischemia in rat hearts. *J Clin Invest* 1994; 93: 951–957.

Camacho SA, Figueredo VM, Brandes R, Weiner MW. Ca^{2+}-dependent fluorescence transients and phosphate metabolism during low-flow ischemia in rat hearts. *Am J Physiol* 1993; 265: H114–H122.

Carroll JD, Hess OM, Hirzel HO, Krayenbuehl HP. Exercise-induced ischemia: the influence of altered relaxation on early diastolic pressures. *Circulation* 1983a; 67: 521–528.

Carroll JD, Hess OM, Hirzel HO, Krayenbuehl HP. Dynamics of left ventricular filling at rest and during exercise. *Circulation* 1983b; 68: 59–67.

Carroll JD, Carroll EP. Diastolic function in coronary artery disease. *Herz* (Germany) 1991; 16: 1–9.

Cheng CP, Igarashi Y, Little WC. Mechanism of augmented rate of left ventricle filling during exercise. *Circ Res* 1992; 70: 9–19.

Cheng CP, Noda T, Nozawa T, Little WC. Effect of heart failure on the mechanism of exercise induced augmentation of mitral valve flow. *Circ Res* 1993; 72: 795–806.

Cobbold PH, Bourne PK. Aequorin measurements of free calcium in single heart cells. *Nature* 1984; 312: 444–446.

Cohen GI, Pietrolungo JF, Thomas JD, Klein AL. A practical guide to assessment of ventricular diastolic function using Doppler echocardiography. *J Am Coll Cardiol* 1996; 27: 1753–1760.

Cross HR, Radda GK, Clarke K. The role of Na^+/K^+ ATPase activity during low flow ischemia in preventing myocardial injury: a ^{31}P, ^{23}Na and ^{87}Rb NMR spectroscopic study. *Magn Reson Med* 1995; 34: 673–685.

Cunningham MJ, Apstein CS, Weinberg EO, et al. Influence of glucose and insulin on exaggerated diastolic and systolic dysfunction of hypertrophied rat hearts during hypoxia. *Circ Res* 1990; 66: 406–415.

Dahloef B, Pennert K, Hansson L. Reversal of left ventricular hypertrophy in hypertensive patients. A meta-analysis of 109 treatment studies. *Am Heart J* 1992; 5: 95–110.

Eberli FR, Apstein CS, Ngoy S, Lorell BH. Exacerbation of left ventricular ischemic diastolic dysfunction by pressure-overload hypertrophy: modification by specific inhibition of cardiac angiotensin converting enzyme. *Circ Res* 1992a; 70: 931–943.

Eberli FR, Ferrell MA, Apstein CS. Role of calcium in diastolic dysfunction. *Circulation* 1990; 82(Suppl III): III-605.

Eberli FR, Ferrell MA, Ngoy S, Apstein CS. Role of calcium and calcium-sodium exchange on diastolic dysfunction. *Circulation* 1991a; 84(Suppl II): II-211.

Eberli FR, Ngoy S, Bernstein E, Apstein CS. More evidence against calcium overload as direct cause of ischemic diastolic dysfunction. *Circulation* 1992b; 86(Suppl I): I-480.

Eberli FR, Ritter M, Schwitter J, et al. Coronary reserve in patients with aortic valve disease before and after successful aortic valve replacement. *Eur Heart J* 1991b; 12: 127–138.

Eberli FR, Weinberg EO, Grice WN, et al. Protective effect of increased glycolytic substrate against systolic and diastolic dysfunction and increased coronary resistance from prolonged global underperfusion and reperfusion in isolated rabbit hearts perfused with erythrocyte suspensions. *Circ Res* 1991c; 68: 466–481.

Fifer MA, Bourdillon PD, Lorell BH. Altered left ventricular diastolic properties during pacing-induced angina in patients with aortic stenosis. *Circulation* 1986; 74: 675–683.

Friedrich SP, Lorell BH, Rousseau MF, et al. Intracardiac angiotensin-converting enzyme inhibition improves diastolic function in patients with left ventricular hypertrophy due to aortic stenosis. *Circulation* 1994; 90: 2761–2771.

Gaasch WH. Diagnosis and treatment of heart failure based on left ventricular systolic or diastolic function. *JAMA* 1994; 271: 1276–1280.

Gaasch WH, Zile MR, Hoshino PK, et al. Tolerance of the hypertrophic heart to ischemia. *Circulation* 1990; 81: 1644–1653.

Grossman W. Diastolic dysfunction in congestive heart failure. *N Engl J Med* 1991; 325: 1557–1564.

Haigney MCP, Miyata H, Lakatta EG, et al. Dependence of hypoxic cellular calcium loading on Na^+- Ca^{2+} exchange. *Circ Res* 1992; 71: 547–557.

Han JW, Thielczek R, Varsanyi M, Herlmeyer LMG. Compartmentalized ATP synthesis in skeletal muscle triads. *Biochemistry* 1992; 31: 377–384.

Hatle L. Doppler echocardiographic evaluation of diastolic function in hypertensive cardiomyopathies. *Eur Heart J* 1993; 14(Suppl J): 88–94.

Hearse DJ, Garlick PB, Humphrey SM. Ischemic contracture of the myocardium: mechanisms and prevention. *Am J Cardiol* 1977; 39: 986–993.

Henderson Y. Volume changes of the heart. *Physiol Rev* 1923; 3: 165–208.

Hess OM, Krayenbuehl HP. Beta-adrenergic receptor blockers and calcium channel blockers in left ventricular hypertrophy. In: Gaasch WH, LeWinter MM, eds. *Left ventricular diastolic dysfunction and heart failure*. Philadelphia: Lea & Febiger, 1994: 455–464.

Hess OM, Murakami T, Krayenbuehl HP. Does verapamil improve left ventricular relaxation in patients with myocardial hypertrophy? *Circulation* 1986; 74: 530–543.

Illingworth JA, Ford WCB, Kobayashi K, Williamson JR. Regulation of myocardial energy metabolism. *Recent Adv Stud Card Struct Metab* 1975; 8: 271–290.

Ishihara K, Zile MR, Nagatsu M, et al. Coronary blood flow after the regression of pressure-overload left ventricular hypertrophy. *Circ Res* 1992; 71: 1472–1481.

Isoyama S. Interplay of hypertrophy and myocardial ischemia. In: Lorell BH, Grossman W, eds. *Diastolic relaxation of the heart*. 2nd ed. Boston: Kluwer Academic Publishers, 1992: 203–211.

Isoyama S, Apstein CS, Wexler LF, et al. Acute decrease in left ventricular diastolic chamber distensibility during simulated angina in isolated hearts. *Circ Res* 1987; 61: 925–933.

Kagaya Y, Weinberg EO, Ito N, et al. Glycolytic inhibition: effects on diastolic relaxation and intracellular calcium handling in hypertrophied rat ventricular myocytes. *J Clin Invest* 1995; 95: 2766–2776.

Katz AM. *Physiology of the heart*. New York: Raven Press, 1992: 178–195.

Katz A, Tada M. The "stone heart:" a challenge to the biochemist. *Am J Cardiol* 1972; 29: 578–580.

Kihara Y, Grossman W, Morgan JP. Direct measurement of changes in [Ca^{2+}]$_i$ during hypoxia, ischemia, and reperfusion of the intact mammalian heart. *Circ Res* 1989; 65: 1029–1044.

Kingsley PB, Sako EY, Yang MQ, et al. Ischemic contracture begins when anaerobic glycolysis stops: a ^{31}P-NMR study of isolated rat hearts. *Am J Physiol* 1991; 261: H469–H478.

Kitzman DW, Higginbotham MB, Cobb FR, et al. Exercise intolerance in patients with heart failure and preserved left ventricular systolic function: failure of the Frank-Starling mechanism. *J Am Coll Cardiol* 1991; 17: 1065–1072.

Koretsune Y, Marban E. Mechanism of ischemic contracture in ferret hearts: relative roles of [Ca^{2+}]$_i$ elevation and ATP depletion. *Am J Physiol* 1990; 258: H9–H16.

Kurganov BI, Sugrobova NP, Mil'man LS. Supramolecular organization of glycolytic enzymes. *J Theor Biol* 1985; 116: 509–526.

Labovitz AJ, Pearson AC. Evaluation of left ventricular diastolic function: clinical relevance and recent Doppler echocardiographic insights. *Am Heart J* 1987; 114: 836–851.

Labovitz AJ, Lewen MK, Kern H, et al. Evaluation of LV systolic and diasolic dysfunctions during transient myocardial ischemia produced by angioplasty. *J Am Coll Cardiol* 1987; 10: 748–755.

Lee HC, Mohabir R, Smith N, et al. Effect of ischemia on calcium-dependent fluorescence transients in rabbit hearts containing Indo-1. *Circulation* 1988; 78: 1047–1059.

Levine HJ, Gaasch WH. Clinical recognition and treatment of diastolic dysfunction and heart failure. In Gaasch WH, LeWinter MM, eds. *Left ventricular diastolic dysfunction and heart failure.* Philadelphia: Lea & Febiger, 1994: 439–454.

Little WC, Cheng CP. Modulation of diastolic dysfunction in the intact heart. In: Lorell BH, Grossman W, eds. *Diastolic relaxation of the heart*. 2nd ed. Boston: Kluwer Academic Publishers, 1994: 167–176.

Lorell BH. Left ventricular hypertrophy: the consequences for diastole. In: Gaasch WH, LeWinter MM, eds. *Left ventricular diastolic dysfunction and heart failure.* Philadelphia: Lea & Febiger, 1994: 345–353.

Lorell BH, Grice WN, Apstein CS. Influence of hypertension with minimal hypertrophy during demand ischemia. *Hypertension* 1989; 13: 36l–370.

Lorell BH, Wexler LF, Momomura S, et al. The influence of pressure overload left ventricular hypertrophy on diastolic properties during hypoxia in isovolumically contracting rat hearts. *Circ Res* 1986; 58: 653–663.

Lowe JE, Jennings RB, Reimer KA. Cardiac rigor mortis in dogs. *J Mol Cell Cardiol* 1979; 11: 1017–1031.

Marban E, Kitakaze M, Kusuoka H, et al. Intracellular free calcium concentration measured with ^{19}F NMR spectroscopy in intact ferret heart. Proc Natl Acad Sci USA 1987; 84: 6005–6009.

Marcus ML, Koyanagi S, Harrison DG, et al. Abnormalities in the coronary circulation that occur as a consequence of cardiac hypertrophy. *Am J Med* 1983; 75: 62–66.

McKenney P, Apstein CS, Mendes LA, et al. Increased left ventricular diastolic chamber stiffness immediately after coronary artery bypass surgery. *J Am Coll Cardiol* 1994a; 24: 1189–1194.

McKenney P, Apstein CS, Mendes LA, et al. Marked diastolic dysfunction immediately after aortic valve replacement for aortic stenosis. *J Am Coll Cardiol* 1994b; Suppl I: 278A.

Miyata H, Lakatta EG, Stern MD, Silverman HS. Relation of mitochondrial and cytosolic free calcium to cardiac myocyte recovery after exposure to anoxia. *Circ Res* 1992; 71: 605–613.

Mochizuki T, Eberli FR, Apstein CS, Lorell BH. Exacerbation of ischemic dysfunction by angiotensin II in red cell-perfused rabbit hearts: effects of coronary flow, contractility, and high-energy phosphate metabolism. *J Clin Invest* 1992; 89: 490–498.

Mohabir R, Lee HC, Kurz RW, Clusin WT. Effects of ischemia and hyperbaric acidosis on myocyte calcium transients, contraction, and pH$_i$ in perfused rabbit hearts. *Circ Res* 1991; 69: 1525–1537.

Nixon JV, Burns CA. Cardiac effects of aging and diastolic dysfunction in the elderly. In: Gaasch WH, LeWinter MM, eds. *Left ventricular diastolic dysfunction and heart failure.* Philadelphia: Lea & Febiger, 1994: 427–435.

Owen P, Dennis S, Opie LH. Glucose flux regulates onset of ischemic contracture in globally underperfused rat hearts. *Circ Res* 1990; 66: 406–415.

Packer M. Abnormalities in diastolic function as a potential cause of exercise intolerance in chronic heart failure. *Circulation* 1990; 81(Suppl III): III-78–III-86.

Paulus WJ, Takashi S, Grossman W. Altered left ventricular diastolic properties during pacing-induced ischemia in dogs with coronary stenoses: potentiation by caffeine. *Circ Res* 1982; 50: 218–227.

Pepine C, Wiener L. Relationship of anginal symptoms to lung mechanics during myocardial ischemia. *Circulation* 1972; 46: 863–869.

Rousseau MF, Gurne O, van Eyll C, et al. Effects of benazeprilat on left ventricular systolic and diastolic function and neurohumoral status in patients with ischemic heart disease. *Circulation* 1990; 81(Suppl III): III-123–III-129.

Schaefer S, Prussel E, Carr LJ. Requirement of glycolytic substrate for metabolic recovery during moderate low flow ischemia. *J Mol Cell Cardiol* 1995; 27: 2167–2176.

Serizawa T, Vogel WM, Apstein CS, Grossman W. Comparison of acute alterations in left ventricular diastolic chamber stiffness induced by hypoxia and ischemia. *J Clin Invest* 1981; 68: 91–102.

Setaro JF, Zaret BL, Schulman DS, et al. Usefulness of verapamil for congestive heart failure associated with abnormal left ventricular diastolic filling and normal left ventricular systolic performance. *Am J Cardiol* 1990; 66: 981–986.

Steenbergen C, Murphy E, Levy L, London RE. Elevation in cytosolic free calcium concentration early in myocardial ischemia in perfused rat heart. *Circ Res* 1987; 60: 700–707.

Tomanek RJ, Wessel TJ, Harrison DG. Capillary growth and geometry during long-term hypertension and myocardial hypertrophy in dogs. *Am J Physiol* 1991; 261: H1011–H1018.

Topol EJ, Traill TA, Fortuin NJ. Hypertensive hypertrophic cardiomyopathy of the elderly. *N Engl J Med* 1985; 312: 277–282.

Vanoverschelde L-J, Janier MF, Bakke JE, et al. Rate of glycolysis during ischemia determines extent of ischemic injury and functional recovery after reperfusion. *Am J Physiol* 1994; 267: H1785–H1794.

Varma N, Eberli FR, Apstein CS. Calcium sensitivity of diastolic dysfunction is dissociated in demand ischemia compared to reperfusion, suggesting differing roles for increased myocyte calcium. *Circulation* 1994; 90(Suppl I):I-432.

Varma N, Eberli FR, Apstein CS. Diastolic dysfunction during demand ischemia is due to a reversible rigor force and is not a calcium activated tension. *J Am Coll Cardiol* 1995a (Suppl A): 27A.

Varma N, Eberli FR, Ngoy S, Apstein CS. Subcellular mechanisms of ischemic diastolic dysfunction: further evidence for rigor force in pathogenesis and not for Ca^{++} activated diastolic tension. *Circulation* 1995b; 92(Suppl I):I-657.

Ventura-Clapier R, Mekhfi H, Vassort G. Role of creatine kinase in chemically skinned rat cardiac muscle. *J Gen Physiol* 1987; 89: 815-837.

Ventura-Clapier R, Veksler V. Myocardial ischemic contracture metabolites affect rigor tension development stiffness. *Circ Res* 1994; 74: 920–929.

Weber KT, Brilla CG. Pathological hypertrophy and cardiac interstitium. *Circulation* 1991; 83: 1849–1865.

Weiss J, Hiltbrand B. Functional compartmentation of glycolytic versus oxidative metabolism in isolated rabbit heart. *J Clin Invest* 1985; 75: 436–447.

Wexler LF, Lorell BH, Momomura S, et al. Enhanced sensitivity to hypoxia-induced diastolic dysfunction in pressure overload hypertrophy in the rat: role of high energy phosphate depletion. *Circ Res* 1988; 62: 766–775.

Wexler LF, Weinberg EO, Ingwall JS, Apstein CS. Acute alterations in diastolic left ventricular chamber distensibility: mechanistic differences between hypoxemia and ischemia in isolated perfused rabbit and rat hearts. *Circ Res* 1986; 59: 515–528.

Yamashita H, Sata M, Sugiura S, et al. ADP inhibits the sliding velocity of fluorescent actin filaments on cardiac and skeletal myosins. *Circ Res* 1994; 74: 1027–1033.

Yellin EL, Nikolic SD. Diastolic suction and the dynamics of left ventricular filling. In: Gaasch WH, LeWinter MM, eds. *Left ventricular diastolic dysfunction and heart failure.* Philadelphia: Lea & Febiger, 1994: 89–102.

CHAPTER 9

"Maimed Myocardium": Incomplete, Delayed Functional Recovery Late after Reperfusion following Acute Myocardial Infarction

William E. Boden

Left ventricular dysfunction following acute coronary occlusion may be reversible or irreversible. The duration of coronary occlusion and the rapidity/extent of reperfusion are the primary determinants of LV salvage and recovery. Brief periods of coronary occlusion (minutes) followed by prompt reperfusion (no biochemical or histological evidence of myocardial necrosis) result either in no LV dysfunction or reversibly injured (stunned) myocardium that, over time, returns completely to normal. Alternatively, prolonged coronary occlusion without reperfusion results typically in severe LV dysfunction and little, if any, salvage or recovery because myocardial segments subtending a persistently occluded infarct-related coronary artery invariably progress to transmural necrosis.

However, reperfusion that occurs late (hours or days) after coronary occlusion may result in incomplete, delayed functional recovery, since partial myocardial necrosis and/or intense myocardial ischemia would be expected to result in intermediate degrees of LV dysfunction. Since *some* myocardial necrosis is inevitable after prolonged coronary occlusion followed by late reperfusion, it is unrealistic to assume that the partial LV recovery that occurs in this context would be quantitatively similar to that which occurs during only brief periods of ischemia without necrosis.

During the last decade, the value of reperfusion late after AMI has become firmly established (Dalen et al., 1988; Finci et al., 1990; ISIS-2 Collaborative Group, 1988; Schroder et al., 1989; Stampfer et al., 1982; Yusuf et al., 1985). Whereas improved survival has been an almost invariable finding following thrombolytic therapy for evolving AMI, the effects on global and regional LV function have been less consistent and more controversial (Rentrop et al., 1989; Sheehan et al., 1988; White et al., 1987). While a number of mechanisms have been suggested to explain the salutary effects of late reperfusion including a reduction in infarct size (Habib et al, 1991; ISAM Study Group, 1986; Simoons et al., 1986), limitation of infarct expansion and LV cavitary dilatation (Eaton & Bulkley, 1981; Force et al., 1988; Hochman & Choo, 1987), changes in LV architecture due to remodeling (McKay et al., 1986), and a decrease in incidence of fatal ventricular arrhythmia (Kersschot et al., 1986), it seems clear that successful reperfusion (and residual patency) of an occluded, infarct-related coronary artery is a pivotal event to improved survival and enhanced ventricular function.

A recent clinical study by Sabia and coworkers (1992) demonstrated that LV myocardium remains viable for a prolonged period in many patients with AMI following coronary artery occlusion, and that late reperfusion may provide clinical benefit by improving residual function of depressed, but viable, myocardium within the infarct zone. Such observations of improved LV function late after reperfusion are consistent with the favorable outcome observed in published thrombolysis trials among patients in whom patency of the infarct-related coronary artery was reestablished late after AMI (Dalen et al., 1988; Finci et al., 1990; ISIS-2 Collaborative Group, 1988; Schroder et al., 1989; Stampfer et al., 1982; Yusuf et al., 1985).

These more recent clinical observations, however, appear at variance with classic physiologic teachings dating back almost 100 years, in which Porter (1895) and subsequently Herrick (1912) first detailed the consequences of occlusion of a major epicardial coronary artery. These seminal observations included the prompt decline in systolic LV pressure and its rate of rise (Porter, 1895), the development of acute myocardial necrosis, and rapid progression to irreversible myocardial damage followed by a failure of LV functional recovery despite reperfusion (Herrick, 1912).

Furthermore, it is now well recognized that severe myocardial contraction abnormalities may occur with brief periods of coronary artery occlusion. Tennant and Wiggers (1935) showed that brief periods of coronary artery occlusion produced myocardial ischemia associated with focal aneurysmal bulging within 60 seconds of coronary ligation. Thereafter, numerous studies, initially dating back to 1969 in our own laboratory (Boden et al., 1978; Hood et al., 1969; Weiner et al., 1976), demonstrated that brief periods (10 minutes) of coronary occlusion resulted in prolonged ischemic contractile impairment even after restoration of antegrade coronary blood flow (Ellis et al., 1983; Heyndrickx et al., 1975, 1978). A consistent observation has been that the rate of LV functional recovery in ischemic segments is, in general, inversely proportional to the duration of coronary occlusion (Hess et al., 1979; Kloner et al., 1983; Preuss et al., 1987). Studies performed in the late 1960s and early 1970s were among the first to report that periods of coronary occlusion less than 20 minutes in duration were not associated with the development of myocardial necrosis. However, it was demonstrated that when the coronary artery occlusion was released, systolic function of the previously ischemic myocardium remained depressed for extended time periods (Boden et al., 1978; Ellis et al., 1983; Kloner et al., 1983; Preuss et al., 1987; Weiner et al., 1976).

RECOVERY OF POSTISCHEMIC LV FUNCTION AND THE CONCEPT OF "MAIMED MYOCARDIUM"

Braunwald and Kloner (1982), over a decade ago, introduced the term *stunned myocardium* to describe this phenomenon of prolonged *postischemic* LV dysfunction that occurred in the aftermath of an acute coronary occlusion *not* of sufficient severity or duration to produce myocardial necrosis. The important concept galvanized our thinking that an acute period of *reversible* myocardial ischemia was attended by delayed functional recovery after the reestablishment of coronary blood flow, and paved the way for our contemporary views that LV function change in certain acute coronary syndromes might not be discernible in the immediate postintervention period.

Braunwald and Kloner further postulated that if myocardium was subjected to repetitive episodes of stunning, it might manifest *chronic*, postischemic contractile impairment (Patel et al., 1988). Rahimtoola (1989) subsequently introduced the term *hibernating myocardium*, which he defined as a state of persistently impaired myocardial function at rest due to reduced coronary blood flow that can be partially or completely restored to normal if the myocardium oxygen supply/demand relationship is favorably altered, either by improving coronary blood flow and/or by reducing demand.

Kloner and colleagues (1989b) summarized the comparative differences in these altered myocardial states in a previous editorial. They emphasized that there are several potential outcomes of myocardial ischemia. When ischemia is severe, myocyte cell death generally occurs and there is no recovery of contractile function in these cells. When myocardial ischemia is less severe but still prolonged, myocytes may remain viable but exhibit chronically depressed contractile function (*hibernating myocardium*), which is postulated to be a protective mechanism whereby myocardium reduces its oxygen demand in response to reduced oxygen supply ((Kloner et al., 1989b). Alternatively, brief periods of myocardial ischemia may be reversed with coronary artery reperfusion resulting in salvage of myocytes. Such viable myocardium may demonstrate relatively prolonged postischemic contractile dysfunction (*stunned myocardium*) (Kloner et al., 1989b), but full recovery of function is the eventual outcome.

While these altered myocardial states imply LV dysfunction in relation to *either* brief periods of coronary occlusion *or* prolonged periods of severely reduced coronary blood flow, they do not occur *in the context of myocardial necrosis*. These reversible alterations in contractile impairment do not adequately characterize all cases of postinfarction LV dysfunction that culminate in late, incomplete recovery of myocardial performance following reperfusion.

The purpose of this review is to introduce a clinical concept that we believe portrays more accurately a third altered myocardial state, namely that which involves incomplete, late functional recovery of severely injured myocardium that has been partially salvaged long after reperfusion. We propose the term *maimed myocardium* to describe the phenomenon of incomplete, delayed functional recovery of myocardial tissue segments late after reperfusion following AMI, and the multiform pathophysiological processes that may contribute to this condition. We postulate that certain acute coronary syndromes, namely non-Q-wave AMI (Gibson et al., 1986; Maisel et al., 1985; Marmor et al., 1981) and evolving infarction treated acutely with thrombolytic therapy (Dalen et al., 1988; Finci et al., 1990; ISIS-2 Collaborative Group, 1988; Schroder et al., 1989; Stampfer et al., 1982; Yusuf et al., 1985), culminate in subepicardial and/or patchy subendocardial myocardial salvage that can be manifest clinically as delayed LV functional recovery. Both of these acute coronary syndromes are clinical conditions that are felt to represent manifestations of "incomplete infarction" following spontaneous or drug-induced coronary reperfusion, respectively (Boden, 1991).

Both the "naturally occurring" non-Q-wave AMI and the evolving infarction treated with thrombolytic therapy share many features anatomically, histologically, angiographically, clinically, and prognostically (Boden, 1991). In brief, these features include subtotal coronary occlusion, partial reperfusion with altered early reflow, contraction band necrosis (Freifeld et al., 1983; Roberts et al., 1983) (the histological hallmark of reperfusion injury), enhanced myocardial salvage (notably in the subepicardium or the lateral subendocardial margins of the infarct [Helfant et al., 1978; Reimer & Jennings, 1979]), and incomplete, delayed LV functional recovery (Feyter et al., 1983; Grines et al., 1989; Stack et al., 1983).

Accordingly, it seems relevant to distinguish the prolonged, but *completely* reversible, *postischemic* LV dysfunction of myocardial stunning and hibernating myocardium from the prolonged, but *incompletely* reversible, *postinfarction* ventricular dysfunction that characterizes certain patients with spontaneous coronary reperfusion (i.e., non-Q-wave AMI) and those whose infarcts are aborted/interrupted because of the early exogenous administration of a thrombolytic agent. These comparative differences are illustrated in Figure 9-1.

Kloner's pioneering work with a reversible experimental model of myocardial stunning has advanced immeasurably our understanding of LV function change following acute coronary occlusion (Braunwald & Kloner, 1982; Patel et al., 1988). However, in their recent review on altered myocardial states, Kloner and colleagues (1989b) cite several examples of acute coronary syndromes as clinical evidence in support of stunned myocardium. These examples include (1) patients undergoing thrombolytic therapy for evolving AMI, (2) patients with unstable angina, (3) patients with exercise-induced angina, (4) patients undergoing angioplasty, and (5) patients requiring inotropic support for the first few days following cardiac surgery (Kloner et al., 1989b).

In all but the first example, ischemia would appear to be the sine qua non of myocardial stunning. Yet, Kloner and

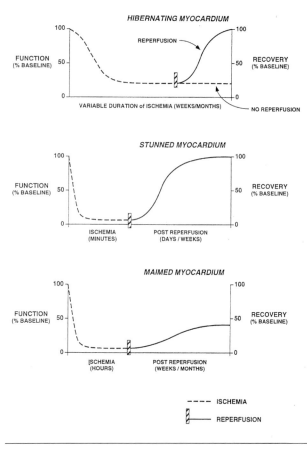

Figure 9-1. Schematic diagram of the time course of left ventricular (LV) function with ischemia and reperfusion, which we postulate occurs in each of the altered myocardial states. The top panel depicts LV function change of hibernating myocardium expressed as the percentage of baseline and recovery during a variable period of ischemia. The center panel depicts LV function change during a brief period of ischemia (minutes) followed by reperfusion, resulting in stunned myocardium. The bottom panel depicts LV function change that occurs during prolonged ischemia (hours) followed by reperfusion, resulting in maimed myocardium. Note the intermediate degree of LV functional recovery.

colleagues cite salvage of myocardium following AMI interrupted by thrombolysis as the "best example" of stunning, despite the fact that this clinical state is characterized by myocardial necrosis—at least in part—which presumably distinguishes the postthrombolysis infarction setting from other "pure" ischemic syndromes where, by definition, necrosis is absent (Kloner et al., 1989b).

While these conditions may be associated with myocardium that recovers completely and therefore may be termed *stunned*, we suggest that other processes may be involved that lead to more delayed and incomplete recovery of function, such as that which occurs following AMI treated with thrombolysis resulting in late reperfusion and delayed myocardial salvage. In fact, we postulate that stunned and maimed myocardium may occur concomitantly in differing myocardial regions in the same patient with an acute coronary syndrome such as non-Q-wave infarction or AMI treated with thrombolytic therapy.

CONSEQUENCES OF PROLONGED CORONARY OCCLUSION ON LV FUNCTION

In order to appreciate better the need for distinguishing *stunned* from *maimed* myocardium, it seems relevant to discuss briefly the fate of myocardium subjected to prolonged coronary occlusion, such as occurs commonly during the non-Q-wave AMI and following thrombolysis for evolving acute infarction. A major assumption, it seems, is that the gradual improvement in regional cardiac function following thrombolytic therapy for evolving AMI (which can range from days to weeks) must indicate the presence of viable myocytes that have been salvaged by reperfusion. While some myocytes presumably have been infarcted, others remain viable despite severe and prolonged ischemia, possibly those myocardial segments within the central zone perfused originally by the infarct-related coronary artery.

A corollary assumption has been that the inevitable result of severe, prolonged ischemia is myocyte cell death with no recovery of contractile function of these cells. Such an all-or-none view of myocardial cell viability post-infarction may be too restrictive physiologically and may represent an inadvertent bias similar to the one that existed until the importance of myocardial stunning was elucidated a decade ago.

The current and prevailing view has been that after sustained coronary occlusion (≥3–4 hours) there is extensive myocardial necrosis and little, if any, functional recovery of those myocardial segments in the center of the infarct zone subtended by the completely occluded coronary artery. Indeed, in a previous editorial, Braunwald (1989) emphasized that after sudden and sustained total coronary occlusion, the course of myocardial necrosis is generally rapid and relentless. (In most cases, the process is completed within 3 to 4 hours of the coronary occlusion, in 6 hours at maximum.) Thus, it has become virtually axiomatic to regard this time window as the obligate point of no return in LV function recovery in the absence of reperfusion.

However, recent studies suggest that these traditional concepts may warrant reappraisal. In particular, the finding that reperfusion is not infrequently associated with a reduction of contractile dysfunction and improved survival (ISIS-2 Collaborative Group, 1988; Stampfer et al., 1982; Yusuf et al., 1985), even beyond the time interval when patency may be expected to salvage myocardium, supports the hypothesis that an "open infarct vessel" is responsible for this clinical benefit. Yet, this may not be the only explanation. Late myocardial salvage may play a role and it may involve not only reversibly injured (stunned), but also more intensely injured and partially infarcted (maimed) myocardial tissue segments—especially if restored patency of the infarct-related coronary artery might enhance antegrade blood flow to severely damaged myocardium that possesses latent viability and the propensity to recover function partially.

DOES REPERFUSION INJURY EXIST IN HUMANS?

Although it has remained controversial for decades, there is still concern that at the time of reperfusion, a further injury to the myocardium occurs with reflow. Theoretically, if this "reperfusion injury" could be identified, favorably altered, or eliminated, the outcome of patients with AMI who have undergone successful reperfusion therapy (thrombolysis or primary angioplasty) might improve further. The concept of reperfusion injury is integrally related to the concept that oxygen free radicals generated at the time of reperfusion cause additional tissue damage (Becker & Ambrosio, 1987; Bolli et al., 1988; Braunwald & Kloner, 1985; Forman & Virmani, 1990; Hearse & Bolli, 1992; McCord, 1988; McCord et al., 1985; Zweier et al., 1987).

Kloner (1993) has described four basic forms of reperfusion injury: lethal reperfusion injury, vascular reperfusion injury, stunned myocardium, and reperfusion arrhythmias. *Lethal reperfusion injury* is described as myocyte cell death due to reperfusion itself, rather than to antecedent ischemia. This concept continues to be controversial in both experimental and clinical studies, but clearly, acceleration of the necrotic process can occur when irreversibly injured myocytes are reperfused (Fishbein, 1990; Kloner et al., 1974b; Whalen et al., 1974). Such myocardial segments display little, if any, potential for recovery and can be considered completely infarcted.

Vascular reperfusion injury refers to progressive damage to the vasculature over time during the phase of reperfusion. Manifestations of vascular reperfusion injury include an expanding zone of no reflow and a deterioration of coronary flow reserve (Kloner, 1993). This form of reperfusion has been documented in animal models and is postulated to occur in humans as a manifestation of *maimed myocardium.*

By contrast, *stunned myocardium* refers to postischemic LV dysfunction of *viable* myocytes, and probably represents a milder form of functional reperfusion compared to maimed myocardium. Stunning myocardium is well documented in both animal models and humans, as noted previously.

Reperfusion arrhythmias represent a fourth form of reperfusion injury, and include ventricular tachycardia and fibrillation that occur within seconds to minutes following restoration of coronary flow after brief (5–15 minutes) episodes of ischemia (Kloner, 1993). Such reperfusion arrhythmias following periods of ischemia too brief to induce myocardial necrosis may coexist mechanically with stunned myocardium and may be a cause of sudden cardiac death in patients with coronary artery spasm. True reperfusion arrhythmias occur only infrequently in AMI patients treated with thrombolytic therapy and may coexist with maimed myocardium. Such occurrences may explain the increased mortality frequently associated with thrombolysis during the initial 24 hours.

THE EXPERIMENTAL BASIS
FOR MAIMED MYOCARDIUM

When the heart is exposed to ischemia and reperfusion, damage occurs not only to the myocytes, but also to the microvasculature. In experimental studies, clamping a proximal coronary artery for 60 to ≥90 minutes, followed by release of the clamp, resulted in persistent subendocardial perfusion defects when tracers such as fluorescent dyes or carbon black were injected into the vasculature. The inability to perfuse previously ischemic tissue has been termed the *no reflow phenomenon* (Kloner et al., 1974a). Electron microscopic examination of zones of no reflow reveal damage to the microvasculature including a loss of pinocytotic vesicles to the endothelium, endothelial blisters or blebs, gaps within the endothelium, and neutrophil infiltration (Engler et al. 1983; Kloner et al., 1974a, 1989a).

Contracture or swelling, or both, of neighboring myocytes may also contribute to the no reflow phenomenon (Engler et al., 1983; Humphrey et al., 1980). Although some of the abnormalities to the endothelium or myocytes that could cause no reflow are present at the end of a period of ischemia (Kloner et al., 1974a), some observations suggest that further damage to the vasculature occurs with progression of reperfusion. For example, one study by Ambrosio and coworkers (1989) described an increase in the size of the no reflow zone with time, after the moment of reperfusion. This abnormality was demonstrated with fluorescent dyes and also by a progressive decrease in regional myocardial blood flow as assessed by radioactive microspheres. One group (Kloner et al., 1991) has reported a deterioration of coronary flow reserve (in response to vasodilators both dependent and not dependent on endothelium-derived relaxing factors) between early reperfusion and several hours later. Several other laboratories ((Ku, 1982; Quillen et al., 1990; Van Benthuysen et al., 1987; Weiss et al., 1986) have observed abnormal vasodilator reserve after reperfusion. The findings of an increase in no reflow and a worsening of vascular reserve with time after reperfusion suggest that some damage to the vasculature occurs during the reperfusion phase and, hence, may represent vascular reperfusion injury. Whether this vascular reperfusion injury directly contributes to myocyte cell death is not known.

Moreover, in the conscious dog, Theroux and associates (1976) were among the first investigators to demonstrate delayed recovery of LV function after a 2-hour period of left anterior descending coronary artery occlusion followed by reperfusion. In their model, postischemic LV dysfunction in hypokinetic regions improved or resolved over a 2- to 3-week period, whereas there was a small but nonetheless discernible improvement observed even in frankly dyskinetic segments that had displayed considerable myocardial necrosis (Theroux et al., 1976).

Similarly, Bush and coworkers (1985) have likewise shown that in conscious dogs subjected to a 4-hour left anterior descending coronary artery occlusion followed by reperfusion, there was a significant recovery of segmental function in the central zone of infarction subtending the occluded artery *at 28 days*. In the most severely injured segments, net systolic thickening declined promptly with reperfusion and was replaced by marked thinning. The administration of the calcium antagonist diltiazem, and the beta-blocker propranolol, prevented the reperfusion-associated decline in segmental function, and was attended by better long-term recovery of segmental function as well (Fig 9-2) (Bush et al., 1985). While this degree of regional LV recovery was not nearly as pronounced as in adjacent, less intensely injured "border zone" segments, the capacity of infarcted myocardium to recover some degree of function was no less striking.

Over a decade ago, it was demonstrated, utilizing postextrasystolic potentiation, that regional mechanical function could be augmented in both border zones and central infarct zones of canine myocardium subjected to a 4-hour left anterior coronary artery occlusion followed by 1 hour of reperfusion (Boden et al., 1980). Despite profound ischemic injury in the center of the infarct zone subtending the occluded coronary artery (78% reduction in regional myocardial blood flow and histological evidence of significant, patchy, nontransmural necrosis confirmed by ntiroblue tetrazolium), both intrinsic and potentiated mechanical function in central infarct segments improved significantly during reperfusion compared with 4 hours of ischemia. Such improvement in regional LV function with postextrasystolic potentiation during coronary occlusion and its augmentation during reperfusion indicates that viable myocardium is present in partially infarcted areas of myocardium, and that recovery of contractile function may occur despite prolonged periods of coronary occlusion (Boden et al., 1980).

Such experimental findings (Boden et al., 1980; Bush et al., 1985; Theroux et al., 1976) of delayed functional recovery likely represent intrinsic latent viability or the presence of maimed myocardium. In contrast, the almost complete return of function in less severely injured border zone segments back to control (baseline) levels indicates that these less intensely ischemic segments are stunned (Bush et al., 1985; Theroux et al., 1976; Weiss et al., 1986). Finally, in a related experiment performed in conscious dogs (Sherman et al., 1979), it was shown that verapamil pretreatment produced improved segment shortening in both border and central ischemic zones during a 2-hour left anterior descending coronary artery occlusion followed by 1 hour of reperfusion. Regional mechanical function was, not unexpectedly, more preserved in the border zone, although there was augmentation in myocardial segments subtending the occluded coronary artery. Postextrasystolic potentiation significantly enhanced regional function in both zones in verapamil- compared with saline-treated control animals, and this was especially so during reperfusion (Sherman et al., 1979). Such data, together with the findings of Bush and colleagues (1985) in a similar model using diltiazem, suggest that severely injured myocardium possesses latent viability that may be unmasked by reperfusion late after coronary occlusion. These experimental studies suggest that myocardial contractile performance may be further increased by pharmacological agents such as calcium channel blockers.

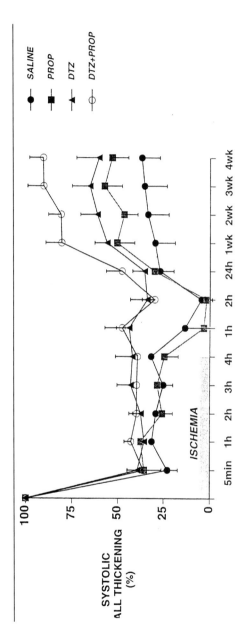

Figure 9-2. Time course of regional LV systolic wall thickening in the central infarct zone subtending a 4-hour total left anterior descending coronary artery occlusion followed by 28 days of reperfusion in conscious dogs. Ischemia is depicted in the shaded area along the abscissa, followed by reperfusion. Systolic wall thickening is expressed as the percent recovery, compared to baseline, for control animals (SALINE), and for animals who received pretreatment with propranolol (PROP), diltiazem (DTZ), and with both PROP and DTZ. Note the gradual return of regional function during reperfusion to a level intermediate between preischemia and early reperfusion.

THE CLINICAL BASIS
FOR MAIMED MYOCARDIUM

As previously noted, Sabia and coworkers (1992) recently reported in the *New England Journal of Medicine* a prospective study that demonstrated that collateral-derived residual flow is present in many patients with a recent AMI and an occluded infarct-related artery. They showed that such blood flow maintained myocardial viability for a prolonged period despite total coronary occlusion, and that restoration of antegrade blood flow as late as 5 weeks after AMI resulted in improvement in regional LV function, even in patients who initially displayed severe regional contraction abnormalities.

In his editorial, Braunwald (1989) outlined several inconsistencies in certain outcome end points, such as LV function and survival following thrombolytic therapy. He cited findings from published studies that indicated that in certain patients *not* treated actively with any reperfusion therapy (i.e., those with evolving Q-wave infarction who presumably exhibit spontaneous reperfusion and a patent coronary artery, confirmed at coronary angiography), there is preserved contractile function compared with patients in whom the infarct artery remained occluded (Feyter et al., 1983; Jeremy et al., 1987; Verheugt et al., 1986).

Such findings are even more commonplace in patients with non-Q-wave AMI who did not receive acute thrombolytic therapy (Gibson et al., 1986; Maisel et al., 1985; Marmor et al., 1981). It is now generally believed that early spontaneous coronary reperfusion (presumably due to a more endogenously active intrinsic fibrinolytic system) is a common pathogenetic finding in non-Q-wave AMI patients that, in part, may explain their more favorable short-term prognosis. However, because these normal intrinsic thrombolytic mechanisms may not come into play sufficiently early (i.e., within the first 3–4 hours after coronary occlusion), it remains unclear precisely what mechanism explains the improvement in contractile performance observed in those patients with patent infarct vessels (Huey et al., 1987).

As noted previously, several published trials utilizing various thrombolytic agents for evolving AMI have demonstrated improved survival and better regional LV function (Fig 9-3A) in patients in whom patency of the infarct-related coronary artery was restored *late* after AMI (Dalen et al., 1988; Finci et al., 1990; ISIS-2 Collaborative Group, 1988; Schroder et al., 1989; Stampfer et al., 1982; Yusuf et al., 1985). It is noteworthy that the benefit of late thrombolytic therapy was discernible well beyond the time period when one would expect an improvement in survival based solely on the delayed reopening of an occluded, infarct-related coronary artery.

Additional evidence in support of the concept of incomplete, delayed functional recovery following AMI is suggested by the previous study of Boden and colleagues (1988) that showed that more than 60% of patients with non-Q-wave AMI who did not receive prior thrombolytic therapy demonstrated late improvement in ejection fraction 10 days after the onset of symptoms. This was particularly promi-

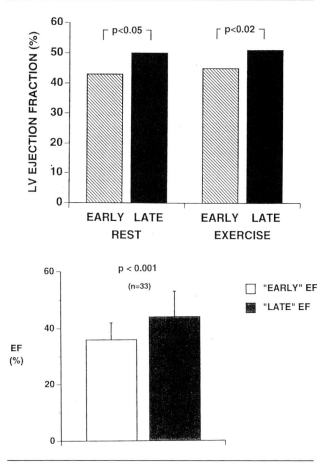

Figure 9-3. *(A) Changes in serial rest and exercise LV ejection fraction observed in postinfarction patients who received intravenous streptokinase. Baseline (early) ejection fraction was obtained during the first 48 hours of acute infarction, and postdischarge (late) ejection fraction was obtained 6 months postinfarction. There was a significant improvement in both rest and exercise ejection fraction over time. (Adapted from Borer and colleagues [1980].) (B) Changes in serial rest LV ejection fraction (EF) in 33 patients with acute non-Q-wave infarction who underwent radionuclide ventriculography 51 hours (early EF) after infarct onset, and who underwent repeat testing 11 days (late EF) after infarct onset. There was a significant increment in ejection fraction between the two studies.*

nent (a 76% incidence of late LV functional recovery) in the subset of non-Q-wave AMI patients whose initial radionuclide ejection fraction was below 50% (Fig 9-3B).

Such clinical observations are reinforced by studies that have examined regional myocardial metabolism and blood flow in patients with Q-wave and non-Q-wave AMI, utilizing positron emission tomography (PET) (Hashimoto et al., 1988). In one such study, Hashimoto and colleagues (1988), utilizing direct in vivo visualization of tissue metabolism with F18-deoxyglucose myocardial imaging, showed that 91% of infarcted regions without Q-waves exhibited metabolic integrity (residual viable tissue) compared to only 36% of 11 infarcted segments with Q-waves. Such increased regional accumulation of F18-deoxyglucose in the infarcted areas of non-Q-wave AMI patients supports the presence of latent viability in certain myocardial segments. These clinical findings suggest that many non-Q-wave infarction patients exhibit reversibly injured tissue with enhanced glucose utilization relative to blood flow. This preserved metabolic integrity observed following non-Q-wave AMI supports the concept that residual viable tissue is capable of exhibiting incomplete, delayed functional recovery of contractile performance.

Finally, a pattern of reverse thallium redistribution late after thrombolytic therapy has been reported in 75% of AMI patients 10 days after receiving intravenous streptokinase. This finding was interpreted as a sign of nontransmural myocardial infarction (Weiss et al., 1986). Weiss and associates (1986) demonstrated that reverse redistribution was associated with patency of the infarct-related coronary artery in all 67 patients (100%), and the authors inferred that this scintigraphic finding was related to the presence of both necrotic and viable myocardium within the reperfused zone. They showed that resting wall motion at day 10 was normal (or near normal) in 80% of segments that displayed marked reverse thallium redistribution, in 54% of segments with mild reverse redistribution, and even in 21% of segments with nonreversible defects (Weiss et al., 1986). Thus, thallium-201 reverse redistribution in AMI patients treated with streptokinase is caused by faster-than-normal thallium-201 washout in the reperfused region and is a sign of successful reopening of the occluded coronary artery—findings that support the presence of partially viable, salvaged myocardial segments within the reperfused zone.

Such scintigraphic observations of reverse thallium redistribution suggest that infarcted myocardial segments have the propensity to recover contractile function late after reperfusion. Accordingly, we believe that intensely injured (partially infarcted) myocardium incompletely salvaged by reperfusion may be maimed rather than irreversibly injured. Less intensely injured (ischemic) myocardial segments that recover contractile performance fully after reperfusion are more likely to have been stunned. Table 9-1 describes the comparative features of stunned, hibernating, and maimed myocardium.

TABLE 9-1. COMPARATIVE FEATURES OF REVERSIBLE MYO-
CARDIAL ISCHEMIC STATES

Features	Stunned myocardium	Hibernating myocardium	Maimed myocardium
Duration of ischemia	Minutes	Weeks/months	Hours
Contractility	Decreased	Decreased	Decreased
Necrosis	Absent	Absent	Patchy (subendocardial)
Reflow	Complete	Variable	Late; incomplete
Reversibility	Complete	Complete	Incomplete
Time course of recovery	Days/weeks	? Months/years	Weeks/months
Experimental models	Definite	Probable	Probable

UNRESOLVED ISSUES CONCERNING MAIMED MYOCARDIUM

If LV function can exhibit late recovery in the context of experimental and clinical subendocardial necrosis, can we be certain that the functional improvement is a direct consequence of delayed latent contractility of myocardial segments that have been partially infarcted? In a previous editorial, Verheugt and colleagues (1986) emphasized that a variety of factors can influence regional mechanical dysfunction. These include the degree and duration of subendocardial ischemia, the percentage of myocardial scar, altered global ventricular loading conditions, changes in regional afterload, effects of transmural "tethering," and interactions with adjacent myocardial segments. Thus, alterations in regional mechanical function can be difficult to define in experimental models. For obvious reasons, regional contractility may be even more problematic to assess clinically, given the dynamic interplay of adjacent dyskinetic, hypokinetic, and hyperkinetic segments.

While maimed myocardium appears to characterize more accurately the clinical state of regional and global LV recovery late after AMI followed by spontaneous or drug-induced reperfusion, it remains unclear at present whether, at the tissue level, this altered myocardial state is a composite of intensely injured (or partially infarcted) segments in series and parallel with normal or residually viable segments. Moreover, it remains unclear whether individual myocytes can be maimed.

In addition, we do not know whether reperfusion is a prerequisite for late myocardial salvage following non-Q-wave AMI or following thrombolysis, or whether maimed myocardium may recover only incompletely. Presumably, partially infarcted myocardial segments would not be expected to recover fully—even weeks or months after reperfusion—although this cannot be stated with complete certainty. Similarly, we do not know whether the presence of intact coronary collaterals may be an important factor in maintaining tissue viability late after AMI, with or without reperfusion.

Clearly, the purpose of this chapter is not to provide the precise cellular, biochemical, histological, and pathophysiological basis of maimed myocardium, rather it is to introduce a new, descriptive clinical concept of late contractile recovery that occurs in intensely injured myocardial segments late after prolonged coronary occlusion followed by reperfusion. We believe that this altered myocardial state—at the cardiac tissue level—differs fundamentally from both stunned and hibernating myocardium that now, after a decade, have been validated at the cellular level. It is important to keep in perspective that when the terms *stunned myocardium* and *hibernating myocardium* were introduced in 1982 (Braunwald & Kloner, 1982) and 1989 (Rahimtoola, 1989), respectively, each concept was described predominantly as a clinical phenomenon.

Accordingly, despite the fact that the term *maimed myocardium* may, at present, represent a more heterogeneous process compared to the more specific forms of reversible *postischemic* regional mechanical dysfunction, it appears that incompletely infarcted segments themselves may have the propensity for intrinsic recovery late following non-Q-wave AMI or postthrombolysis, and that such myocardium salvaged long after reperfusion should be conceptualized as fundamentally dissimilar from altered myocardial states (i.e., stunned or hibernating myocardium) in which necrosis, by definition, is absent.

Finally, it is unknown whether remodeling may be a feature of maimed myocardium. Late reperfusion of the infarct-related artery may prevent or limit infarct expansion/dilatation and may facilitate remodeling. Clearly such mechanisms come into play during the recovery phase following AMI (Hutchins & Bulkley, 1987; McKay et al., 1986; Pfeffer et al., 1985; Ross, 1986), but it is uncertain whether remodeling alone is sufficient to explain the presence of residual myocardial viability within the infarct zone late after AMI.

IMPLICATIONS FOR FUTURE RESEARCH AND THERAPY

It is possible that we need not only to expand our views regarding the importance of the open-artery hypothesis, but may likewise need to consider the possibility that (1) the time limit for irreversible damage to regions of the left ventricle subjected to acute coronary occlusion may be longer than currently conceived; (2) the propensity of maimed myocardium to recover partial function *late* after coronary occlusion followed by reperfusion—in a setting where there has been, by definition, some degree of subendocardial necrosis—is fundamentally dissimilar from the complete functional recovery of stunned myocardium, which results from ischemia too brief in duration to cause cellular necrosis; and (3) improvement in contractile function and survival late after reperfusion may result from salvage of severely injured myocardium, separate from the process of remodeling. Figure 9-4 illustrates the proposed spectrum of changes in contractility that we postulate as a continuum that varies according to the severity and duration of coronary occlusion with and without reperfusion.

We believe that it would be important to investigate the intrinsic properties of myocardium subjected to prolonged coronary blood flow deprivation that is of sufficient severity and duration to produce partial myocardial necrosis. It would be of further interest to determine whether reperfusion is essential to even partial contractile recovery and, if so, what is the time course of eventual recovery. Such studies would seem crucial to clarifying the pathophysiological basis of late functional recovery following AMI.

Clearly the time course of myocardial cell survival after acute coronary occlusion remains ill defined. Even in the center of an experimental infarct, where coronary blood flow has been completely interrupted, there is discernible residual myocardial blood flow—although it is severely attenuated. Previous experimental (Boden et al., 1980; Bush et al., 1985; Sherman et al., 1979; Theroux et al., 1976) and re-

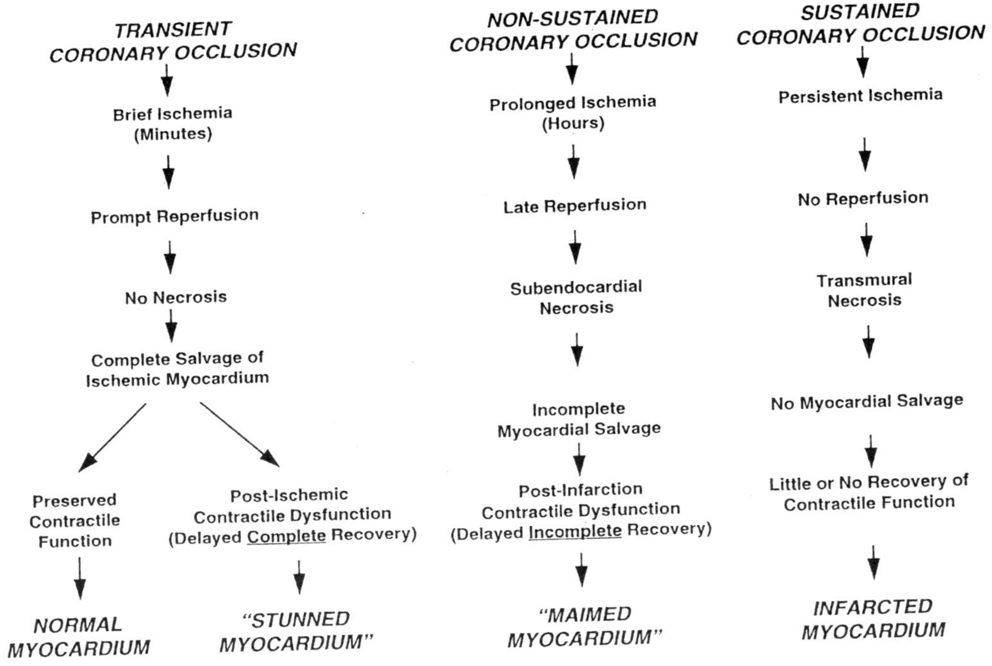

Figure 9-4. Schematic diagram detailing the four possible consequences of myocardial ischemia. Transient coronary occlusion may result in normal LV function or may result in delayed complete recovery (stunned myocardium). Nonsustained coronary occlusion with delayed incomplete recovery may result in maimed myocardium. Sustained coronary occlusion is generally associated with little or no LV functional recovery and results in completely infarcted myocardium.

cent clinical (Habib et al., 1991; Rentrop et al., 1989; Sabia et al., 1992) data indicate that decreased myocardial blood flow (presumably from collaterals recruited from adjacent vascular beds) may be sufficient to preserve tissue viability, particularly in the subepicardium. Such collaterals may be vital to maintaining tissue integrity and may be crucial to the subsequent improvements in regional mechanical function of ischemic myocytes. The role and recruitment of collaterals appears to be a subject for continued future research.

There is a need to investigate and reexplore the intrinsic state of myocardium subjected to prolonged coronary blood flow deprivation that is of sufficient severity and duration to produce partial myocardial necrosis. It is also necessary to better determine the precise role of reperfusion and whether it is obligate to maimed myocardium. Studies of completely and partially reversible changes in isolated myocardial preparations may represent an important scientific approach to answering these questions. Comparative studies should be undertaken in isolated papillary muscle preparations and in in vivo preparations using conscious animals with coronary blood flow characteristics similar to humans (e.g., pigs). Finally, the role of ventricular remodeling including the development of myocardial fibrosis and hypertrophy needs to be further clarified. Single-cell experiments may shed light on whether individual myocytes subjected to profound injury retain the capacity to recover partial function. Such studies would be essential to clarifying the pathophysiological basis of late LV functional recovery following AMI.

From a clinical perspective, the therapeutic implications of maimed myocardium are no less important. Revascularization strategies aimed at opening the infarct-related coronary artery—and keeping it patent—might be conceivably expanded or refined, if certain patient subsets were shown to benefit from delayed, albeit incomplete, LV function recovery. Pump failure remains the single-most important and life-threatening complication following AMI, and aggressive efforts (both pharmacological [ACE inhibitors, nitrates, etc.] and mechanical [angioplasty, atherectomy, etc.]) directed toward late myocardial salvage may result in enhanced overall survival. Indeed, earlier experimental observations (Bush et al., 1985; Sherman et al., 1979) suggest that calcium antagonists administered as adjunctive therapy with reperfusion might be an appropriate strategy to employ in the clinical setting of AMI treated with thrombolysis, particularly if additional late myocardial salvage could be achieved as an additional benefit of such combination therapy.

CONCLUSIONS

Accordingly, it seems appropriate to consider introducing a new concept (*maimed myocardium*) that describes more accurately the incomplete, delayed recovery of LV function that may occur late after reperfusion following AMI. It has been demonstrated previously that myocardium remains viable for a prolonged period in many patients with nonsustained coronary occlusion, despite the occurrence of myocardial necrosis. Thus, late reperfusion may result in myocardial salvage not only in reversibly ischemic (stunned) segments (*complete recovery*), but in intensely injured (maimed) segments that display partial return of LV function over time (*incomplete recovery*). Such an intermediate level of incomplete LV functional recovery would parallel conceptually the vascular reperfusion injury model that Kloner (1993) has postulated as one of the four basic forms of reperfusion injury.

Experimentally, delayed LV functional recovery has been reported in animal models in which prolonged coronary occlusion (hours/days) followed by reperfusion is associated with late recovery of regional LV function in myocardial segments subtending both border (stunned) zones and central infarct (maimed) zones. In both animal and human studies, postextrasystolic potentiation and pharmacological inotropic interventions may augment both maimed and stunned segments, although the magnitude of regional contractile reserve that can be unmasked with these interventions is quantitatively less in the maimed than in stunned segments.

Clinically, the basis for maimed myocardium is the observation that delayed LV functional recovery may occur in partially infarcted segments where there has been an antecedent ischemic insult of sufficient duration to result in some degree of myocardial necrosis. Certain acute coronary syndromes characterized by nonsustained coronary occlusion followed by spontaneous reperfusion (e.g., non-Q-wave AMI) or drug-induced reperfusion induced by the exogenous administration of thrombolytic therapy are associated with incomplete, delayed recovery of LV function as detected clinically by partial improvement in serial radionuclide ejection measurement, enhanced metabolic integrity of cardiac tissue utilizing F18-deoxyglucose myocardial imaging, and scintigraphic findings of reverse thallium redistribution—findings that support the presence of partially viable myocardium that has been incompletely salvaged during reperfusion late after AMI.

The propensity of intensely injured/partially infarcted LV segments to display intermediate functional recovery following reperfusion late after coronary occlusion suggests that even severely depressed but residually viable cardiac muscle can be salvaged incompletely over time. It is suggested that the new clinical term *maimed myocardium* be adopted to describe the latent viability of these partially infarcted tissue segments, and that such partial, delayed LV functional recovery should be distinguished from altered myocardial states in which complete contractile recovery occurs following a coronary occlusion too brief in duration to elicit myocardial necrosis (stunned myocardium).

REFERENCES

Ambrosio G, Weisman HF, Mansini JA, Becker LC. Progressive impairment of regional myocardial perfusion after initial restoration of postischemic blood flow. *Circulation* 1989; 80: 1846–1861.

Becker LC, Ambrosio G. Myocardial consequences of reperfusion. *Prog Cardiovasc Dis* 1987; 30: 23–44.

Boden WE. Electrocardiographic correlates of reperfusion status after thrombolysis: is the "incomplete" or "interrupted" infarction a non-Q-wave infarction? *Am J Cardiol* 1991; 68: 520–524.

Boden WE, Chang-Seng L, Hood Jr WB. Postextrasystolic potentiation of regional mechanical performance during prolonged myocardial ischemia in the dog. *Circulation* 1980; 61(6): 1063–1070.

Boden WE, Fenton SH, Beller GA, et al. Spontaneous improvement in left ventricular function during the early course of non-Q-wave acute myocardial infarction: evidence for "stunned myocardium?" *J Am Coll Cardiol* 1988; 11: 188A.

Boden WE, Liang C, Apstein CS, Hood Jr WB. Experimental myocardial infarction. XVI. The detection of inotropic contractile reserve with postextrasystolic potentiation in acutely ischemic myocardium. *Am J Cardiol* 1978; 41: 523.

Bolli R, Patel BS, Jeroudi MO, et al. Demonstration of free radical generation in "stunned" myocardium of intact dogs with the use of the spin traps alpha-phenyl N-tert-butyl nitrone. *J Clin Invest* 1988; 82: 476–485.

Braunwald E. Myocardial reperfusion, limitation of infarct size, reduction of left ventricular dysfunction, and improved survival. *Circulation* 1989; 79(2): 441–444.

Braunwald E, Kloner RA. The stunned myocardium: prolonged, postischemic ventricular dysfunction. *Circulation* 1982: 66(6): 1146–1149.

Braunwald E, Kloner RA. Myocardial reperfusion: a double-edged sword? *J Clin Invest* 1985; 76: 1713–1719.

Bush LR, Buja ML, Tilton G, et al. Effects of propranolol and diltiazem alone and in combination on the recovery of left ventricular segmental function after temporary coronary occlusion and long-term reperfusion in conscious dogs. *Circulation* 1985; 72: 413–430.

Dalen JE, Gore JM, Braunwald E, et al. Six- and twelve-month follow-up of the phase I thrombolysis in myocardial infarction (TIMI) trial. *Am J Cardiol* 1988; 62: 179–185.

Eaton LW, Bulkley BH. Expansion of acute myocardial infarction: its relationship to infarct morphology in a canine model. *Circ Res* 1981; 49: 80–88.

Ellis SG, Henschke CI, Sandor T, et al. Time course of functional and biochemical recovery of myocardium salvaged by reperfusion. *J Am Coll Cardiol* 1983; 1: 1047–1055.

Engler RL, Schmid-Schonbein GW, Pavelec RS. Leukocyte capillary plugging in myocardial ischemia and reperfusion in the dog. *Am J Pathol* 1983; 111: 98–111.

Feyter PJ, Van Eenige MJ, Van der Wall EE. Effects of spontaneous and streptokinase induced recanalization on left ventricular function in acute myocardial infarction. *Circulation* 1983: 67: 1039–1044.

Finci L, Meier B, Favre J, et al. Long-term results of successful and failed angioplasty for chronic total coronary artery occlusion. *Am J Cardiol* 1990; 66: 660–662.

Fishbein MC. Reperfusion injury. *Clin Cardiol* 1990; 13: 213–217.

Force T, Kemper A, Leavitt M, Parisi AF. Acute reduction in functional infarct expansion with late coronary reperfusion: assessment with quantitative two-dimensional echocardiography. *J Am Coll Cardiol* 1988; 11: 192–200.

Forman MB, Virmani R. Pathogenesis and modification of myocardial reperfusion injury. In: Gersh BJ, Rahimtoola SH, eds. *Acute myocardial infarction*. New York: Elsevier, 1990: 349–370.

Freifeld AG, Schuster EH, Bulkley BH. Nontransmural versus transmural myocardial infarction. *Am J Med* 1983; 75: 423–429.

Gibson RS, Beller GA, Gheorghiade M, et al. The prevalence and clinical significance of residual myocardial ischemia 2 weeks after uncomplicated non-Q-wave infarction: a prospective natural history study. *Circulation* 1986; 6: 1186–1198.

Grines CL, Topol EJ, Califf RM, et al. Prognostic implications and predictors of enhanced regional wall motion of the noninfarct zone after thrombolysis and angioplasty therapy of acute myocardial infarction. *Circulation* 1989; 80: 245–253.

Habib GB, Heibig J, Forman SA, et al. Influence of coronary collateral vessels on myocardial infarct size in humans: results of phase I thrombolysis in myocardial infarction (TIMI) trial. *Circulation* 1991; 83: 739–746.

Hashimoto T, Kambara H, Fudo T, et al. Non-Q-wave vs. Q-wave myocardial infarction: regional myocardial metabolism and blood flow assessed by positron emission tomography. *J Am Coll Cardiol* 1988; 12: 88–93.

Hearse DJ, Bolli R. Reperfusion induced injury: manifestations, mechanisms, and clinical relevance. *Cardiovasc Res* 1992; 26: 101–108.

Helfant RH, Banka VS, Bodenheimer MM. Perplexities and complexities concerning the myocardial infarction border zone and its salvage. *Am J Cardiol* 1978; 41: 345—352.

Herrick JB. Clinical features of sudden obstruction of the coronaries. *JAMA* 1912; 59: 2015–2021.

Hess ML, Barnhart GR, Crute S, et al. Mechanical and biochemical effects of transient myocardial ischemia. *J Surg Res* 1979; 26: 19–27.

Heyndrickx GR, Baig H, Nellens P, et al. Depression of regional blood flow and wall thickening after brief coronary occlusions. *Am J Physiol* 1978; 234: H653–H659.

Heyndrickx GR, Millard RW, McRitchie RJ, et al. Regional myocardial function and electrophysiological alterations after brief coronary artery occlusion in conscious dogs. *J Clin Invest* 1975; 56: 978–985.

Hochman JS, Choo H. Limitation of myocardial infarct expansion by reperfusion independent of myocardial salvage. *Circulation* 1987: 75: 299–306.

Hood Jr WB, Covelli VH, Abelmann WH, Norman JC. Persistence of contractile behavior in acutely ischemic myocardium. *Cardiovasc Res* 1969; 3: 249–255.

Huey BL, Gheorghiade M, Crampton RS, et al. Acute non-Q-wave myocardial infarction associated with early ST-segment elevation: evidence for spontaneous coronary reperfusion and implications for thrombolytic trials. *J Am Coll Cardiol* 1987; 9: 18–25.

Humphrey SM, Gavin JB, Herdson PB. The relationship of ischemic contracture to vascular reperfusion in the isolated rat heart. *J Mol Cell Cardiol* 1980; 12: 1397–1406.

Hutchins GM, Bulkley BH. Infarct expansion versus extension: two different complications of acute myocardial infarction. *Am J Cardiol* 1978; 41: 1127–1132.

ISAM Study Group. A prospective trial of intravenous streptokinase in acute myocardial infarction (ISAM): mortality, morbidity, and infarct size at 21 days. *N Engl J Med* 1986; 314: 1465–1471.

ISIS-2 (Second International Study of Infarct Survival) Collaborative Group. Randomized trial of intravenous streptokinase, oral aspirin, both, or neither among 17,187 cases of suspected acute myocardial infarction: ISIS-2. *Lancet* 1988; 2: 349–360.

Jeremy RW, Hackworthy RA, Bautovich G, et al. Infarct artery perfusion and changes in left ventricular volume in the month after acute myocardial infarction. *J Am Coll Cardiol* 1987; 9: 989–995.

Kersschot IE, Brugada P, Ramentol M, et al. Effects of early reperfusion in acute myocardial infarction on arrhythmias induced by programmed stimulation: a prospective, randomized study. *J Am Coll Cardiol* 1986; 7: 1234–1242.

Kloner RA. Does reperfusion injury exist in humans? *J Am Coll Cardiol* 1993; 21: 537–545.

Kloner RA, Alker K, Campbell C, et al. Does tissue-type plasminogen activator have direct beneficial effects on the myocardium independent of its ability to lyse intracoronary thrombi? *Circulation* 1989a; 79: 1125–1136.

Kloner RA, Ellis SG, Lange R, Braunwald E. Studies of experimental coronary artery reperfusion: effects of infarct size, myocardial function, biochemistry, ultrastructure, and microvascular damage. *Circulation* 1983; 68(Suppl I): 8–15.

Kloner RA, Ganote CE, Jennings RB. The "no-reflow" phenomenon following temporary coronary occlusion in the dog. *J Clin Invest* 1974a; 54: 1496–1508.

Kloner RA, Ganote CE, Whalen D, Jennings RB. Effect of a transient period of ischemia on myocardial cells. II. Fine structure during the first few minutes of reflow. *Am J Pathol* 1974b; 74: 399–422.

Kloner RA, Giacomelli F, Alker KJ, et al. Influx of neutrophils into the walls of large epicardial coronary arteries in response to ischemia/reperfusion. *Circulation* 1991; 84: 1758–1772.

Kloner RA, Przyklenk K, Patel B. Altered myocardial states: the stunned and hibernating myocardium. *Am J Med* 1989b; 86(Suppl 1A): 14–22.

Ku DD. Coronary vascular reactivity after myocardial ischemia. *Science* 1982; 218: 576–578.

Maisel AS, Ahnve S, Gilpin E, et al. Prognosis after extension of myocardial infarct: the role of Q-wave or non-V-wave infarction. *Circulation* 1985; 71: 211–217.

Marmor A, Sobel BE, Roberts R. Factors presaging early recurrent myocardial infarction ("extension"). *Am J Cardiol* 1981; 48: 603–610.

McCord JM. Free radicals and myocardial ischemia: overview and outlook. *Free Rad Biol Med* 1988; 4: 9–14.

McCord JM, Roy RS, Schaffer SW. Free radicals in myocardial ischemia. The role of xanthine oxidase. *Adv Myocardiol* 1985; 5: 183–189.

McKay RG, Pfeffer MA, Pasternak RC. Left ventricular remodeling after myocardial infarction: corollary to infarct expansion. *Circulation* 1986; 74(4): 693–702.

Patel B, Kloner RA, Przyklenk K, Braunwald E. Postischemic myocardial "stunning:" a clinically relevant phenomenon. *Ann Intern Med* 1988; 108: 626–628.

Pfeffer JM, Pfeffer MA, Braunwald E. Influence of chronic captopril therapy on the infarcted left ventricle of the rat. *Circ Res* 1985; 57: 84–95.

Porter T. On the results of ligation of the coronary arteries. *J Physiol (Lond)* 1895; 15: 121–124.

Preuss KC, Gross GJ, Brooks HL, Warltier DC. Time course of recovery of "stunned" myocardium following variable periods of ischemia in conscious and anesthetized dogs. *Am Heart J* 1987; 114: 696–703.

Quillen JE, Sellke FW, Brooks LA, Harrison DG. Ischemia-reperfusion impairs endothelium-dependent relaxation of coronary microvessels but does not affect large arteries. *Circulation* 1990; 82: 586–594.

Rahimtoola SH. The hibernating myocardium. *Am Heart J* 1989; 117: 211–221.

Reimer KA, Jennings RB. The "wavefront phenomenon" of myocardial ischemic cell death. II. Transmural progression of necrosis within the framework of ischemic (myocardium at risk) and collateral flow. *Lab Invest* 1979; 40: 633–644.

Rentrop KP, Feit F, Sherman W, et al. Late thrombolytic therapy preserves left ventricular function in patients with collateralized total coronary occlusion: primary end point findings of the second Mount Sinai-New York University reperfusion trial. *J Am Coll Cardiol* 1989: 14: 58–64.

Roberts CS, Maclean D, Braunwald E, et al. Topographic changes in the left ventricle after experimentally induced myocardial infarction in the rat. *Am J Cardiol* 1983; 51: 872–876.

Ross Jr J. Assessment of ischemic regional myocardial dysfunction and its reversibility. *Circulation* 1986; 74(6): 1186–1190.

Sabia PJ, Powers ER, Ragosta M, et al. An association between collateral blood flow and myocardial viability in patients with recent myocardial infarction. *N Engl J Med* 1992; 327: 1825–1831.

Schroder R, Neuhaus KL, Linderer T, et al. Impact of late coronary artery reperfusion on left ventricular function one month after acute myocardial infarction (results from the ISAM study). *Am J Cardiol* 1989; 64: 878–884.

Sheehan FH, Doerr R, Schmidt WG, et al. Early recovery of left ventricular function after thrombolytic therapy for acute myocardial infarction: an important determinant of survival. *J Am Coll Cardiol* 1988; 12: 289–300.

Sherman LG, Liang CS, Boden WE, Hood Jr WB. Effects of verapamil on performance of ischemic myocardium in conscious dogs. *Circulation* 1979; 60(2): 29–38.

Simoons ML, Serruys PW, van den Brand M, et al. Early thrombolysis in acute myocardial infarction: limitation of infarct size and improved survival. *J Am Coll Cardiol* 1986; 7: 717–728.

Stack RS, Phillips III HR, Grierson DS. Functional improvement of jeopardized myocardium following intracoronary streptokinase infusion in acute myocardial infarction. *J Clin Invest* 1983; 72: 84–95.

Stampfer MJ, Goldhaber SZ, Yusuf S, et al. Effect of intravenous streptokinase on acute myocardial infarction: pooled results from randomized trials. *N Engl J Med* 1982; 307: 1180–1182.

Tennant T, Wiggers CJ. Effect of coronary occlusion on myocardial contraction. *Am J Physiol* 1935; 112: 351.

Theroux P, Ross Jr J, Franklin D, et al. Coronary arterial reperfusion. III. Early and late effects on regional myocardial function and dimensions in conscious dogs. *Am J Cardiol* 1976; 38: 599.

Van Benthuysen KM, McMurty IF, Horwitz LD. Reperfusion after coronary occlusion in dogs impairs endothelium dependent relaxation to acetylcholine and augments contractile reactivity in vitro. *J Clin Invest* 1987; 79: 265–274.

Verheugt FWA, Visser FC, van der Wall EE, et al. Prediction of spontaneous coronary reperfusion in myocardial infarction. *Postgrad Med J* 1986; 62: 1007–1010.

Weiner JM, Apstein CS, Arthur JH, et al. Persistence of myocardial injury following brief periods of coronary occlusion. *Cardiovasc Res* 1976; 10: 678.

Weiss AT, Maddahi J, Lew AS, et al. Reverse redistribution of thallium-201: a sign of nontransmural myocardial infarction with patency of the infarct-related coronary artery. *J Am Coll Cardiol* 1986; 7: 61–67.

Whalen DA, Hamilton DG, Ganote CE, Jennings RB. Effect of a transient period of ischemia on myocardial cells. I. Effects on cell volume regulation. *Am J Pathol* 1974; 74: 381–398.

White HD, Norris RM, Brown MA, et al. Effect of intravenous streptokinase on left ventricular function and early survival after acute myocardial infarction. *N Engl J Med* 1987; 317: 850–855.

Yusuf S, Collins R, Peto R. Intravenous and intracoronary fibrinolytic therapy in acute myocardial infarction: overview of results on mortality, reinfarction and side-effects from 33 randomized controlled trials. *Eur Heart J* 1985; 6: 556–585.

Zweier JL, Rayburn BK, Flaherty JT, Weisfeldt ML. Recombinant superoxide dismutase reduces oxygen free radical concentrations in reperfused myocardium. *J Clin Invest* 1987; 80: 1728–1734.

CHAPTER 10

"Stunned" Myocardium in the Clinical Setting: Occurrence, Diagnosis, and Treatment

Marcus F. Stoddard
Roberto Bolli

The prolonged, but ultimately reversible, impairment of mechanical function that occurs after an episode of myocardial
ischemia, or "stunned" myocardium (Braunwald & Kloner,
1982), is increasingly being accepted as an important determinant of global cardiac function and presumably symptoms in
patients with coronary artery disease (Bolli, 1992; Bolli et al.,
1991). Although the phenomenon of myocardial stunning
was described 20 years ago by Heyndrickx and colleagues
(1975) in a conscious canine model, its potential clinical importance has only recently been appreciated by practicing clinicians. Part of the reason for this lag is that myocardial
stunning is a sequela of reperfusion, which in the 1970s was
not thought to be a common clinical occurrence. In the 1990s,
however, this view has changed dramatically. The relatively
recent widespread use of reperfusion treatments, such as
thrombolytic therapy and PTCA, for acute myocardial ischemia and the appreciation that spontaneous reperfusion is
indeed a common feature of many coronary syndromes have
been powerful factors in kindling the interest of practicing
cardiologists in the phenomenon of stunned myocardium.

Although our knowledge regarding the pathogenesis
and pathophysiology of myocardial stunning in the experimental setting has grown very rapidly (Bolli, 1990), progress
in the clinical area has been slow. There continues to be considerable uncertainty regarding virtually every aspect of
myocardial stunning in patients, including the very existence
of this phenomenon, its prevalence, the optimal diagnostic
approaches for identifying it, and the effective treatment
modalities for either preventing it or reversing it. To the practicing cardiologist, the diagnosis of stunned myocardium remains elusive, being often based on circumstantial or
retrospective evidence. As a result, cardiologists cannot assess the actual prevalence and importance of this form of
ventricular dysfunction or implement specific therapies.

Even when the presence of stunned myocardium seems very probable, the cardiologist wonders whether this syndrome requires any specific management (and if so, which one) or even why stunned myocardium is important at all.

Although many of these issues await further investigation to be resolved, some progress has been made in recent years, particularly with regard to the diagnosis of stunning and the recognition of its occurrence. The existing body of knowledge pertaining to myocardial stunning in the clinical arena is sufficiently developed that we believe it is important for the practicing cardiologist to be aware of it. It is important to keep in mind that we are only at the beginning of a wave of clinical investigations of stunning and that considerably more progress will likely take place in the next few years.

This chapter is specifically aimed at the practicing cardiologist. It is our intent to review critically the current evidence suggesting the occurrence of stunned myocardium in various clinical settings, the usefulness and limitations of the techniques used for the clinical diagnosis of "stunning," the potential clinical importance of the phenomenon, and its impact on decision making in patient management.

STUNNED VERSUS HIBERNATING MYOCARDIUM

Definition of myocardial stunning

A clear definition is essential to avoid confusion, particularly because the term *stunning* is sometimes loosely applied to situations that are not relevant to this phenomenon. *Stunned myocardium can be defined as myocardium exhibiting persistent mechanical dysfunction after reperfusion despite the absence of irreversible damage and despite restoration of normal or near-normal flow* (Fig 10-1) (Bolli, 1990). Implicit in this definition is that myocardial stunning is a fully reversible abnormality, provided of course that sufficient time is allowed for the myocardium to recover. The diagnosis of myocardial stunning in humans requires two major points: (1) demonstration that the abnormality is reversible and (2) demonstration that contractile function is abnormal despite normal or near-normal flow (i.e., a perfusion-contraction mismatch) (see Fig 10-1). The first point is usually documented in clinical studies, but only rarely has the second point been demonstrated in humans.

Definition of myocardial hibernation

Myocardial hibernation could be defined as a persistent (at least several hours) contractile dysfunction that is caused by a persistently reduced coronary flow and is associated with preserved myocardial viability (see Fig 10-1). Hibernating myocardium has been postulated to be an adaptive response to decrease myocardial oxygen demands and thereby maintain myocyte viability in the face of limited oxygen supply (Braunwald & Rutherford, 1986; Rahimtoola, 1985, 1989; Ross, 1991; Tillisch et al., 1986). Hibernating myocardium has been proposed to occur in patients with chronic contrac-

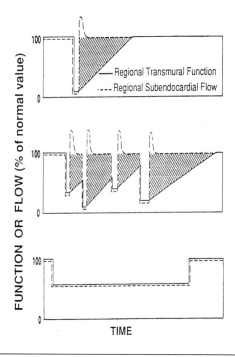

Figure 10-1. *Schematic illustration of several possible scenarios that could occur in a patient with a fixed critical coronary stenosis sufficient to blunt reactive hyperemia. Stunning is indicated by the hatched areas. The* upper panel *denotes a brief episode of ischemia (caused by thrombosis and /or vasoconstriction) followed by rapid restoration of flow and by stunning (i.e., by a perfusion-contraction "mismatch"). The* middle panel *shows recurrent brief episodes of silent ischemia (caused by recurrent thrombosis and/or vasoconstriction). Each ischemic episode is followed by stunning (i.e., by a flow-function mismatch). Note that because the myocardium cannot recover fully between one ischemic episode to the next, recurrent ischemia results in "chronic" stunning. The* lower panel *indicates hibernation in a patient with severe, fixed coronary stenosis. According to current views, hibernating myocardium is characterized by a steady, low coronary flow, as depicted in this panel. Function is down-regulated to match flow and recovers immediately after restoration of flow. (Reproduced with permission of the American Heart Association, from Bolli [1992].)*

tile abnormalities associated with reduced perfusion that reverses after coronary revascularization (Braunwald & Rutherford, 1986; Rahimtoola, 1985, 1989; Ross, 1991; Tillisch et al., 1986).

Thus, stunned and hibernating myocardium have in common the fact that in both cases the myocardium is viable and the LV dysfunction is reversible. *The major difference is that blood flow is normal or near-normal in stunned myocardium, whereas it is reduced in hibernating myocardium.* Because regional myocardial flow is not usually measured in clinical studies, a positive distinction between stunned and hibernating myocardium is frequently not possible in humans. Indeed, the most vexing problem in the clinical diagnosis of stunned myocardium has been the distinction between this situation and hibernating myocardium or silent myocardial ischemia (Bolli, 1992). Conclusive demonstration of myocardial stunning requires simultaneous measurements of regional myocardial function and flow (Bolli, 1992). In addition, it is conceivable that the clinical situation may be very complex, and that stunned and hibernating myocardium may coexist (Bolli, 1992). Accordingly, even with measurements of regional myocardial flow, distinguishing stunned from hibernating myocardium may not always be possible in clinical situations.

EXPERIMENTAL MODELS AND PATHOGENESIS OF STUNNED MYOCARDIUM

There are several experimental settings in which myocardial stunning has been described and is well characterized (Bolli, 1990) (Table 10-1). They include the following: (1) a completely reversible ischemic episode (i.e., a coronary occlusion lasting less than 20 minutes), (2) a partly irreversible ischemic episode (subendocardial infarction) (i.e., a coronary occlusion lasting longer than 20 minutes, but less than 2 hours), (3) exercise-induced ischemia, and (4) global ischemia. Each of these experimental settings has a clinical equivalent (Bolli, 1992).

The pathophysiology and pathogenesis of myocardial stunning are beyond the scope of this chapter (Table 10-2). In brief, it appears that the mechanism of myocardial stunning involves two major processes: (1) generation of oxygen-derived free radicals after reperfusion as a result of reintroduction of oxygen into previously ischemic tissue and (2) perturbations of calcium homeostasis, and particularly a decreased sensitivity of contractile filaments to calcium (Bolli, 1990). These two processes may be interrelated, as oxygen radicals may damage contractile proteins, resulting in impaired responsiveness to calcium (Bolli, 1990).

TABLE 10-1. EXPERIMENTAL MODELS OF MYOCARDIAL STUNNING AND POTENTIAL CLINICAL EQUIVALENTS

Experimental model	Clinical equivalent
Regional ischemia	
Completely reversible ischemic episode (coronary occlusion ≤20 minutes	Percutaneous transluminal coronary angioplasty; unstable angina; variant angina
Partly irreversible ischemic episode (subendocardial infarction, >20 minutes to ≤2 hours)	Acute myocardial infarction with early reperfusion
Exercise-induced ischemia with coronary stenosis without coronary stenosis (hypertrophy)	Exercise-induced ischemia with coronary stenosis without coronary stenosis (hypertrophy)
Global ischemia	
Cardioplegic arrest	Cardiac surgery; cardiac transplantation; cardiac arrest

TABLE 10-2. PROPOSED MECHANISMS OF MYOCARDIAL STUNNING

Most likely mechanisms

Generation of oxygen-derived free radicals
Decreased responsiveness of myofilaments to calcium
Excitation-contraction uncoupling due to sarcoplasmic reticulum dysfunction
Calcium overload*

Other proposed mechanisms

Insufficient energy production by mitochondria
Impaired energy use by myofibrils
Impairment of sympathetic neural responsiveness
Impairment of myocardial perfusion
Damage of the extracellular collagen matrix

* For detailed analysis and data regarding this hypothesis, see Opie L.H., *Circulation* 1989; 80: 1049; Opie L.H., *Cardiovasc Drugs and Therapy* 1991; 5:895–900; Marban et al., *Circ Res* 1995; 75: 1036–1048.

CLINICAL EVIDENCE OF STUNNED MYOCARDIUM

A variety of clinical conditions exists in which transient myocardial ischemia is followed by reperfusion. These common clinical situations are potentially associated with stunned myocardium and include AMI with early reperfusion, unstable angina, exercise-induced ischemia, variant or Prinzmetal's angina, cardiac surgery, cardiac transplantation, cardiac arrest, and PTCA.

Acute myocardial infarction with early reperfusion

Numerous studies assessing the recovery of LV function in the setting of an AMI after thrombolysis and/or PTCA have uniformly shown that systolic function does not improve immediately after reperfusion. Instead, the improvement is usually delayed for several days, a time course similar to that observed in experimental animals (Anderson et al., 1983, 1984; Bateman et al., 1983; Bolli, 1990; Charuzi et al., 1984; Erbel et al., 1986; Reduto et al., 1981b; Schroeder et al., 1983; Serruys et al., 1986; Stack et al., 1983; Topol et al., 1985). The precise time course of the recovery of myocardial function has varied (Bourdillon et al., 1989; Schmidt et al., 1989; Zaret et al., 1992; Zoghbi et al., 1990). Bourdillon and colleagues (1989) found that the majority of improvement in regional LV function (assessed by two-dimensional echocardiography) occurred within the first 3 days after reperfusion; only modest additional improvement occurred by 7 days. In contrast, Schmidt and associates (1989) noted only modest improvement of regional systolic function (measured by contrast ventriculography) in the first 3 days after reperfusion, and a considerably greater recovery between 3 days and 6 months. Others have noted improvement in regional or global LV function beyond 9 to 10 days (Zoghbi et al., 1990), although the observation has not been a consistent one (Zaret et al., 1992).

Several factors may explain the variability in the rate of recovery of LV function after reperfusion therapy in acute myocardial infarction (Bourdillon et al., 1989; Schmidt et al., 1989; Zaret et al., 1992; Zoghbi et al., 1990), including the duration of ischemia before reperfusion, the degree of perfusion by collateral vessels, the severity of residual coronary stenosis after thrombolysis, the size of the ischemic region, and the methodology used for assessing LV function. Although it is clear that most of the improvement takes place within the first 7 to 10 days after reperfusion, it is still not clear when the recovery can be considered complete. Longitudinal studies extending beyond 7 to 10 days are needed to resolve this issue. One of the best studies addressing this issue was by Ito and coworkers (1993), who studied patients successfully reperfused (TIMI grade 3 and no reocclusion) within 6 hours from the onset of anterior myocardial infarction. In this study, there was a progressive improvement in regional myocardial function from day 1 to day 14, but no significant change between day 14 and day 28. On average, wall-motion abnormalities (assessed by echocardiography) decreased by 28% between day 1 and day 14, suggesting that almost one third of the dysfunction observed immediately after thrombolysis is due to myocardial stunning, although in individual cases this percentage was larger (Ito et al., 1993).

It is not unexpected that the recovery of diastolic function is also delayed after AMI with reperfusion. Williamson and colleagues (1990) showed that LV diastolic filling (assessed by Doppler echocardiography) was significantly improved at 7 days as compared to 24 hours after AMI, suggesting the existence of diastolic stunning in patients who are successfully reperfused.

Unstable angina

Since by definition unstable angina is characterized by transient myocardial ischemia without necrosis, this syndrome would be expected to be associated with stunned myocardium. Indeed, echocardiographic studies evaluating LV function in unstable angina (Bolli et al., 1991; de Zwaan et al., 1991; Jeroudi et al., 1994; Nixon et al., 1982) give support to the notion that myocardial stunning is common in this setting. In a study by Nixon and colleagues (1982) 11 of 19 patients with unstable angina were found to have regional LV contractile abnormalities by two-dimensional echocardiography at the time of presentation. In 5 of these 11 patients, however, contractile function improved or normalized after 7 to 10 days of medical therapy. de Zwaan and associates (1991) reported similar findings in 18 patients with unstable angina treated with medical therapy. These studies (de Zwaan et al., 1991; Nixon et al., 1982), however, measured wall motion only at two time points, so that it was not possible to assess whether the time course of recovery of function followed the pattern of progressive improvement that is characteristic of stunned myocardium in experimental animals (Bolli, 1990). Recently, Jeroudi and associates (1994) used two-dimensional echocardiography to assess the time course of wall-motion abnormalities after an episode of chest pain at rest in 6 patients with unstable angina. The wall-motion abnormalities exhibited a gradual improvement. They resolved within 2 hours in some patients but persisted for as long as 24 hours after the chest pain in other subjects, despite the fact that no patient had evidence of AMI or recurrent ischemia. This delayed, gradual recovery of LV function lasting several hours after the resolution of the chest pain is consistent with myocardial stunning, although simultaneous measurements of function and flow would have been necessary to establish this diagnosis unequivocally.

The repeated observations of improvement in LV function after revascularization with coronary artery bypass graft (CABG) surgery or PTCA in patients with unstable angina further support the existence of stunned myocardium in this syndrome (Kolibask et al., 1979; Priest et al., 1978; Renkin et al., 1990). Potentially important to the practicing cardiologist are the findings by Renkin and coworkers (1990) and de Zwaan and colleagues (1991) that inverted T-waves in the precordial leads identify a subset of patients with unstable angina that is more likely to show reversibility of anterior wall-motion abnormalities after PTCA. It is also noteworthy that results with PET using F18-fluorodeoxy-glucose have demonstrated increased glucose uptake in the absence of perfusion abnormalities in patients with unstable angina, supporting the presence of stunned myocardium (Camici et al., 1986).

Although the studies reviewed here (Bolli et al., 1991; de Zwaan, 1991; Jeroudi et al., 1994; Kolibask et al., 1979; Nixon et al., 1982; Priest et al., 1978; Renkin et al., 1990) support the concept that stunned myocardium occurs commonly in patients with unstable angina, definitive proof is still lacking because alternative explanations for the persistent LV dysfunction, such as recurrent episodes of silent ischemia or hibernating myocardium, cannot be excluded (Bolli, 1992). *A conclusive diagnosis of stunned myocardium, as opposed to hibernating myocardium or silent ischemia, in patients with unstable angina will require the simultaneous measurement of regional myocardial perfusion and function.*

Exercise-induced ischemia

Several two-dimensional echocardiographic studies have documented the persistence of regional and global LV dysfunction after exercise-induced ischemia (Kloner et al., 1991; Robertson et al., 1983; Scognamiglio et al., 1991; Stoddard et al., 1992). Robertson and coworkers (1983) were the first to report persisting wall-motion abnormalities 30 minutes after exercise-induced ischemia in 6 of 16 patients (38%) with coronary artery disease. Kloner and associates (1991) noted new regional wall-motion abnormalities in 18 of 19 patients (95%) at 15 minutes and in 19 of 21 patients (90%) at 30 minutes after exercise-induced ischemia. Scognamiglio and colleagues (1991) found a decline in LV ejection fraction 30 minutes after exercise-induced ischemia as compared to rest in 22 of 26 patients (84%) undergoing testing. In keeping with these prior studies, Stoddard and associates (1992) reported that, 2 hours after exercise-induced ischemia, there was a new systolic wall-motion abnormality in 9 of 52 patients (17%), which was associated with a decrease in peak early filling velocity, peak early/atrial filling velocity ratio, and mean deceleration rate of early filling, and an increase in percent atrial contribution to filling (assessed by Doppler echocardiography). The peak early/peak atrial filling velocity ratio decreased in 45 of 52 patients (87%) 2 hours after exercise-induced ischemia. These findings (Stoddard et al., 1992) are consistent with the concept that myocardial stunning provoked by exercise-induced ischemia involves both the systolic and the diastolic properties of the myocardium. The frequent occurrence of impaired LV diastolic filling (Stoddard et al., 1992) suggests that after exercise-induced ischemia diastolic dysfunction occurs more commonly than systolic dysfunction.

Although these studies (Kloner et al., 1991; Robertson et al., 1983; Scognamiglio et al., 1991; Stoddard et al., 1992) are consistent with the presence of stunned myocardium after exercise-induced ischemia in humans, they are not conclusive because reversibility of wall-motion abnormalities was not shown and myocardial ischemia possibly due to a transmural maldistribution or coronary flow after exercise was not excluded. A recent preliminary report by Ambrosio and colleagues (1993) fulfills these requirements and thus strongly supports the occurrence of exercise-induced myocardial stunning in humans. In this study, 7 patients showed a simultaneous reduction in LV thickening by two-dimensional echocardiography and normal myocardial perfusion by Tc-99m sestamibi scan 30 minutes after exercise-induced ischemia.

In contrast to these echocardiographic studies (Ambrosio et al., 1993; Kloner et al., 1991; Robertson et al., 1983; Scognamiglio et al., 1991; Stoddard et al., 1992), several radionuclide angiographic studies (Dymond et al., 1984; Marzullo et al., 1993b; Schneider et al., 1986) have failed to demonstrate a protracted delay in recovery of global or regional LV systolic function after exercise-induced ischemia. It is possible that the variance in the results of echocardiographic versus radionuclide studies relates to differences in the techniques for the assessment of LV systolic function. Although radionuclide angiography is an excellent method to assess global LV systolic function by determination of ejection fraction, two-dimensional echocardiography allows for a better delineation of regional LV wall motion and myocardial thickening.

Variant angina

Support for the presence of stunned myocardium in variant angina is anecdotal (Fournier et al., 1991; Mathias et al., 1987; Takatsu et al., 1986). For example, Mathias and associates (1987) described a patient with recurrent episodes of variant angina who demonstrated akinesis of the LV anteroseptal and apical segments that almost completely resolved after 10 days. Importantly, in this patient myocardial perfusion was normal, as demonstrated by resting thallium-201 scintigraphy, at the time when the wall-motion abnormalities were noted. In contrast to these case reports (Fournier et al., 1991; Mathias et al., 1987; Takatsu et al., 1986), Distante and coworkers (1984a, 1984b) were unable to demonstrate persistent LV wall-motion abnormalities after episodes of variant angina in 12 patients by M-mode echocardiography (Distante et al., 1984b) or in 20 patients by two-dimensional echocardiography (Distante et al., 1984a). It should be noted that multiple recurrent episodes of ischemia occurred in the patients reported in the case studies

(Fournier et al., 1991; Mathias et al., 1987; Takatsu et al., 1986), which may have had a cumulative effect in depressing LV systolic function after the last episode of angina, while Distante and coworkers (1984a) studied LV function after a single episode of variant angina.

These results (Fournier et al., 1991; Mathias et al., 1987; Takatsu et al., 1986), would suggest that a single episode of variant angina, if short lived, does not usually cause postischemic systolic dysfunction. However, it is plausible that frequent, severe, or protracted variant anginal episodes might lead to prolonged LV dysfunction after resolution of ischemia.

Cardiac surgery

Since during cardiac surgery the heart is exposed to global ischemia followed by reperfusion, one would expect stunned myocardium to be present in this setting. Indeed, a transient ventricular dysfunction, peaking a few hours after CABG and resolving by 24 to 48 hours, has been well described (Ballantyne et al., 1987; Bolli et al., 1990; Breisblatt et al., 1990; Cunningham et al., 1979; Czer et al., 1983; Fremes et al., 1984, 1985; Gray et al., 1979; Hartley et al., 1989; Mangano, 1985; Reduto et al., 1981a; Roberts et al., 1980, 1981). For example, Breisblatt and associates (1990) demonstrated a decrease in mean LV ejection from 58% before surgery to 37% after CABG, which was associated with a decrease in right ventricular ejection fraction, cardiac index, and LV stroke work index. LV function decreased in 23 of 24 patients (96%); on average, the most striking decline occurred at approximately 4 hours after surgery and completely recovered within 24 to 48 hours (Breisblatt et al., 1990). A dramatic example of life-threatening but ultimately reversible LV dysfunction after CABG was reported by Ballantyne and colleagues (1987). Recently, highly accurate measurements of LV systolic wall thickening were obtained by Hartley and coworkers (1989) and Bolli and associates (1990) in 31 patients undergoing CABG. These authors used pulsed Doppler ultrasonic probes sutured on the epicardial surface, which have accuracy and sensitivity superior to any other clinically available method. In keeping with previous results, these studies (Bolli et al., 1990; Hartley et al., 1989) showed that LV wall thickening decreased after surgery, reached a nadir at 2 to 6 hours, and then progressively improved, approaching baseline levels by 24 to 48 hours.

On the basis of the aforementioned studies (Ballantyne et al., 1987; Bolli et al., 1990; Breisblatt et al., 1990; Cunningham et al., 1979; Czer et al., 1983; Fremes et al., 1984, 1985; Gray et al., 1979; Hartley et al., 1989; Mangano, 1985; Reduto et al., 1981a; Roberts et al., 1980, 1981), there is little doubt that myocardial stunning occurs commonly after cardiac surgery and thus contributes to the low-output syndrome observed postoperatively in some patients.

Cardiac transplantation

During cardiac transplantation the donor heart is subjected to global ischemia followed by reperfusion. Several reports support the concept that myocardial stunning may occur in the cardiac donor heart (Cabrol et al., 1989; Uretsky, 1990; Wicomb et al., 1984). For example, Wicomb and coworkers (1984) noted in 2 patients who received heterotopic heart transplants that the donor heart functioned poorly postoperatively and was unable to support the circulation; however, a dramatic recovery occurred 20 hours after surgery and at 36 hours the donor heart was able to support the circulation.

Cardiac arrest

In a bevy of young patients resuscitated after cardiac arrest secondary to ventricular fibrillation, Deantonio and colleagues (1990) noted a profoundly depressed LV function with an ejection fraction of <30%. Subsequent echocardiograms demonstrated virtually complete resolution of LV dysfunction 2 weeks later. None of the patients had evidence of myocardial infarction by cardiac enzymes. Since the cardiac arrest led to transient global myocardial ischemia followed by reperfusion after successful resuscitation, it is possible that the initial depression and subsequent normalization of ventricular function were due to stunned myocardium, although the effects of electric shock and metabolic acidosis cannot be ruled out.

PTCA

During PTCA, transient myocardial ischemia is induced during occlusion of a coronary artery by balloon inflation, followed by myocardial reperfusion on balloon deflation. Although in theory PTCA could be a cause of stunned myocardium, numerous clinical studies have confirmed that LV systolic function recovers fully within a few minutes after the procedure (Alam et al., 1986; Doorey et al., 1985; Hauser et al., 1985; Labovitz et al., 1987; Serruys et al., 1984; Visser et al., 1986; Wolfgelernter, 1986). Diastolic function, however, may remain impaired, as suggested by Wijns and associates (1986), who found that regional myocardial stiffness in the distribution of the dilated coronary artery was increased 12 minutes after the last balloon deflation. Using Doppler echocardiographic indexes of LV filling as measures of diastolic function, Labovitz and coworkers (1987) demonstrated a return to normal LV filling within 15 seconds after deflation following the first balloon inflation. The different findings in these studies (Labovitz et al., 1987; Wijns et al., 1986) may relate to the magnitude and duration of ischemia provoked. Patients were studied after a single balloon inflation by Labovitz and coworkers (1987), and after multiple inflations by Wijns and associates (1986). In addition, Doppler echocardiographic indexes are indirect measures of LV diastolic function and do not exclude the possibility that LV compliance may be impaired after PTCA.

It would appear that the episodes of ischemia associated with PTCA are too short to cause protracted impairment of LV systolic function, but may provoke prolonged abnormalities of diastolic function. This is not surprising, since experimental studies have demonstrated that coronary occlusions lasting ≤2 minutes do not cause appreciable myocardial stunning (Bolli, 1990). In one study (Sheiban et al., 1993) the duration of balloon inflation was unusually long (5.5 $\pm$ 1.1 min); however, both systolic and diastolic function were found to remain depressed for at least 24 hours and to normalize by 3 days, clearly documenting the occurrence of stunning.

TECHNIQUES TO DIAGNOSE STUNNED MYOCARDIUM

The development of practical approaches for the diagnosis of stunned myocardium is essential to further our understanding of the prevalence and clinical impact of this condition. The ideal diagnostic method to detect stunned myocardium would be reliable, widely applicable, inexpensive, and would allow for prospective detection of viable myocardium and differentiation of stunned from hibernating myocardium. Multiple approaches are presently being investigated for this purpose, which emphasizes that no one approach has been found to be ideal. The existing techniques being employed to diagnose stunned myocardium assess one of its two fundamental properties, namely, inotropic responsiveness and adequacy of perfusion. Table 10-3 summarizes the current diagnostic techniques for assessing stunned myocardium. Listed for each technique are the property of stunned myocardium being assessed, the advantages and disadvantages of the technique, and the potential ability to differentiate stunned from hibernating myocardium.

Positron emission tomography

Positron emission tomography (PET) is probably the "gold standard" for the detection of stunned myocardium, since it enables one to measure absolute regional myocardial blood flow and therefore can distinguish stunned myocardium (in which flow is normal or near normal) from hibernating or ischemic myocardium (in which flow is decreased). This technique is a relatively new imaging modality that allows for the quantitative assessment of regional myocardial metabolism and perfusion (Camici et al., 1989). Fatty acids are the primary substrate for the production of high-energy phosphates in normal myocardium (Neely et al., 1972). However, during myocardial ischemia oxygen deprivation reduces the utilization of fatty acids and the myocyte increases utilization of glucose for high-energy phosphate production (Camici et al., 1989).

To determine myocardial viability by PET, F18-fluorodeoxyglucose is used as a metabolic marker of glucose utilization. Although F18-fluorodeoxyglucose is not a metabolic substrate, it is taken up by viable myocytes and "trapped" within the cell by phosphorylation. As an alternative, C-11-acetate can be used to evaluate regional myocardial metabolism. This agent is taken up in proportion to blood flow. Its washout rate is related to the oxidative tricarboxylic acid cycle flux (Armbrecht et al., 1990). Measurement of blood flow during PET is made with nitrogen-13-labeled ammonia or oxygen-15-labeled water. An irreversibly damaged myocardial region on PET imaging is characterized by a matched reduction in perfusion and glucose uptake, whereas viable myocardium is characterized by intact glu-

TABLE 10-3. CURRENTLY USED TECHNIQUES TO DIAGNOSE STUNNED MYOCARDIUM

Technique	Property assessed	Advantages	Limitations/disadvantages	Able to differentiate stunned from hibernating myocardium
PET	Metabolism/perfusion	Measures absolute RMBF	High cost/no LVF	Yes
Thal-201 scan	Membrane integrity/perfusion	Widely available	Expensive/no LVF, only relative RMBF	Undetermined
Tc-99m scan	Membrane integrity/perfusion	Measures both RMBF (relative) and LVF	Expensive, only relative RMBF	Undetermined
Dobuta-echo	Contractile reserve	Widely available/less expensive	No perfusion	Doubtful
Dobuta-TEE	Contractile reserve	Superior image quality	Expensive/no perfusion	Doubtful

Dobuta-echo = dobutamine transthoracic echocardiography; Dobuta-TEE = dobutamine transesophageal echocardiography; LVF = left ventricular function; PET = positron emission tomography; RMBF = regional myocardial blood flow; Tc-99m scan = technetium-99m isonitrile scintigraphy; Thal-201 scan = thallium-201 scintigraphy.

cose uptake. Stunned and hibernating myocardium would both demonstrate this characteristic feature of viable myocardium, so that increased glucose uptake, in itself, may not suffice to distinguish the two. In theory, PET could differentiate between stunned and hibernating myocardium by demonstrating normal perfusion in the former and reduced blood flow in the latter. Identification of the most accurate positron emission tomographic index of stunned myocardium will require further investigation.

The positive predictive value of PET for improvement in myocardial function in asynergic segments after revascularization has been between 75 and 85% (Schwaiger & Hicks, 1991; Tamaki et al., 1989; Tillisch et al., 1986). However, these results may not be applicable to predicting recovery of stunned myocardium because hypoperfusion of myocardial regions demonstrating viability was present in these studies (Schwaiger & Hicks, 1991; Tamaki et al., 1989; Tillisch et al., 1986). Although PET is useful in identifying viable myocardium, it is unknown if this technique will adequately predict recovery in function of stunned myocardial segments. The absence of metabolic activity by PET identifies 78 to 92% of asynergic segments, which will not improve after revascularization (Tamaki et al., 1989; Tillisch et al., 1986).

PET is an excellent technique to determine viability of myocardium, but it has several important limitations. The technique is not widely available. Cyclotrons are needed to generate the metabolic tracers, therefore its cost is exorbitant. Lastly, PET does not assess LV function. This necessitates an additional diagnostic test to evaluate myocardial function.

Thallium-201 single photon emission computed tomography

Myocardial uptake of thallium-201, a potassium analog, for imaging by SPECT is dependent on myocardial blood flow, and uptake and retention of thallium by myocytes (Grunwald et al., 1981; Weich et al., 1977). The ability of viable myocardium to retain thallium-201 as compared to necrotic myocytes, which have a rapid washout of the isotope, distinguishes it from nonviable myocardium when imaging by SPECT. Unlike PET, which depends on intermediary metabolism, thallium-201 SPECT simply depends on integrity of the cell membrane for the potassium analog to determine viability.

TABLE 10-4.   THALLIUM-201 PROTOCOLS FOR ASSESSMENT OF POTENTIALLY VIABLE MYOCARDIUM

Protocol	Advantage	Disadvantage
Stress-early (3- to 4-hr) redistribution	Assesses ischemia/ convenient	Underestimates viability
Stress-late (8- to 24-hr) redistribution	Assesses ischemia/ better sensitivity	Inconvenient (three scans)
Rest-stress-reinjection	Comparable to PET	Inconvenient (three scans)
Rest-redistribution	Good sensitivity	No assessment of ischemia

PET = positron emission tomography.

The optimal protocol for detection of viable myocardium using thallium-201 SPECT remains undetermined. Listed in Table 10-4 are several of the protocols used for the assessment of dysfunctional but potentially viable myocardium by thallium-201 imaging. Injection of thallium-201 at peak exercise followed but scintigraphic imaging immediately after stress (i.e., stress imaging) and 3 to 4 hours after exercise (i.e., early redistribution imaging) is a commonly used protocol to detect viable myocardium (i.e., stress-early redistribution protocol). After the initial uptake of thallium-201 by myocytes during stress, exchange of thallium between viable myocardium and the blood pool continues after exercise, a process called *redistribution*. In dyskinetic, akinetic, or severely hypokinetic myocardial segments, the presence of thallium redistribution in the stress-early redistribution protocol is indicative of viable myocardium. Although the presence of redistribution on the stress-early redistribution thallium protocol is a reliable index of myocardial viability, the lack of redistribution does not necessarily reflect nonviable myocardium (Grunwald et al., 1981). Forty-five percent of defects without evidence of redistribution during stress-early redistribution imaging demonstrate improved thallium uptake consistent with viability after CABG surgery (Grunwald et al., 1981). Additional studies have also shown that 38 to 58% of persistent defects on exercise thallium imaging show evidence of F18-fluorodeoxyglucose uptake on PET (Fig 10-2) (Bonow et al., 1991; Brunken et al., 1987; Tamaki et al., 1988).

Additional protocols using thallium-201 scintigraphy have been developed to improve the detection of viable myocardium. These include 8- to 24-hour delayed redistribution imaging; imaging after reinjection of thallium; and 3-to 4-hour rest-redistribution imaging (see Table 10-3). These protocols have significantly improved the detection of viable myocardium using thallium-201 scintigraphy as compared with the stress-early redistribution protocol. The equilibration of thallium between the blood pool and viable myocardial segments may take greater than 3 to 4 hours and, therefore, delayed imaging at 8 to 24 hours during redistribution improves the detection of viable myocardium. Redistribution on 24-hour images but not on 4-hour images has been reported in 20 to 60% of defects (Kiat et al., 1988; Yang et al., 1990). Segments that demonstrate redistribution at 24 hours are likely to show improved function after revascularization (Dilsizian & Bonow, 1992). Yang and associates (1990) demonstrated late redistribution of thallium in the absence of early redistribution in 22% of myocardial segments (Fig 10-3). Importantly, the presence of late redistribution on thallium imaging predicts recovery of regional function in 95% of segments after revascularization (Kiat et al., 1988). Unfortunately, myocardial segments that failed to demonstrate redistribution at 24 hours may remain viable. Thirty-seven percent of segments without redistribution at 24 hours improved after revascularization (Kiat et al., 1988). Although late thallium redistribution imaging improves identification of viable myocardium, the frequency of myocardial necrosis may be overestimated.

Reinjection of thallium and repeat imaging after a stress-early redistribution protocol improves detection of viable

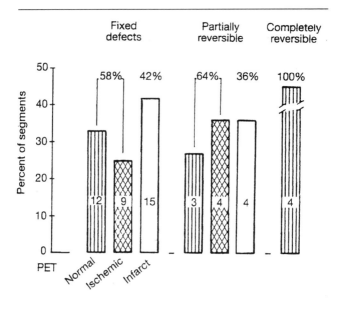

Figure 10-2. *Histogram showing percent of myocardial segments with thallium scans demonstrating fixed defects, partial reversibility, and complete reversibility stratified on the basis of positron emission tomography (PET) imaging results demonstrating normal myocardium* (vertical lines), *ischemia* (cross-hatched lines), *and nonviability* (open bars). *The majority of segments showing a fixed or partially reversible thallium defect are viable on PET imaging. (From Brunken and colleagues [1987], with permission of the* Journal of the American College of Cardiology.)

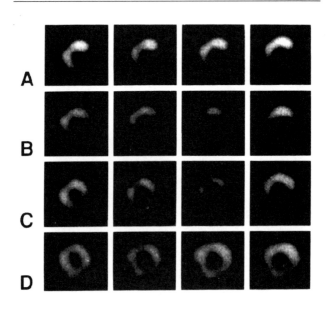

Figure 10-3. *A series of short-axis thallium tomograms demonstrating detection of reversible thallium abnormalities by late redistribution imaging. The large lateral and inferior thallium defect on stress images (A) persist on 4-hour redistribution images (B) but reverse at 24 hours (C). Stress images after coronary artery bypass graft surgery (D) showed normal thallium uptake and confirmed viability of the inferior and lateral segments. (From Yang and colleagues [1990], with permission from the* Journal of the American College of Cardiology.)

Stress

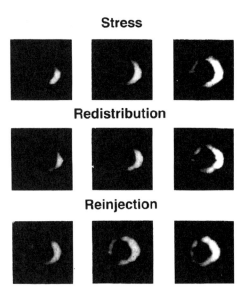

Redistribution

Reinjection

Figure 10-4. Short-axis thallium tomograms demonstrating a large anterior and septal defect on the immediate postexercise images (Stress) that persisted on 3- to 4-hour redistribution images (Redistribution) but improved significantly on reinjection (Reinjection) images. (From Dilsizian and coworkers [1990], with permission from the New England Journal of Medicine.)

myocardium. Approximately 30 to 50% of myocardial segments that show persistent defects and no redistribution at 3 to 4 hours demonstrate additional thallium uptake after reinjection (Fig 10-4) (Bonow et al., 1991; Ohtani et al., 1990; Rocco et al., 1990). Approximately 87% of such segments will demonstrate improved regional function after PTCA (Dilsizian et al., 1990). The thallium reinjection protocol was comparable to PET in differentiating viable from nonviable myocardium (Bonow et al., 1991). Imaging at 24 hours does not improve the sensitivity or specificity of the thallium reinjection protocol for detecting viable myocardium (Dilsizian et al., 1992).

Thallium-201 can be injected at rest and images obtained at 10 minutes and 3 to 4 hours afterward (i.e., rest-redistribution imaging). Thallium uptake and redistribution in dysfunctional myocardial segments identifies viable myocardium that frequently improves function after revascularization (Iskandrian et al., 1983, 1986). Iskandrian and colleagues (1983) showed that rest-redistribution scans indicative of viable myocardium predicted improvement of global LV function after CABG surgery in 12 of 16 patients (75%). Eight of 10 patients (80%) with fixed defects on rest-redistribution scans failed to improve ventricular function after surgery (Iskandrian et al., 1983).

Although thallium-201 scintigraphy is a useful method of detecting viable myocardium, it is uncertain that this technique can reliably differentiate stunned from hibernating myocardium. Experimental canine models of stunned myocardium have shown normal myocardial extraction and washout kinetics of thallium-201 (Moore et al., 1990; Sinusas et al., 1989).

Although thallium-201 scintigraphy is an important technique for the assessment of viable and potentially stunned myocardium, it has several practical limitations. Reinjection protocols require three sets of images and considerably adds to the time to perform the test. Twenty-four-hour redistribution images may be inconvenient to patients. The rest-redistribution protocol does not allow for an evaluation of myocardial ischemia. Although less costly than PET, thallium scintigraphy is expensive, particularly when additional reinjection imaging is needed. Lastly, thallium-201 SPECT cannot assess LV function and requires an additional diagnostic test to evaluate myocardial function when used to delineate potentially viable myocardium.

Technetium-99m isonitrile scintigraphy

Newer radionuclide isotopes such as technetium-99m (Tc-99m) isonitrile have been developed and used to determine myocardial viability. In experimental models, uptake of Tc-99m isonitrile is only severely decreased in areas of myocardial necrosis (Sinusas et al., 1990). Clinical studies have shown that Tc-99m isonitrile can be used to identify viable myocardium. However, it underestimates the presence of viable myocardium (Rocco et al., 1989). Sixty-one percent of myocardial segments with severely decreased Tc-99m isonitrile uptake preoperatively manifest improved uptake after CABG surgery, demonstrating viability (Rocco et al., 1989). It is unknown if Tc-99m isonitrile can differentiate stunned from hibernating myocardium. Theoretically, the limited amount of redistribution of Tc-99m isonitrile could lead to an underestimation of viable myocardium in segments that are dysfunctional due to chronic decrease in blood flow.

A potential advantage of Tc-99m isonitrile over thallium-201 is its better physical characteristics for gamma camera imaging, which improves image quality. LV function may be potentially assessed used Tc-99m isonitrile. However, Tc-99m isonitrile scintigraphy has substantial cost.

Dobutamine echocardiography

Experimental studies have shown that stunned myocardium can be identified by demonstrating a return in or improvement of regional contractile myocardial function after exposure to inotropic stimulants such as dopamine, isoproterenol, dobutamine, and premature extrasystolic beats (i.e., postextrasystolic potentiation) (Becker et al., 1986; Bolli et al., 1985; Dyke et al., 1975; Ellis et al., 1984; Hood et al., 1969; Mercier et al., 1982). Human studies also support the notion that stunned myocardium may be identified using inotropic stimulants (Barilla et al., 1991; Piérard et al., 1990; Previtali et al., 1993; Salustri et al., 1994; Satler et al., 1986; Smart et al., 1993; Watada et al., 1994). To determine the usefulness of low-dose (i.e., 10 μg per kilogram per minute) dobutamine transthoracic two-dimensional echocardiography (DE) for differentiating stunned myocardium from necrotic tissue, Piérard and colleagues (1990) studied 17 patients an average of 7 days after receiving thrombolytic therapy within the first 3 hours of an acute anterior myocardial infarction. In myocar-

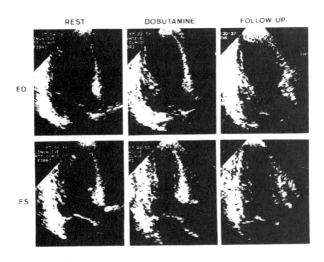

Figure 10-5. *Two-dimensional, apical, long-axis echocardiographic views from end diastole (ED) and end systole (ES) obtained at rest, during low-dose dobutamine infusion, and at follow-up. In the rest study, akinesia of the anteroseptum (arrows) is present, which normalizes during dobutamine infusion and remains normal at follow-up. (From Piérard and colleagues [1990], with permission of the* Journal of the American College of Cardiology.)

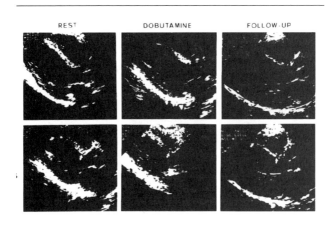

Figure 10-6. *Two-dimensional, parasternal, long-axis echocardiographic views at end diastole (ED) and end systole (ES) obtained at rest, during low-dose dobutamine infusion, and at follow-up. The septum is akinetic at rest (arrow) and is not improved during dobutamine infusion or at follow-up. (From Piérard and colleagues [1990], with permission from the* Journal of the American College of Cardiology.)

dial segments that showed improvement in systolic function during low-dose DE restoration in function occurred 2 months later (Fig 10-5). In addition, myocardial segments that did not respond to dobutamine remained dyskinetic or akinetic 2 months after thrombolysis (Fig 10-6). Similar to this earlier study, Watada and coworkers (1994) showed that low-dose DE performed 3 days after an acute anterior myocardial infarction treated with angioplasty had a sensitivity of 83% (55 of 66 segments) and a specificity of 86% (43 of 50 seg-

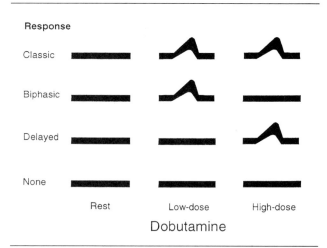

Figure 10-7. Schematic representation of the response of stunned myocardium to dobutamine at low and high dose. The classic response (Classic) as illustrated by the **top** panel *shows a sustained enhancement of wall motion. However, in the face of a critically stenosed coronary artery myocardial ischemia is provoked at the high dose and creates a biphasic response (Biphasic). Importantly, the low dose may be inadequate and a high dose may be necessary to demonstrate enhanced wall motion (Delayed). Stunned segments may not respond to dobutamine (None).*

ments) for the detection of stunned myocardium as confirmed by recovery of regional myocardial function at a mean of 25 days after myocardial infarction. Subsequent studies using low-dose DE have confirmed that it is equally useful for the detection of stunned myocardium in segments other than the anterior wall (Previtali et al., 1993; Salustri et al., 1994; Smart et al., 1993). Smart and associates (1993) demonstrated that low-dose DE was equally sensitive and specific for the detection of stunned myocardium of the anterior wall versus the inferior, posterior, or lateral wall. It remains undetermined if high-dose (i.e., 20–40 µg per kilogram per minute) DE will increase the sensitivity of low-dose protocols for the detection of stunned myocardium. Although high-dose dobutamine infusion would lead to myocardial ischemia and deterioration of regional myocardial function in the distribution of a critically stenosed coronary artery, it is plausible that enhanced myocardial function of stunned myocardium supplied by a patent coronary artery will be detectable at the high dose as opposed to the low dose of dobutamine in selected patients. A schematic diagram detailing the potential responses of stunned myocardium to low-dose and high-dose dobutamine, and the influence of coronary artery patency on the responses is shown in Figure 10-7.

Several studies have demonstrated that DE can be used to identify hibernating myocardium (Afridi et al., 1995; Charney et al., 1994; Cigarroa et al., 1993; La Canna et al., 1994; Mariani et al., 1995). The response in contractile function of hibernating myocardium to low-dose and high-dose dobutamine is similar to that of stunned myocardium, namely function may improve at low dose and deteriorate at high dose, show sustained improvement at low and high dose, improve only at high dose, or worsen at low dose

(Afridi et al., 1995). Given the heterogeneous and overlapping responses of stunned and hibernating myocardium to dobutamine, it is unlikely that DE could reliably differentiate these forms of viable myocardium. Future studies addressing this issue are needed.

The majority of studies have utilized a return in segmental function with or without revascularization as criteria for viable myocardium when assessing the sensitivity and specificity of DE for the identification of stunned myocardium (Barilla et al., 1991; Piérard et al., 1990; Previtali et al., 1993; Salustri et al., 1994; Satler et al., 1986; Smart et al., 1993; Watada et al., 1994). However, Piérard and colleagues (1990) have shown an excellent agreement between DE and PET for the detection of stunned myocardium. Additional studies have shown that DE compares favorably to thallium-201 scintigraphy for the detection of viable myocardium (Charney et al., 1994; Foster et al., 1995; Marzullo et al., 1993a; Panza et al., 1995).

Dobutamine echocardiography has several advantages for the assessment of viable myocardium as compared to PET, thallium-201, or Tc-99m isonitrile scintigraphy, such as lower cost, widespread availability, portability, convenience, and ability to monitor ventricular function on-line during pharmacological infusions. However, DE cannot directly assess perfusion of dysfunctional but potentially viable myocardial segments. Also, technically adequate, transthoracic, two-dimensional echocardiographic studies are not feasible in all patients. A recent study has shown that dobutamine two-dimensional transesophageal echocardiography (TEE) has a sensitivity of 81% and a specificity of 97% for the detection of viable myocardium using F18-fluorodeoxyglucose PET to determine myocardial viability (Baer et al., 1994). Dobutamine TEE may play an important adjunctive role to DE for the detection of viable and potentially stunned myocardium.

Dipyridamole echocardiography

Experimental studies support the notion that dipyridamole selectively enhances function of stunned myocardium as opposed to necrotic tissue by augmenting coronary flow (Stahl et al., 1986). Picano and coworkers (1992) demonstrated a sensitivity of 81% and a specificity of 96% for dipyridamole echocardiography in the identification of viable but potentially stunned myocardium using thallium-201 scintigraphy as the standard for viability. Dipyridamole echocardiography shows promise but additional studies confirming these results will need to be performed to determine its ultimate role in the assessment of potentially stunned myocardium.

Dipyridamole thallium-201 scintigraphy

Dipyridamole thallium-201 scintigraphy may be useful for the detection of viable myocardium (Simek et al., 1993). Simek and colleagues (1993) showed a sensitivity of 98% for dipyridamole thallium-201 scintigraphy for the detection of viable myocardium. Additional studies are needed confirming the potential role of dipyridamole thallium-201 imaging for the assessment of stunned myocardium.

Myocardial contrast echocardiography

Myocardial contrast echocardiography (MCE) uses air-filled microbubbles, ranging in size from 4 to 6 microns, that scatter ultrasound. Microbubbles traverse the myocardial microvasculature after injection into coronary arteries and produce ultrasonic opacification of myocardial segments on two-dimensional echocardiography. If microvascular integrity is intact, microbubbles will remain within the intravascular space as they traverse the myocardium. Myocardial segments with no flow or <15% of normal resting flow fail to show opacification during MCE (Kaul et al., 1989). Ragosta and associates (1994) demonstrated that the presence of microvascular integrity as assessed by MCE was the best predictor of recovery in LV segmental function after AMI in patients with revascularization of the infarct-related artery. Sabia and coworkers (1992) showed that the demonstration of collateral blood flow by MCE to a recently infarcted segment was associated with return of function and predictive of viable or stunned myocardium. MCE appears promising in the assessment of stunned myocardium. However, additional studies particularly in other clinical conditions are needed to determine its ultimate role.

Electrocardiography

Although the ECG is insensitive for the detection of stunned myocardium, certain electrocardiographic changes occurring during specific coronary artery syndromes may suggest the presence of stunned myocardium (de Zwaan et al., 1991; Hirota et al., 1992; Renkin et al., 1990; Stack et al., 1983). Inverted T-waves in the precordial electrocardiographic leads identify a subset of patients with unstable angina more likely to show reversibility of anterior wall-motion abnormalities several months after revascularization (de Zwaan et al., 1991; Renkin et al., 1990). Similarly, patients with acute anterior myocardial infarction and inverted T-waves with QT prolongation of the precordial leads may show a return to normal function of the anterior wall 4 to 8 weeks after successful PTCA. Q-waves are not necessarily synonymous with irreversibly injured myocardium (Bateman et al., 1983). Although the ECG may be useful in certain select situations, cardiac imaging modalities will remain the mainstay for the diagnosis of stunned myocardium.

CLINICAL IMPORTANCE AND TREATMENT

Although stunned myocardium is by definition reversible and will eventually disappear spontaneously, there are several reasons that make this abnormality important for the practicing cardiologist. First, it is conceivable that in those patients who experience frequent bouts of ischemia (often painless) in the same territory, repetitive episodes of stunning may result in persistent or even chronic ventricular dysfunction mimicking myocardial hibernation (Bolli, 1992). This is an intriguing scenario that is being actively investigated. Second, stunned myocardium is likely to be a major cause of viable but dysfunctional myocardial segments. Enhancement of LV function after revascularization is associated with improved survival (Alderman et al., 1983; Nesto et al., 1982; Pigott et al., 1985). Therefore, the prospective differentiation of viable from nonviable myocardium in patients with coronary artery disease and impaired LV function is of significant clinical importance in the modern era of myocardial revascularization. In some patients, the decision to perform revascularization is predominantly based on the presence and extent of viable myocardium. However, the importance of establishing viability of dysfunctional myocardial segments on decisions regarding revascularization should not be overstated. In most patients with coronary artery disease and anatomy technically suitable for PTCA or CABG surgery, management decisions regarding the appropriateness of revascularization can be adequately made by determining the presence and severity of myocardial ischemia, and the status of resting LV function.

Although stunned and hibernating myocardium may coexist in some cases (Bolli, 1992), and although the ultimate treatment for repetitive stunning and hibernation is the same (i.e., coronary revascularization), differentiating viable myocardium as predominantly stunned or hibernating may be clinically important in specific situations. For example, in patients with severely impaired cardiac function due to stunned myocardium that is not supplied by a critically stenosed coronary artery, the use of inotropic medications may enhance the function of viable myocardium, and help to improve and stabilize the hemodynamic state. On the other hand, inotropic agents may increase myocardial oxygen demand and upset the precarious balance between oxygen demand and supply in hibernating myocardium, thereby worsening LV function. Although hibernating myocardium may initially respond to inotropic agents, this response can be transient and later followed by a deterioration due to the increased myocardial oxygen demands and worsening ischemia (Schulz et al., 1992).

A better understanding of the mechanisms of stunned myocardium in humans may allow for the development of pharmacological agents that hasten the functional recovery of viable but dysfunctional tissue. Therapies aimed at preventing the development of stunned myocardium would be of great importance. Several groups of drugs have been shown to attenuate myocardial stunning in experimental animals, including antioxidants, calcium antagonists, ACE inhibitors, adenosine and adenosine modulators, and ATP-dependent potassium channel blockers (Bolli, 1990). Clinical trials with these agents, however, are still lacking.

Finally, repeated episodes of myocardial stunning may result in protracted or even chronic LV dysfunction, as postulated (Bolli, 1992) (see Fig 10-1). Because regional blood flow is rarely measured in patients with coronary artery disease, repetitive stunning resulting in chronic LV dysfunction (with normal or near-normal perfusion) can be easily misinterpreted as chronic hibernation with decreased perfusion (Bolli, 1992). The concept that many instances of so-called chronic hibernation actually represent chronic stunning caused by repetitive bouts of ischemia (with no or minimal decrease in perfusion) is now supported both by experimental (Shen & Vatner, 1995) and clinical (Marinho et al., 1996; Vanoverschelde et al., 1993) evidence.

These studies (Marinho et al., 1996; Shen & Vatner, 1995; Vanoverschelde et al., 1993) have shown that prolonged, reversible ventricular dysfunction is observed in settings in which coronary flow is normal or near normal, but coronary flow reserve is markedly decreased, resulting in a propensity to the development of ischemic episodes in conjunction with increased myocardial oxygen demands.

The clinical importance of stunned myocardium varies widely among patients and is influenced by the specific clinical situation. Therefore, the significance and possible treatment of stunned myocardium will be discussed separately for each clinical setting.

Cardiac surgery

Experimental studies have shown that stunned myocardium is exquisitely sensitive to inotropic stimulation and afterload manipulations (Bolli, 1990). Thus, the true frequency and severity of stunned myocardium after cardiac surgery may not be fully appreciated because most patients are treated postoperatively with inotropes and vasodilators, which improve cardiac function and probably mask myocardial stunning. Among all of the clinical situations, cardiac surgery is the one in which myocardial stunning is likely to have the most serious impact on outcome, because it involves the entire heart and therefore causes global (as opposed to regional) dysfunction. In most cases, postoperative stunning is well tolerated and does not require any specific treatment. In a minority of patients, however, postoperative myocardial stunning can profoundly depress LV function and cause hemodynamic instability that requires intensive and prolonged treatment with inotropes, vasoactive agents, and/or mechanical circulatory assist devices. This occurrence is particularly common in patients with baseline depression of ventricular function, in those who undergo prolonged aortic cross-clamping, in those who are operated on in conditions of unstable angina, and in those with left main coronary disease. In these situations, the development of stunned myocardium can have a major impact on the prognosis and can be a cause of morbidity and mortality. Indeed, stunning is probably the most frequent cause of low cardiac output syndrome after CABG. Even when myocardial stunning is masked by intravenous inotropic or vasodilator therapy, its presence is likely to prolong the intensive care unit stay, thereby causing significant additional costs.

In view of these considerations, treatments that can prevent or attenuate myocardial stunning after cardiac surgery are needed and are being investigated. Experimental studies have shown that antioxidants and adenosine can enhance recovery of function after cardiopulmonary bypass in animals (Bolli, 1990). Clinical studies are still lacking. Johnson and associates (1991) performed a randomized, placebo-controlled study investigating the potential of allopurinol to protect cardiac function after CABG surgery. Allopurinol is a xanthine oxidase inhibitor that blocks the production of reactive oxygen species by this enzyme. Since oxygen radicals contribute to stunning (Bolli, 1990), it was postulated that allopurinol would limit myocardial stunning due to cardiac surgery. Johnson and associates (1991) reported that hospital mortality was lower and cardiac function better preserved in patients who received allopurinol compared with placebo. Additional approaches, such as adenosine, are being investigated and are likely to impact the future management of patients undergoing cardiac surgery. Magnesium could also be beneficial. Even if "antistunning" therapies do not affect postoperative mortality, they may decrease the need for inotropic, vasodilator, and /or mechanical support, and thus shorten the stay in intensive care units. This would be a significant result, particularly in view of current efforts to minimize health-care expenditures.

Acute myocardial infarction with early reperfusion

The development of myocardial stunning after reperfusion therapy for AMI can be a cause of morbidity and mortality in those patients who have a preexisting impairment of cardiac function (i.e., patients with prior infarction) or in whom the size of the ischemic region is large (e.g., patients with proximal LAD lesions). In these subjects, the persistence of postischemic stunning may cause hemodynamic instability requiring intensive monitoring, pharmacological and/or mechanical support, and urgent revascularization under suboptimal conditions. As in the case of cardiac surgery, the development of stunning will also likely prolong the intensive care unit stay, with its attendant financial implications. Furthermore, clinicians must be cognizant of the fact that the benefits of thrombolysis cannot be appreciated soon after reperfusion because the recovery of function in the viable but stunned tissue may require several days or possibly even longer. This necessitates careful assessment of patients who are in cardiogenic shock or severe LV failure after reperfusion. In these patients, the usefulness of maintaining circulatory support for extended periods of time obviously depends on whether the ventricular dysfunction is reversible, which requires a distinction between infarcted and stunned myocardium. A similar distinction must also be made in order to decide whether to proceed with PTCA when an akinetic/hypokinetic region is perfused by a critically stenotic vessel in patients treated with thrombolytic therapy. In this latter case DE may be helpful.

Given the inevitable delay in the initiation of treatment, it is unlikely that medications administered along with reperfusion therapy for AMI will entirely prevent the development of stunned myocardium. Even in experimental animals, it is unclear whether myocardial stunning can be attenuated by antioxidants after subendocardial infarction (Bolli, 1990). Experimental studies (Bolli et al., 1989) suggest that radical scavengers must be delivered into ischemic myocardial tissue before reperfusion in order to attenuate the development of stunned myocardium, which would make the peripheral venous administration of antioxidants ineffective. Clinical studies are lacking. Werns and coworkers (1989) were unable to show benefit on LV systolic function with the administration of SOD, an antioxidant enzyme, in patients undergoing PTCA for an AMI; however, this study was not designed to evaluate stunning soon after reperfusion. Additional agents that may be of benefit in the attenuation of myocardial stunning due to myocardial infarction include ACE inhibitors, calcium antagonists, beta adrenergic blockers, adenosine, and ATP-dependent potassium channel openers. However, no data with these agents are yet available.

Exercise-induced ischemia

Exercise is probably the most common cause of ischemia in patients with coronary artery disease. Many of these ischemic episodes are clinically silent. Therefore, if stunned myocardium due to exercise-induced ischemia is confirmed as suggested by recent echocardiographic studies (Kloner et al., 1991; Robertson et al., 1983; Scognamiglio et al., 1991; Stoddard et al., 1992), this phenomenon would have a significant clinical impact. Furthermore, if repetitive episodes of exercise-induced ischemia have a cumulative effect (as noted in experimental animals [Homans et al., 1989]) and chronically depress LV systolic and/or diastolic function, the clinical implications of stunned myocardium would be of even greater importance. Prevention of postischemic LV dysfunction due to exercise-induced ischemia is primarily focused on eliminating ischemic episodes by pharmacological or interventional therapies. No medication specifically designed to attenuate postischemic myocardial stunning associated with exercise-induced ischemia has been developed yet.

Unstable angina

The recognition that ischemic episodes due to unstable angina may cause protracted postischemic LV dysfunction is clinically relevant for patient management. Although anti-ischemic, antiplatelet, and anticoagulant medications play an important role in the treatment of patients with unstable angina, revascularization by PTCA is indicated when there are large regions of dysfunctional but viable myocardium. Several investigators have demonstrated improvement of LV function after PTCA in patients with unstable angina (de Feyter et al., 1987; de Zwaan et al., 1991; Renkin et al., 1990). On the other hand, the use of inotropic agents to recruit dysfunctional but viable myocardial segments in patients with unstable angina and heart failure may be problematic, for these drugs can potentially induce arrhythmias and precipitate or aggravate ischemia distal to a severe coronary stenosis. Thus, the cardiologist must be aware of the existence of stunned myocardium in unstable angina and use tests to distinguish dysfunctional, necrotic myocardium from dysfunctional, stunned myocardium, since in the former case PTCA is not indicated, whereas in the latter it can be extremely helpful. No therapies have been tested to prevent myocardial stunning in unstable angina.

Congestive heart failure

In patients with congestive heart failure due to coronary artery disease and LV systolic dysfunction, revascularization by CABG surgery is an effective treatment to enhance cardiac function, increase functional status, and improve survival. However, mortality from CABG surgery increases with worsening resting LV dysfunction. Patients with profound LV dysfunction are at particularly high risk. In these patients, demonstration of large zones of viable myocardium with considerable contractile reserve (possibly secondary to repetitive stunning) may weigh heavily in the final decision to pursue revascularization. It is anticipated that studies confirming the importance of identifying viable myocardium in such patients will be forthcoming in the near future.

SUMMARY

Numerous clinical observations suggest that stunned myocardium occurs in various settings in which the myocardium is subjected to transient ischemia, such as AMI with early reperfusion, unstable angina, exercise-induced ischemia, variant angina, cardiac surgery, and cardiac transplantation. Potentially of major importance is the possibility that frequent episodes of ischemia, particularly in the ambulatory setting, may have a cumulative effect and cause protracted or even chronic postischemic LV dysfunction. This could be mistakenly diagnosed as hibernating myocardium when in fact it is a result of repetitive stunning. The clinical significance of stunned myocardium is beginning to be appreciated by clinicians. Recognition of this phenomena is important from a practical standpoint and may impact patient management. Diagnostic imaging techniques now allow for a prospective diagnosis of stunned myocardium. Although the ideal diagnostic technique has yet to be developed, existing modalities such as thallium-201 scintigraphy or dobutamine echocardiography are available and should be applied in the appropriate clinical setting. Although the mechanism of stunned myocardium in humans is not yet known, experimental models of stunning are useful in guiding future clinical investigations. Perhaps such investigations will ultimately lead to the development of medications that can prevent or attenuate the occurrence of stunned myocardium and/or hasten its recovery.

ACKNOWLEDGMENTS

The excellent secretarial assistance of Sandy Dunaway is gratefully acknowledged. The work reported here was supported in part by NIH grants HL-43151 and HL-55757.

REFERENCES

Afridi I, Kleiman NS, Raizner AE, Zoghbi WA. Dobutamine echocardiography in myocardial hibernation: optimal dose and accuracy in predicting recovery of ventricular function after coronary angioplasty. *Circulation* 1995; 91: 663–670.

Alam M, Khaja F, Brymer J, et al. Echocardiographic evaluation of left ventricular function during coronary artery angioplasty. *Am J Cardiol* 1986; 57: 20–25.

Alderman EL, Fisher LD, Litwin P, et al. Results of coronary artery surgery in patients with poor left ventricular function (CASS). *Circulation* 1983; 68: 785–795.

Ambrosio G, Losi MA, Perrone Filardi P, et al. Persistence of contractile impairment in the absence of flow abnormalities after exercise: evidence for myocardial stunning in patients with stable angina [abstract]. *Circulation* 1993; 88(Suppl I): I-646.

Anderson JL, Marshall HW, Askins JC, et al. A randomized trial of intravenous and intracoronary streptokinase in patients with acute myocardial infarction. *Circulation* 1984; 70: 606–618.

Anderson JL, Marshall HW, Bray BE, et al. A randomized trial of intracoronary streptokinase in the treatment of acute myocardial infarction. *N Engl J Med* 1983; 308: 1313–1318.

Armbrecht JJ, Buxton DB, Schelbert HR. Validation of [1-^{11}C] acetate as a tracer for noninvasive assessment of oxidative metabolism with positron emission tomography in normal, ischemic, postischemic, and hyperemic canine myocardium. *Circulation* 1990; 81: 1594–1605.

Baer FM, Voth E, Deutsch HJ, et al. Assessment of viable myocardium by dobutamine transesophageal echocardiography and comparison with fluorine-18 fluorodeoxyglucose positron emission tomography. *J Am Coll Cardiol* 1994; 24: 343–353.

Ballantyne CM, Verani MS, Short HD, et al. Delayed recovery of severely "stunned" myocardium with the support of a left ventricular assist device after coronary artery bypass graft surgery. *J Am Coll Cardiol* 1987; 10: 710–712.

Barilla F, Gheorghiade M, Alam M, et al. Low-dose dobutamine in patients with acute myocardial infarction identifies viable but not contractile myocardium and predicts the magnitude of improvement in wall motion abnormalities in response to coronary revascularization. *Am Heart J* 1991; 122: 1522–1531.

Bateman TM, Czer LSC, Gray RJ, et al. Transient pathologic Q waves during acute ischemic events: an electrocardiographic correlate of stunned but viable myocardium. *Am Heart J* 1983; 6: 1421–1426.

Becker LC, Levine JH, Di Paula AF, et al. Reversal of dysfunction in postischemic stunned myocardium by epinephrine and postextrasystolic potentiation. *J Am Coll Cardiol* 1986; 7: 580–589.

Bolli R. Mechanism of myocardial "stunning." *Circulation* 1990; 82: 723–738.

Bolli R. Myocardial "stunning" in man. *Circulation* 1992; 86: 1671–1691.

Bolli R, Hartley CJ, Chelly JE, et al. An accurate nontraumatic ultrasonic method to monitor myocardial wall thickening in patients undergoing cardiac surgery. *J Am Coll Cardiol* 1990; 15: 1055–1065.

Bolli R, Hartley CJ, Rabinovitz RS. Clinical relevance of myocardial "stunning." *Cardiovasc Drugs Ther* 1991; 5: 877–890.

Bolli R, Jeroudi MO, Patel BS, et al. Marked reduction of free radical generation and contractile dysfunction by antioxidants therapy begun at the time of reperfusion. *Circ Res* 1989; 65: 607–622.

Bolli R, Zhu WO, Myers ML, et al. Beta-adrenergic stimulation reverses postischemic myocardial dysfunction without producing subsequent functional deterioration. *Am J Cardiol* 1985; 56: 964–968.

Bonow RO, Dilsizian V, Cuocolo A, Bacharach SL. Identification of viable myocardium in patients with chronic coronary artery disease and left ventricular dysfunction. Comparison of thallium scintigraphy with reinjection and PET imaging with ^{18}F-fluorodeoxyglucose. *Circulation* 1991; 83: 26–37.

Bourdillon PDV, Broderick TM, Williams ES, et al. Early recovery of regional left ventricular function after reperfusion in acute myocardial infarction assessed by serial two-dimensional echocardiography. *Am J Cardiol* 1989; 63: 641–646.

Braunwald E, Kloner RA. The stunned myocardium: prolonged, postischemic ventricular dysfunction. *Circulation* 1982; 66: 1146–1149.

Braunwald E, Rutherford JD. Reversible ischemic left ventricular dysfunction: evidence for the "hibernating myocardium." *J Am Coll Cardiol* 1986; 8: 1467–1470.

Breisblatt WM, Stein KL, Wolfe CJ, et al. Acute myocardial dysfunction and recovery: a common occurrence after coronary bypass surgery. *J Am Coll Cardiol* 1990; 15: 1261–1269.

Brunken R, Schwaiger M, Grover-McKay M, et al. Positron emission tomography detects tissue metabolic activity in myocardial segments with persistent thallium perfusion defects. *J Am Coll Cardiol* 1987; 10: 557–567.

Cabrol C, Grandjbakhch I, Pavie A, et al. Current problems in cardiac transplantation. *Biomed Pharmacother* 1989; 43: 87–92.

Camici P, Araujo L, Spinks T, et al. Myocardial glucose utilization in ischemic heart disease: preliminary results with F18-fluorodeoxyglucose and positron emission tomography. *Eur Heart J* 1986; 7(Suppl C): 19–23.

Camici P, Gerrannini E, Opie LH. Myocardial metabolism in ischemic heart disease: basic principles and application to imaging by positron emission tomography. *Prog Cardiovasc Dis* 1989; 32: 217–238.

Charney R, Schwinger ME, Chun J, et al. Dobutamine echocardiography and resting-redistribution thallium-201 scintigraphy predicts recovery of hibernating myocardium after coronary revascularization. *Am Heart J* 1994; 128: 864–869.

Charuzi Y, Beeder C, Marshall LA, et al. Improvement in regional and global left ventricular function after intracoronary thrombolysis: assessment with two-dimensional echocardiography. *Am J Cardiol* 1984; 53: 662–665.

Cigarroa CG, deFilippi CR, Brickner E, et al. Dobutamine stress echocardiography identifies hibernating myocardium and predicts recovery of left ventricular function after coronary revascularization. *Circulation* 1993; 88: 430–436.

Cunningham Jr JN, Adams PX, Knopp EA, et al. Preservation of ATP, ultrastructure, and ventricular function after aortic cross-clamping and reperfusion: clinical use of blood potassium cardioplegia. *J Thorac Cardiovasc Surg* 1979; 78: 708–720.

Czer L, Hamer A, Murphy F, et al. Transient hemodynamic dysfunction after myocardial revascularization: temperature dependence. *J Thorac Cardiovasc Surg* 1983; 86: 226–234.

Deantonio HJ, Kaul S, Lerman BB. Reversible myocardial depression in survivors of cardiac arrest. *PACE* 1990; 13: 982–985.

de Feyter PJ, Suryapranata H, Serruys PW, et al. Effects of successful percutaneous transluminal coronary angioplasty on global and regional left ventricular function in unstable angina pectoris. *Am J Cardiol* 1987; 60: 993–997.

de Zwaan C, Cheriex EC, Braat SHJG, et al. Improvement of systolic and diastolic left ventricular wall motion by serial echocardiograms in selected patients treated for unstable angina. *Am Heart J* 1991; 121: 789–797.

Dilsizian V, Bonow RO. Differential uptake and apparent thallium-201 washout after thallium reinjection. Options regarding early redistribution imaging before reinjection or late redistribution imaging after reinjection. *Circulation* 1992; 85: 1032–1038.

Dilsizian V, Rocco TP, Freedman NMT, et al. Enhanced detection of ischemic but viable myocardium by the reinjection of thallium after stress-redistribution imaging. *N Engl J Med* 1990; 323: 141–146.

Distante A, Rovai D, Picano E, et al. Transient changes in left ventricular mechanics during attacks of Prinzmetal angina: a two-dimensional echocardiographic study. *Am Heart J* 1984a; 108: 440–446.

Distante A, Rovai D, Picano E, et al. Transient changes in left ventricular mechanics during attacks of Prinzmetal's angina: an M-mode echocardiographic study. *Am Heart J* 1984b; 107: 465–473.

Doorey AJ, Mehmel HC, Schwartz FX, Kuble W. Amelioration by nitroglycerin of left ventricular ischemia induced by percutaneous transluminal coronary angioplasty: assessment by hemodynamic variables and left ventriculography. *J Am Coll Cardiol* 1985; 6: 267–274.

Dyke SH, Urschel CW, Sonnenblick EH, et al. Detection of latent function in acutely ischemic myocardium in the dog: comparison of pharmacologic inotropic stimulation and postextrasystolic potentiation. *Circ Res* 1975; 36: 490–497.

Dymond DS, Foster C, Grenier RP, et al. Peak exercise and immediate postexercise imaging for the detection of left ventricular function abnormalities in coronary artery disease. *Am J Cardiol* 1984; 53: 1532–1537.

Ellis SG, Wynne J, Braunwald E, et al. Response of reperfusion-salvaged stunned myocardium to inotropic stimulation. *Am Heart J* 1984; 107: 13–19.

Erbel R, Pop T, Henrichs K, et al. Percutaneous transluminal coronary angioplasty after thrombolytic therapy: a prospective controlled randomized trial. *J Am Coll Cardiol* 1986; 8: 485–495.

Foster E, O'Kelly B, LaPidus A, et al. Segmental analysis of resting echocardiographic function and stress scintigraphic perfusion: implications for myocardial viability. *Am Heart J* 1995; 129: 7–14.

Fournier C, Boujon B, Hebert JL, et al. Stunned myocardium following coronary spasm. *Am Heart J* 1991; 121: 593–595.

Fremes SE, Christakis GT, Weisel RD, et al. A clinical trial of blood and crystalloid cardioplegia. *J Thorac Cardiovasc Surg* 1984; 88: 725–741.

Fremes SE, Weisel RD, Mickle DAG, et al. Myocardial metabolism and ventricular function following cold potassium cardioplegia. *J Thorac Cardiovasc Surg* 1985; 89: 531–546.

Gray R, Maddhai J, Berman D, et al. Scintigraphic and hemodynamic demonstration of transient left ventricular dysfunction immediately after uncomplicated coronary artery bypass grafting. *J Thorac Cardiovasc Surg* 1979; 77: 504–510.

Grunwald AM, Watson DD, Holzgrefe HH, et al. Myocardial thallium-201 kinetics in normal and ischemic myocardium. *Circulation* 1981; 64: 610–618.

Hartley CJ, Rabinovitz RS, Lee HS, et al. Postoperative measurements of ventricular function in man using an implantable ultrasonic sensor. In: West AI, ed. *Catheter-based sensing and imaging technology*. Proc SPIE 1989; 1068: 53–58.

Hauser AM, Gangadharan V, Ramos RG, et al. Sequence of mechanical, electrocardiographic and clinical effects of repeated coronary artery occlusion in human beings: echocardiographic observations during coronary angioplasty. *J Am Coll Cardiol* 1985; 5: 193–197.

Heyndrickx GR, Millard RW, McRitchie RJ, et al. Regional myocardial functional and electrophysiological alterations after brief coronary artery occlusion in conscious dogs. *J Clin Invest* 1975; 56: 978–985.

Hirota Y, Kita Y, Tsuji R, et al. Prominent negative T waves with QT prolongation indicate reperfusion injury and myocardial stunning. *J Cardiol* 1992; 22: 325–340.

Homans DC, Laxson DD, Sublett E, et al. Cumulative deterioration of myocardial function after repeated episodes of exercise-induced ischemia. *Am J Physiol* 1989; 256: H1462–H1471.

Hood WB, Covell VH, Abelman WH, Norman JC. Persistence of contractile behavior in acutely ischemic myocardium. *Cardiovasc Res* 1969; 3: 249–260.

Iskandrian AS, Hakki A, Kane S. Resting thallium-201 myocardial perfusion patterns in patients with severe left ventricular dysfunction: differences between patients with primary cardiomyopathy, chronic coronary artery disease, or acute myocardial infarction. *Am Heart J* 1986; 111: 760–767.

Iskandrian AS, Hakki A, Kane SA, et al. Rest and redistribution thallium-201 myocardial scintigraphy to predict improvement in left ventricular function after coronary arterial bypass grafting. *Am J Cardiol* 1983; 51: 1312–1316.

Ito H, Tomooka T, Sakai N, et al. Time course of functional improvement in stunned myocardium in risk area in patients with reperfused anterior infarction. *Circulation* 1993; 87: 355–362.

Jeroudi MO, Cheirif J, Habib G, Bolli R. Prolonged wall motion abnormalities after chest pain at rest in patients with unstable angina: a possible manifestation of myocardial stunning. *Am Heart J* 1994; 127: 1241–1250.

Johnson WD, Kayser KL, Brenowitz JB, Saedi SF. A randomized controlled trial of allopurinol in coronary artery bypass surgery. *Am Heart J* 1991; 121: 20–24.

Kaul S, Kelly P, Oliner JD, et al. Assessment of regional myocardial blood flow with myocardial contrast two-dimensional echocardiography. *J Am Coll Cardiol* 1989; 13: 468–482.

Kiat H, Berman DS, Maddahi J, et al. Late reversibility of tomographic myocardial thallium-201 defects: an accurate marker of myocardial viability. *J Am Coll Cardiol* 1988; 12: 1456–1463.

Kloner RA, Allen J, Cox TA, et al. Stunned left ventricular myocardium after exercise treadmill testing in coronary artery disease. *Am J Cardiol* 1991; 68: 329–334.

Kolibask AJ, Goodenow JS, Busk CA, et al. Improvement of myocardial perfusion and left ventricular function after coronary artery bypass grafting in patients with unstable angina. *Circulation* 1979; 59: 66–74.

Labovitz AJ, Lewen MK, Kern M, et al. Evaluation of left ventricular systolic and diastolic dysfunction during transient myocardial ischemia produced by angioplasty. *J Am Coll Cardiol* 1987; 10: 748–755.

La Canna G, Alfieri O, Giubbini R, et al. Echocardiography during infusion of dobutamine for identification of reversible dysfunction in patients with chronic coronary artery disease. *J Am Coll Cardiol* 1994; 23: 617–626.

Mangano DT. Biventricular function after myocardial revascularization in humans: deterioration and recovery patterns during the first 24 hours. *Anesthesiology* 1985; 62: 571–577.

Mariani MA, Palagi C, Donatelli F, et al. Identification of hibernating myocardium: a comparison between dobutamine echocardiography and study of perfusion and metabolism in patients with severe left ventricular dysfunction. *Am J Card Imaging* 1995; 9: 1–8.

Marinho NVS, Keogh BE, Costa DC, et al. Pathophysiology of chronic left ventricular dysfunction: new insights from the measurement of absolute myocardial blood flow and glucose utilization. *Circulation* 1996; 93: 737–744.

Marzullo P, Parodi O, Reisenhofer B, et al. Value of rest thallium-201/technetium-99m sestamibi scans and dobutamine echocardiography for detecting myocardial viability. *Am J Cardiol* 1993a; 71: 166–172.

Marzullo P, Parodi O, Sambuceti G, et al. Does the myocardium become "stunned" after episodes of angina at rest, angina on effort, and coronary angioplasty? *Am J Cardiol* 1993b; 71: 1045–1051.

Mathias P, Kerin NZ, Blevins RD, et al. Coronary vasospasm as a cause of stunned myocardium. *Am Heart J* 1987; 113: 383–385.

Mercier JC, Lando U, Kanmatsuse K, et al. Divergent effects of inotropic stimulation on the ischemic and severely depressed reperfused myocardium. *Circulation* 1982; 66: 397–400.

Moore CA, Cannon J, Watson DD, et al. Thallium-201 kinetics in stunned myocardium characterized by severe postischemic systolic dysfunction. *Circulation* 1990; 81: 1622–1632.

Neely JR, Rovetto MJ, Oram JF. Myocardial utilization of carbohydrate and lipids. *Prog Cardiovasc Dis* 1972; 15: 289–329.

Nesto RW, Chon LH, Collin Jr JJ, et al. Inotropic contractile reserve: a useful predictor of increased 5-year survival and improved postoperative left ventricular function in patients with coronary artery disease and reduced ejection fraction. *Am J Cardiol* 1982; 50: 39–44.

Nixon JV, Brown CN, Smitherman TC. Identification of transient and persistent segmental wall motion abnormalities in patients with unstable angina by two-dimensional echocardiography. *Cirulation* 1982; 65: 1497–1503.

Ohtani H, Tamaki N, Yonekura Y, et al. Value of thallium-201 reinjection after delayed SPECT imaging for predicting reversible ischemia after coronary artery bypass grafting. *Am J Cardiol* 1990; 66: 394–399.

Panza JA, Dilsizian V, Laurienzo JM, et al. Relation between thallium uptake and contractile response to dobutamine: implications regarding myocardial viability in patients with chronic coronary artery disease and left ventricular dysfunction. *Circulation* 1995; 91: 990–998.

Picano E, Marzullo P, Gigli G, et al. Identification of viable myocardium by dipyridamole-induced improvement in regional left ventricular function assessed by echocardiography in myocardial infarction and comparison with thallium scintigraphy at rest. *Am J Cardiol* 1992; 70: 703–710.

Piérard LA, De Lansheere CM, Berthe C, et al. Identification of viable myocardium by echocardiography during dobutamine infusion in patients with myocardial infarction after thrombolytic therapy: comparison with positron emission tomography. *J Am Coll Cardiol* 1990; 15: 1021–1031.

Pigott JD, Kouchoukos NT, Oberman A, Cutter GR. Late results of surgical and medical therapy for patients with coronary artery disease and depressed left ventricular function. *J Am Coll Cardiol* 1985; 5: 1036–1045.

Previtali M, Poli A, Lanzarini L, et al. Dobutamine stress echocardiography for assessment of myocardial viability and ischemia in acute myocardial infarction treated with thrombolysis. *Am J Cardiol* 1993; 72: 124G–130G.

Priest MF, Curry GC, Smith LR, et al. Changes in left ventricular segmental wall motion following randomization to medicine or surgery in patients with unstable angina. *Circulation* 1978; 58(Suppl I): I-62–I-68.

Ragosta M, Camarano G, Kaul S, et al. Microvascular integrity indicates myocellular viability in patients with recent myocardial infarction: new insights using myocardial contrast echocardiography. *Circulation* 1994; 89: 2562–2569.

Rahimtoola SH. A perspective on the three large multicenter randomized clinical trials of coronary bypass surgery for chronic stable angina. *Circulation* 1985; 75(Suppl V): V-123–V-135.

Rahimtoola SH. The hibernating myocardium. *Am Heart J* 1989; 117: 211–221.

Reduto LA, Lawrie GM, Reid JW, et al. Sequential postoperative assessment of left ventricular performance with gated cardiac blood pool imaging following aortocoronary bypass surgery. *Am Heart J* 1981a; 101: 59–66.

Reduto LA, Smalling RW, Freund GC, Gould KL. Intracoronary infusion of streptokinase in patients with acute myocardial infarction: effects of reperfusion on left ventricular performance. *Am J Cardiol* 1981b; 48: 403–409.

Renkin J, Wijns W, Ladha Z, Col J. Reversal of segmental hypokinesis by coronary angioplasty in patients with unstable angina, persistent T wave inversion, and left anterior descending coronary artery stenosis: additional evidence for myocardial stunning in humans. *Circulation* 1990; 82: 912–921.

Roberts AJ, Spies M, Meyers SN, et al. Early and long term improvement in left ventricular performance following coronary bypass surgery. *Surgery* 1980; 88: 467–475.

Roberts AJ, Spies M, Sanders JH, et al. Serial assessment of left ventricular performance following coronary artery bypass grafting. *J Thorac Cardiovasc Surg* 1981; 81: 69–84.

Robertson WS, Feigenbaum H, Armstrong WF, et al. Exercise echocardiography: a clinical practical addition in the evaluation of coronary artery disease. *J Am Coll Cardiol* 1983; 6: 1085–1089.

Rocco TP, Dilsizian V, McKusick KA, et al. Comparison of thallium redistribution with rest "reinjection" imaging for the detection of viable myocardium. *Am J Cardiol* 1990; 66: 158–163.

Rocco TP, Dilsizian V, Strauss HW, Boucher CA. Technetium-99m isonitrile myocardial uptake at rest. II. Relation to clinical markers of potential viability. *J Am Coll Cardiol* 1989; 14: 1678–1684.

Ross Jr J. Myocardial perfusion-contraction matching: implications for coronary heart disease and hibernation. *Circulation* 1991; 83: 1076–1083.

Sabia PJ, Powers ER, Ragosta M, et al. An association between collateral blood flow and myocardial viability in patients with recent myocardial infarction. *N Engl J Med* 1992; 327: 1825–1831.

Salustri A, Elhendy A, Garyfallydis P, et al. Prediction of improvement of ventricular function after first acute myocardial infarction using low-dose dobutamine stress echocardiography. *Am J Cardiol* 1994; 74: 853–856.

Satler LF, Kent KM, Fox LM, et al. The assessment of contractile reserve after thrombolytic therapy for acute myocardial infarction. *Am Heart J* 1986; 111: 821–825.

Schmidt WG, Sheehan FH, von Essen R, et al. Evolution of left ventricular function after intracoronary thrombolysis for acute myocardial infarction. *Am J Cardiol* 1989; 63: 497–502.

Schneider RM, Weintraub WS, Klein LW, et al. Rate of left ventricular function recovery by radionuclide angiography after exercise in coronary artery disease. *Am J Cardiol* 1986; 57: 927–932.

Schroeder R, Biamino G, von Leitner E-R, et al. Intravenous shortterm infusion of streptokinase in acute myocardial infarction. *Circulation* 1983; 67: 536–548.

Schulz R, Guth BD, Pieper K, et al. Recruitment of an inotropic reserve in moderately ischemic myocardium at the expense of metabolic recovery. *Circ Res* 1992; 70: 1282–1295.

Schwaiger M, Hicks R. The clinical role of metabolic imaging of the heart by positron emission tomography. *J Nucl Med* 1991; 32: 565–578.

Scognamiglio R, Ponchia A, Fasoli G, et al. Exercise-induced left ventricular dysfunction in coronary heart disease: a model for studying the stunned myocardium in man. *Eur Heart J* 1991; 12 (Suppl G): 16–19.

Serruys PW, Simoons ML, Suryapranata H, et al. Preservation of global and regional left ventricular function after early thrombolysis in acute myocardial infarction. *J Am Coll Cardiol* 1986; 7: 729–742.

Serruys PW, Wijns W, van den Brand M, et al. Left ventricular performance, regional blood flow, wall motion and lactate metabolism during transluminal angioplasty. *Circulation* 1984; 70: 24–36.

Sheiban I, Tonni S, Benussi P, et al. Left ventricular dysfunction following transient ischemia induced by transluminal coronary angioplasty. Beneficial effects of calcium antagonists against post-ischemic myocardial stunning. *Eur Heart J* 1993; 14(Suppl A): 14–21.

Shen Y-T, Vatner SF. Mechanism of impaired myocardial function during progressive coronary stenosis in conscious pigs: hibernation versus stunning? *Circ Res* 1995; 73: 479–488.

Simek CL, Watson DD, Smith WH, et al. Dipyridamole thallium-201 imaging versus dobutamine echocardiography for the evaluation of coronary artery disease in patients unable to exercise. *Am J Cardiol* 1993; 72: 1257–1262.

Sinusas AJ, Trautman KA, Bergin JD, et al. Quantification of area at risk during coronary occlusion and degree of myocardial salvage after repercussion with technetium-99m methoxyisobutyl isonitrile. *Circulation* 1990; 82: 1424–1437.

Sinusas AJ, Watson DD, Cannon JM, Beller GA. Effect of ischemia and postischemic dysfunction on myocardial uptake of technetium-99m-labeled methoxyisobutyl isonitrile and thallium-201. *J Am Coll Cardiol* 1989; 14: 1785–1793.

Smart SC, Sawada S, Ryan T, et al. Low-dose dobutamine echocardiography detects reversible dysfunction after thrombolytic therapy of acute myocardial infarction. *Circulation* 1993; 88: 405–415.

Stack RS, Phillips III HR, Grierson DS, et al. Functional improvement of jeopardized myocardium following intracoronary streptokinase infusion in acute myocardial infarction. *J Clin Invest* 1983; 72: 84–95.

Stahl LD, Aversano TR, Becker LC. Selective enhancement of function of stunned myocardium by increased flow. *Circulation* 1986; 74: 843–851.

Stoddard MF, Johnstone J, Dillon S, Kupersmith J. The effect of exercise-induced myocardial ischemia on postischemic left ventricular diastolic filling. *Clin Cardiol* 1992; 15: 265–273.

Takatsu F, Suzuki A, Nagaya T. Variant angina pectoris with prolonged electrical and mechanical stunning. *Am J Cardiol* 1986; 58: 647–649.

Tamaki N, Yonekura Y, Yamashita K, et al. Positron emission tomography using fluorine-18deoxyglucose in evaluation of coronary artery bypass grafting. *Am J Cardiol* 1989; 64: 860–865.

Tamaki N, Yonekura Y, Yamashita K, et al. Relation of left ventricular perfusion and wall motion with metabolic activity in persistent defects on thallium-201 tomography in healed myocardial infarction. *Am J Cardiol* 1988, 62: 202–208.

Tillisch J, Brunken R, Marshall R, et al. Reversibility of cardiac wall-motion abnormalities predicted by positron tomography. *N Engl J Med* 1986; 314: 884–888.

Topol EJ, Weiss JL, Brinker JA, et al. Regional wall motion improvement after coronary thrombolysis with recombinant tissue plasminogen activator: importance of coronary angioplasty. *J Am Coll Cardiol* 1985; 6: 426–433.

Uretsky BF. Physiology of the transplanted heart. In: Brest AN, ed. *Cardiovascular clinics*. Philadelphia: FA Davis, 1990: 23–56.

Vanoverschelde J-LJ, Wijns W, Depre C, et al. Mechanism of chronic regional postischemic dysfunction in humans: new insights from the study of noninfarcted collateral-dependent myocardium. *Circulation* 1993; 87: 1513–1523.

Visser CA, David GK, Kan G, et al. Two-dimensional echocardiography during percutaneous transluminal coronary angioplasty. *Am Heart J* 1986; 111: 1035–1046.

Watada H, Ito H, Oh H, et al. Dobutamine stress echocardiography predicts reversible dysfunction and quantitates the extent of irreversibly damaged myocardium after reprefusion of anterior myocardial infarction. *J Am Coll Cardiol* 1994; 24: 624–630.

Weich HF, Strauss HW, Pitt B. The extraction of thallium-201 by the myocardium. *Circulation* 1977; 56: 188–191.

Werns S, Brinker J, Gruber J, et al. A randomized, double-blind trial of recombinant human superoxide dismutase in patients undergoing PTCA for acute myocardial infarction. *Circulation* 1989; 80: 113.

Wicomb WN, Cooper DKC, Novitzky D, Barnard CN. Cardiac transplantation following storage of the donor heart by a portable hypothermic perfusin system. *Ann Thorac Surg* 1984; 37: 243–248.

Wijns W, Serruys PW, Slager CJ, et al. Effect of coronary occlusion during percutaneous transluminal angioplasty in humans on left ventricular chamber stiffness and regional diastolic pressure-radius relations. *J Am Coll Cardiol* 1986; 7: 455–461.

Williamson BD, Lim MJ, Buda AJ. Transient left ventricular filling abnormalities (distolic stunning) after acute myocardial infarction. *Am J Cardiol* 1990; 12: 897–903.

Wolfgelernter D, Cleman M, Highman HA, et al. Regional myocardial dyfunction during coronary angioplasty: evaluation by two-dimensional echocardiography and 12 lead electrocardiography. *J Am Coll Cardiol* 1986; 7: 1245–1254.

Yang LD, Berman DS, Kiat H, et al. The frequency of late reversibility in SPECT thallium-201 stress-redistribution studies. *J Am Coll Cardiol* 1990; 15: 334–340.

Zaret BL, Wackers FJT, Terrin ML, et al. Assessment of global and regional left ventricular performance at rest and during exercise after thrombolytic therapy for acute myocardial infarction: results of the thrombolysis in myocardial infarction (TIMI) II study. *Am J Cardiol* 1992; 69: 1–9.

Zoghbi WA, Marion A, Cheirif JB, et al. Time course of recovery of regional function following thrombolysis in acute myocardial infarction (TIMI): preliminary observatoins for the TIMI trial phase II [Abstract]. *J Am Coll Cardiol* 1990; 15: 233A.

CHAPTER 11

Characterization of Short-term Hibernating Myocardium

Gerd Heusch
Rainer Schulz

DEFINITION OF THE TERM HIBERNATING MYOCARDIUM

On the basis of clinical observations in patients with coronary artery disease and chronically depressed LV function that normalized on coronary revascularization, Rahimtoola (1985) coined the term *myocardial hibernation*: a state of chronic contractile dysfunction over months and possibly years that is reversible on reperfusion.

The term *hibernation* has been borrowed from zoology and implies that the observed reduction in contractile function is an adaptive and regulatory event acting to preserve viability. This concept has subsequently gained support from experimental studies, which were well controlled, however confined to an observation period of only a few hours. Therefore, Ross (1989, 1991) proposed the term *short-term myocardial hibernation*.

Since it is still unclear whether or not short-term myocardial hibernation progresses into long-term myocardial hibernation, as observed in the clinical setting, these two phenomena should be treated as separate entities at present.

TIME SEQUENCE OF EVENTS FOLLOWING ACUTE ISCHEMIA

On acute coronary artery occlusion, contractile function in the ischemic region rapidly ceases. Within a few cardiac cycles systolic segment shortening and systolic wall thickening are reduced (hypokinesis), later abolished (akinesis), and within 30 seconds to 2 minutes replaced by paradoxic systolic segment lengthening and systolic wall thinning (dyskinesis, bulging) (Theroux et al., 1974, 1976). Electrophysiological changes in the surface ECG occur only after the loss of systolic wall excursion, and changes in the local subendocardial ECG occur even later than those in the surface ECG (Battler et al., 1980). During more moderate regional contractile dysfunction distal to a coronary artery stenosis, ischemic changes become apparent in the local ECG, but not in the surface ECG (Battler et al., 1980). Thus, loss of regional contractile activity is a rapid, sensitive, and important consequence of regional myocardial ischemia.

MECHANISMS OF ACUTE ISCHEMIC CONTRACTILE DYSFUNCTION

ATP is well accepted as the ultimate source of energy for the contractile process. Understandably then, the reduced concentration of ATP has been proposed as the mechanism of acute ischemic contractile dysfunction (Hearse, 1979). A causal link between the appearance of regional ischemic contractile dysfunction and the loss of regional myocardial ATP, however, has never been proven experimentally. In the inner myocardial layers of anesthetized swine, ATP is reduced within 15 cardiac cycles following an acute reduction in myocardial blood flow. However, contractile dysfunction occurs prior to changes in myocardial ATP (Arai et al., 1992). A further and compelling argument against ATP loss as the mediator of acute ischemic contractile failure is that the result of ATP loss should be rigor of the myofibrils rather than the observed loss of wall tension (Katz, 1973). This apparent discrepancy can be at least partially reconciled if the early ATP loss acts not as a primary energy depletion, but through a modulatory mechanism that could interfere with excitation-contraction coupling (Kübler & Katz, 1977).

Activation of ATP-dependent potassium channels by an ischemia-induced decrease in myocardial ATP, an increase in the intracellular proton or lactate concentrations, or by activation of adenosine A_1 receptors could increase potassium efflux, thereby reducing the action potential duration and subsequently calcium influx into the myocyte (Noma, 1983). Such decreased intracellular calcium concentration could then reduce contractile function and ATP consumption. Indeed, blockade of ATP-dependent potassium channels abolishes the hypoxia-induced reduction of global LV function in saline-perfused rat hearts (Decking et al., 1995). In contrast, in anesthetized swine in situ, blockade of ATP-dependent potassium channels does prevent the ischemic reduction of action potential duration, but does not alter ischemic contractile dysfunction or the myocardial ATP concentration (Schulz et al., 1995).

Apart from changes in the absolute concentration of myocardial ATP, a decrease in the free energy change of ATP hydrolysis could be responsible for the decrease in contractile function. Indeed the reduction in the free energy change of ATP hydrolysis correlates well with the onset of contractile dysfunction in isolated saline perfused hearts (Kammermeier et al., 1982).

Other mediators that have been proposed to be involved in the development of early ischemic contractile dysfunction are the accumulation of lactate (Jacobus et al., 1982), a decrease in the intracellular pH (Jacobus et al.,1982), or a disturbance in the calcium handling of the SR (Krause & Hess, 1984; Kübler & Katz, 1977). Also, collapse of the coronary arteries has been suggested to be responsible for the decrease in contractile function early during ischemia (Koretsune et al., 1991). The accumulation of inorganic phosphate resulting from the ischemic breakdown of myocardial creatine phosphate and ATP, however, is the most likely candidate responsible for the early ischemic decrease in contractile function (Kusuoka et al., 1986). The increase in inorganic phosphate could reduce contractile function by direct binding to contractile proteins (Rüegg et al., 1971), an uncoupling of the myofibrillar ATPase activity (Schmidt-Ott et al., 1990), or by desensitization of myofibrils for calcium (Kentish, 1986).

To summarize, potential mechanisms of acute ischemic contractile dysfunction are as follows:

- Reduction in myocardial ATP concentration (Hearse, 1979)
- Reduction of free energy change of ATP hydrolysis (Kammermeier et al., 1982)
- Accumulation of inorganic phosphate (Kübler & Katz, 1977; Kusuoka et al., 1986)
- Accumulation of protons and lactate (Jacobus et al., 1982)
- Disturbance in calcium handling of the SR (Krause & Hess, 1984; Kübler & Katz, 1977)
- Desensitization of myofibrils to calcium (Kentish, 1986; Kusuoka et al., 1986)
- Collapse of coronary arteries (Koretsune et al., 1991)

TRANSITION FROM AN IMBALANCE BETWEEN SUPPLY AND DEMAND TOWARD SHORT-TERM MYOCARDIAL HIBERNATION

Within the first few seconds following an acute reduction of myocardial blood flow, energy demand of the hypoperfused myocardium clearly exceeds the reduced energy supply. However, this imbalance between energy supply and demand is an inherently unstable condition since ischemia induces mechanisms that reduce contractile function and thus energy demand (Guth et al., 1993). In the subsequent steady-state condition, the amount of contractile dysfunction is in proportion to the reduction of myocardial blood flow (Gallagher et al., 1980; Vatner, 1980)—in other words, a state of perfusion-contraction matching exists (Ross, 1989, 1991). The characterization of short-term hibernating myocardium is as follows:

- Balance between the reduced regional myocardial blood flow and the reduced contractile function (perfusion-contraction matching) (Matsuzaki et al., 1983; Ross, 1989, 1991)
- Recovery of contractile function during reperfusion (Downing & Chen, 1992; Matsuzaki et al., 1983)
- Recovery of metabolic parameters (creatine phosphate, lactate) during persistent ischemia (Arai et al., 1991; Downing & Chen, 1990; Fedele et al., 1988; Pantely et al., 1990; Schulz et al., 1992)

- Recruitable inotropic reserve at the expense of metabolic recovery (Schulz et al., 1992, 1993)

In chronically instrumented, conscious dogs, a reduction in myocardial blood flow associated with a decrease in regional contractile function by 40% can be maintained for 5 hours without the development of necroses within the dysfunctional myocardium. Regional contractile function recovers during reperfusion, but full recovery requires 7 days (Matsuzaki et al., 1983).

METABOLISM OF SHORT-TERM HIBERNATING MYOCARDIUM

Within the first 5 minutes of an acute coronary inflow reduction, coronary venous pH and lactate extraction are reduced and coronary venous pCO_2 increases. These parameters, however, gradually return to control values during continued moderate ischemia (Fedele et al., 1988). Likewise, during constant moderate ischemia myocardial creatine phosphate concentration is significantly decreased immediately after the onset of ischemia, but gradually recovers over time to control values, whereas regional contractile function is persistently reduced (Arai et al., 1991; Pantely et al., 1990; Schulz et al., 1992).

These studies are consistent with the idea that there is only a transient phase of an energetic supply/demand imbalance during early myocardial ischemia. The ensuing reduction in regional myocardial function may induce a down-regulation of energy demand and allow stabilization at a new metabolic level characterized again by an energetic balance, as indicated by the recovery of metabolic markers.

RECRUITMENT OF AN INOTROPIC RESERVE AT THE EXPENSE OF METABOLIC RECOVERY IN SHORT-TERM HIBERNATING MYOCARDIUM

Although baseline contractile function is depressed, the hypoperfused myocardium retains its responsiveness to an inotropic challenge (Schulz et al., 1992). When, after 85 to 90 minutes of sustained moderate ischemia in anesthetized pigs, dobutamine is infused selectively into the ischemic region, contractile function increases, although regional blood flow remains reduced (Fig. 11-1). Thus, energy is available in the ischemic myocardium that is not used to maintain baseline function, but permits the increase in contractile function on an inotropic challenge. These results suggest that the decrease in contractile function secondary to a reduction in myocardial blood flow is not simply the consequence of an energetic deficit, but rather reflects an active adaptive process of the myocardium. Imposition of an inotropic stimulus on the short-term hibernating myocardium disrupts this adaptive process, as indicated by the once more decreased myocardial creatine phosphate concentration and increased lactate production.

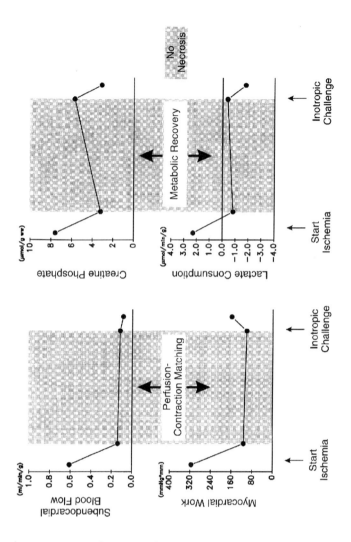

Figure 11-1. *Within the first few seconds following an acute reduction of myocardial blood flow, energy demand of the hypoperfused myocardium clearly exceeds the reduced energy supply, resulting in a reduction in myocardial creatine phosphate content and a reversal of lactate consumption into net lactate production. However, this imbalance between energy supply and demand is an inherently unstable condition since ischemia induces mechanisms that reduce contractile function and thus energy demand in proportion to the reduction of myocardial blood flow (i.e., a state of perfusion-contraction matching exists). With the extension of ischemia, in a situation of perfusion-contraction matching, lactate production is attenuated and myocardial creatine phosphate content recovers to control values. Infusion of dobutamine increases regional contractile function at an unchanged subendocardial blood flow, thereby disrupting the adaptive state of the myocardium, as indicated by renewed increased lactate production and renewed decreased myocardial creatine phosphate content. (Data adapted from Schulz and colleagues [1992].)*

A similar disruption of the developing metabolic balance after prolonged moderate ischemia is observed on a chronotropic challenge (Arai et al., 1991). Increasing heart rate by atrial pacing in this particular study, however, increased the severity of ischemia and reduced regional myocardial blood flow, function, and creatine phosphate content, and increased lactate production. Since the severity of ischemia was increased, the observed metabolic deterioration during pacing does not conclusively demonstrate active adaptation of energy demand during the preceding more moderate ischemia.

ENERGETIC LIMITATIONS OF SHORT-TERM HIBERNATION

As already stated, the development of such a delicate balance between regional myocardial blood flow and function during early ischemia is disturbed by unfavorable alterations in supply and demand. When, in anesthetized pigs after 5 minutes of ischemia, at a blood flow reduction compatible with the development of myocardial hibernation over 90 minutes, energy supply is further reduced by an additional reduction of myocardial blood flow, necroses develop. The lower limit of myocardial blood flow compatible with the development of myocardial hibernation amounts to approximately 25% of baseline in the experimental setting (Schulz et al., 1993).

Also, a further increase in energy demand by continuous inotropic stimulation with dobutamine induces necrosis (Schulz et al., 1993). Thus, both the further reduction in energy supply by an increasing severity of ischemia and an enhanced energy expenditure by continuous inotropic stimulation impair the development of short-term myocardial hibernation and precipitate myocardial infarction.

MECHANISMS OF SHORT-TERM HIBERNATING MYOCARDIUM

The mechanisms responsible for the development of short-term myocardial hibernation remain unclear at present. Alterations in the beta-adrenoceptor density or affinity as the underlying mechanism of such an adaptive process have been excluded (Schulz et al., 1993).

As mentioned earlier, the ischemia-induced activation of ATP-dependent potassium channels might increase potassium efflux, thereby reducing the action potential duration and subsequently the calcium influx into the cardiomyocyte. Such decreased intracellular calcium concentration could then reduce contractile function and ATP consumption, thus finally allowing the development of myocardial hibernation. Indeed, monophasic action potential duration shortens during ischemia, and this shortening is prevented by a blockade of ATP-dependent potassium channels with glibenclamide. However, complete blockade of ATP-dependent potassium channels neither alters contractile function, metabolic parameters, nor myocardial viability. Obviously, activation of ATP-dependent potassium channels is therefore not involved in the development of short-term myocardial hibernation (Schulz et al., 1995).

Endogenous adenosine (which is released during ischemia) might, through a number of secondary mechanisms (such as inhibition of adenylate cyclase activity, inhibition of norepinephrine release from sympathetic nerve endings, or inhibition of L-type calcium channels), attenuate the decrease in myocardial energy-rich phosphates and the increase in intracellular calcium concentration, thereby preserving myocardial viability during ischemia. However, a role for endogenous adenosine in the development of hibernation has been excluded, since neither contractile function, metabolic parameters, nor viability are altered by increased catabolism of endogenous adenosine by infusion of adenosine deaminase (Schulz et al., 1995).

In short-term hibernating myocardium, regional contractile function is decreased without apparent alterations in the calcium sensitivity. In anesthetized pigs after 90 minutes of ischemia, at a time when lactate production is attenuated and creatine phosphate is restored to a value no longer significantly different from the respective control value, the maximal responses to graded intracoronary calcium infusion and postextrasystolic potentiation are decreased. However, the relationships between the fractional increases in regional contractile function and dose of added intracoronary calcium and the postextrasystolic time interval, respectively, are not different (Heusch et al., 1996).

PROGRESSION OF SHORT-TERM HIBERNATION TO LONG-TERM HIBERNATION

It is still unclear whether or not short-term myocardial hibernation progresses to long-term myocardial hibernation. Whereas short-term hibernation is well characterized in animal experiments, the existence of hibernation over weeks or months (long-term hibernation) can only be inferred from clinical studies. Hibernation, as defined by Rahimtoola, is a state of chronic contractile dysfunction secondary to coronary artery disease that is fully reversible on reperfusion. In long-term hibernating myocardium morphological alterations occur. In myocardial biopsies from patients with prolonged contractile dysfunction that was reversible after bypass surgery, myofibrils are reduced in number and disorganized. Myocardial glycogen content as well as the extracellular collagen network are increased (Flameng et al., 1981). Thus, despite the fact that the myocardium remains viable during persistent ischemia and contractile dysfunction is reversible on reperfusion (Rahimtoola, 1985), there are severe morphological alterations. Understandably, full functional recovery following reperfusion can therefore require weeks or even months (Rahimtoola, 1985). The reasons for the morphological alterations (degeneration [Elsässer & Schaper, 1995] or dedifferentiation [Borgers & Ausma, 1995]) are not clear at present.

It is still under debate whether chronic contractile dysfunction occurs during persistent mild ischemia (i.e., true long-term myocardial hibernation) or is the result of repetitive episodes of ischemia and reperfusion (i.e., stunning). In patients with a complete occlusion of a major coronary artery but extensive collateral circulation (Vanoverschelde et al., 1993), as well as in pigs with a chronic coronary artery stenosis (Shen & Vatner, 1995), chronic contractile dysfunction is observed at normal (Shen & Vatner, 1995) or almost-normal (Vanoverschelde et al., 1993) resting myocardial blood flows. At normal or almost-normal resting blood flow but impaired coronary reserve, there could indeed be repetitive episodes of exercise-induced ischemia and reperfusion inducing stunning, which then result in chronic contractile dysfunction. Nevertheless, these studies do not rule out the existence of true myocardial hibernation—a situation of chronic contractile dysfunction during persistent ischemia.

There are a few experimental studies that tried to investigate the transition process from short-term hibernation to long-term hibernation by subjecting swine to a partial coronary artery stenosis for 1 day (Chen et al., 1995), 4 to 7 days (Bolukoglu et al., 1992; Liedtke et al., 1994, 1995), or even up to 32 weeks (Mills et al., 1994). These studies, however, failed to monitor continuously myocardial blood flow and contractile function over the entire time period of coronary hypoperfusion. When resting regional myocardial blood flow was measured (Chen et al., 1995; Liedtke, 1995; Mills et al., 1994), it was found to be reduced at the beginning and the end of the stenosis protocol (Chen et al., 1995; Mills et al., 1994), except for one study where it was almost normal at the beginning and the end of the stenosis protocol (Liedtke et al., 1995). Changes in the severity of ischemia between these two measurements could not be ruled out, and therefore these studies do not prove or disprove the existence of true myocardial hibernation.

RELEVANCE TO CLINICIANS

In contrast to dysfunctional, irreversibly damaged myocardium, the hibernating myocardium retains an inotropic reserve. To further distinguish hibernating from stunned myocardium, either regional myocardial blood flow must be measured or the metabolic changes associated with an inotropic challenge must be analyzed.

Demonstration of a perfusion-contraction match (i.e., decreased contraction in the face of decreased perfusion)

- PET (^{13}N, ^{15}O)
- Thallium-201 scintigraphy, in particular with redistribution or reinjection
- Tc-99m sestamibi scintigraphy, in particular with redistribution or reinjection
- Techniques requiring concurrent assessment of function by other methods, including ventriculography and echocardiography

Demonstration of a perfusion-metabolism mismatch (i.e., increased glycolytic metabolism in the face of decreased perfusion)

- PET ([18]FDG, ^{13}N, ^{15}O)

Demonstration of an inotropic reserve at the expense of worsening of myocardial metabolism

- Dobutamine echocardiography
- Postextrasystolic potentiation during contrast ventriculography or echocardiography
- Techniques requiring concurrent assessment of myocardial metabolism by other methods include PET and coronary sinus lactate

The recruitment of an inotropic reserve in hibernating myocardium is at the expense of metabolic recovery (Schulz et al., 1992, 1993), while in stunned myocardium no metabolic deterioration occurs during inotropic stimulation (Görge et al., 1990).

Also, the extent of postsystolic wall thickening in the ischemic myocardium allows a distinction to be made between irreversibly damaged and viable short-term hibernating myocardium. The extent of postsystolic wall thickening at the end of a 90-minute ischemic period correlates inversely to the extent of necroses, and positively to myocardial creatine phosphate concentration, the dobutamine-recruitable inotropic reserve, and the functional recovery on reperfusion. Thus, the greater the postsystolic wall thickening, the more myocardium is successfully hibernating (Rose et al., 1993).

Hibernating myocardium, although exhibiting a number of cardioprotective features, is nevertheless ischemic and therefore a pathological condition. Thus, the only causal therapy of hibernating myocardium is to restore blood flow to the hypoperfused tissue.

OPEN QUESTIONS RELATED TO MYOCARDIAL HIBERNATION

1. How long can the ischemic myocardium maintain its metabolic integrity? It is possible that the metabolic status of short-term hibernating myocardium once again deteriorates over time. In this scenario, the decrease in contractile function during persistent, moderate ischemia is only a temporary mechanism to prolong myocardial viability but is inherently time limited. On the other hand, it is possible that the successfully adapted myocardium can maintain such a state indefinitely and will proceed to long-term hibernation.
2. What are the mechanisms responsible for the transition from an initial supply/demand imbalance to a state of perfusion-contraction matching?
3. How long can the ischemic myocardium respond to an inotropic stimulation? A progressive loss of myofibrils in ischemic myocardium may result in a reduction and finally loss of response to an inotropic challenge. Thus, the identification of viable, long-term hibernating myocardium by an inotropic challenge may eventually be lost.
4. Does chronic contractile dysfunction in patients reflect true hibernation (i.e., a situation of chronic con-

tractile dysfunction during persistent ischemia) or repetitive episodes of ischemia and reperfusion (i.e., repetitive stunning)?
5. Can myocardial hibernation be induced or reinforced? This is a challenging therapeutic goal, as it would extend the time frame for reperfusion interventions in patients with acute ischemic syndromes. In this respect, short-term myocardial hibernation (i.e., an endogenous cardioprotective mechanism during acute ischemic syndromes) may be a much more common and important phenomenon than long-term myocardial hibernation (Schulz & Heusch, 1995).

SUMMARY

Within a few seconds after a sudden reduction of coronary blood flow, regional contractile dysfunction ensues. The mechanisms responsible for the rapid reduction in contractile function during acute myocardial ischemia remain unclear, but may involve a rise in inorganic phosphate. When severe ischemia, such as resulting from a sudden and complete coronary artery occlusion, is prolonged for more than 20 to 40 minutes, myocardial infarction develops and there is irreversible loss of contractile function. When myocardial ischemia is less severe but nevertheless prolonged, the myocardium is dysfunctional but can remain viable.

In such ischemic and dysfunctional myocardium, contractile function is reduced in proportion to the reduction in regional myocardial blood flow (i.e., a state of perfusion-contraction matching or short-term myocardial hibernation exists). The metabolic status of such short-term hibernating myocardium improves over the first few hours as myocardial lactate production is attenuated and creatine phosphate, after an initial reduction, returns to control values. The hibernating myocardium can respond to an inotropic stimulation with increased contractile function, however, at the expense of a renewed worsening of the metabolic status. This situation of an increased regional contractile function at the expense of metabolic recovery during inotropic stimulation can be used to identify short-term hibernating myocardium. When inotropic stimulation is prolonged, the development of short-term hibernation is impaired and myocardial infarction develops. The mechanisms responsible for the development of short-term myocardial hibernation remain unclear at present; a significant involvement of adenosine and of activation of ATP-dependent potassium channels has been excluded.

REFERENCES

Arai AE, Pantely GA, Anselone CG, et al. Active downregulation of myocardial energy requirements during prolonged moderate ischemia in swine. *Circ Res* 69: 1991; 1458–1469.

Arai AE, Pantely GA, Thoma WJ, et al. Energy metabolism and contractile function after 15 beats of moderate myocardial ischemia. *Circ Res* 1992; 70: 1137–1145.

Battler A, Froelicher VF, Gallagher KP, et al. Dissociation between regional myocardial dysfunction and ECG changes during ischemia in the conscious dog. *Circulation* 1980; 62: 735–744.

Bolukoglu H, Liedtke AJ, Nellis SH, et al. An animal model of chronic coronary stenosis resulting in hibernating myocardium. *Am J Physiol* 1992; 263: H20–H29.

Borgers M, Ausma J. Structural aspects of the chronic hibernating myocardium in man. *Basic Res Cardiol* 1995; 90: 44–46.

Chen C, Li L, Chen LL, et al. Incremental doses of dobutamine induce a biphasic response in dysfunctional left ventricular regions subtending coronary stenoses. *Circulation* 1995; 92: 756–766.

Decking UKM, Reffelmann T, Schrader J, Kammermeier H. Hypoxia-induced activation of K_{ATP} channels limits energy depletion in the guinea pig heart. *Am J Physiol* 1995; 269: H734–H742.

Downing SE, Chen V. Myocardial hibernation in the ischemic neonatal heart. *Circ Res* 1990; 66: 763–772.

Downing SE, Chen V. Acute hibernation and reperfusion of the ischemic heart. *Circulation* 1992; 85: 699–707.

Elsässer A, Schaper J. Hibernating myocardium: adaptation or degeneration? *Basic Res Cardiol* 1995; 90: 47–48.

Fedele FA, Gewirtz H, Capone RJ, et al. Metabolic response to prolonged reduction of myocardial blood flow distal to a severe coronary artery stenosis. *Circulation* 1988; 78: 729–735.

Flameng W, Suy R, Schwarz F, et al. Ultrastructural correlates of left ventricular contraction abnormalities in patients with chronic ischemic heart disease: determinants of reversible segmental asynergy postrevascularization surgery. *Am Heart J* 1981; 102: 846–857.

Gallagher KP, Kumada T, Koziol JA, et al. Significance of regional wall thickening abnormalities relative to transmural myocardial perfusion in anesthetized dogs. *Circulation* 1980; 62: 1266–1274.

Görge G, Papageorgiou I, Lerch R. Epinephrine-stimulated contractile and metabolic reserve in postischemic rat myocardium. *Basic Res Cardiol* 1990; 85: 595–605.

Guth BD, Schulz R, Heusch G. Time course and mechanisms of contractile dysfunction during acute myocardial ischemia. *Circulation* 1993; 87(Suppl IV): IV-35–IV-42.

Hearse DJ. Oxygen deprivation and early myocardial contractile failure: a reassessment of the possible role of adenosine triphosphate. *Am J Cardiol* 1979; 44: 1115–1121.

Heusch G, Rose J, Skyschally A, et al. Calcium responsiveness in regional myocardial short-term hibernation and stunning in the in situ porcine heart—inotropic responses to postextrasystolic potentiation and intracoronary calcium. *Circulation* 1996; 93: 1556–1566.

Jacobus WE, Pores IH, Lucas SK, et al. Intracellular acidosis and contractility in normal and ischemic hearts examined by 31P NMR. *J Mol Cell Cardiol* 1982; 14: 13–20.

Kammermeier H, Schmidt P, Jüngling E. Free energy change of ATP-hydrolysis: a causal factor of early hypoxic failure of the myocardium? *J Mol Cell Cardiol* 1982; 14: 267–277.

Katz AM. Effects of ischemia on the contractile processes of heart muscle. *Am J Cardiol* 1973; 32: 456–460.

Kentish JC. The effects of inorganic phosphate and creatine phosphate on the force production in skinned muscle from rat vesicle. *J Physiol* 1986; 370: 585–604.

Koretsune Y, Corretti MC, Kusuoka H, Marban E. Mechanism of early ischemic contractile failure. *Circ Res* 1991; 68: 255–262.

Krause S, Hess ML. Characterization of cardiac sarcoplasmic reticulum dysfunction during short-term, normothermic, global ischemia. *Circ Res* 1984; 55: 176–184.

Kübler W, Katz AM. Mechanism of early "pump" failure of the ischemic heart: possible role of adenosine triphosphate depletion and inorganic phosphate accumulation. *Am J Cardiol* 1977; 40: 467–471.

Kusuoka H, Weisfeldt ML, Zweier JL, et al. Mechanism of early contractile failure during hypoxia in intact ferret heart: evidence for modulation of maximal Ca-activated force by inorganic phosphate. *Circ Res* 1986; 59: 270–282.

Liedtke AJ, Renstrom B, Nellis SH, et al. Mechanical and metabolic functions in pig hearts after 4 days of chronic coronary stenosis. *J Am Coll Cardiol* 1995; 26: 815–828.

Liedtke AJ, Renstrom B, Nellis SH, Subramanian R. Myocardial function and metabolism in pig hearts after relief from chronic partial coronary stenosis. *Am J Physiol* 1994; 267: H1312–H1319.

Matsuzaki M, Gallagher KP, Kemper WS, et al. Sustained regional dysfunction produced by prolonged coronary stenosis: gradual recovery after reperfusion. *Circulation* 1983; 68: 170–182.

Mills I, Fallon JT, Wrenn D, et al. Adaptive responses of coronary circulation and myocardium to chronic reduction in perfusion pressure and flow. *Am J Physiol* 1994; 266: H447–H457.

Noma A. ATP-regulated K+ channels in cardiac muscle. *Nature* 1983; 305: 147–148.

Pantely GA, Malone SA, Rhen WS, et al. Regeneration of myocardial phosphocreatine in pigs despite continued moderate ischemia. *Circ Res* 1990; 67: 1481–1493.

Rahimtoola SH. A perspective on the three large multicenter randomized clinical trials of coronary bypass surgery for chronic stable angina. *Circulation* 1985; 72(Suppl V): V-123–V-135.

Rose J, Schulz R, Martin C, Heusch G. Post-ejection wall thickening as a marker of successful short term hibernation. *Cardiovasc Res* 1993; 27: 1306–1311.

Ross Jr J. Mechanisms of regional ischemia and antianginal drug action during exercise. *Prog Cardiovasc Dis* 1989; 31: 455–466.

Ross Jr J. Myocardial perfusion-contraction matching. Implications for coronary heart disease and hibernation. *Circulation* 1991; 83: 1076–1083.

Rüegg JC, Schädler M, Steiger GJ, Müller G. Effect of inorganic phosphate on the contractile mechanism. *Pflügers Arch* 1971; 325: 359–364.

Schmidt-Ott SC, Bletz C, Vahl C, et al. Inorganic phosphate inhibits contractility and ATPase activity in skinned fibers from human myocardium. *Basic Res Cardiol* 1990; 85: 358–366.

Schulz R, Guth BD, Pieper K, et al. Recruitment of an inotropic reserve in moderately ischemic myocardium at the expense of metabolic recovery: a model of short-term hibernation. *Circ Res* 1992; 70: 1282–1295.

Schulz R, Heusch G. Acute adaptation to ischemia: short-term myocardial hibernation. *Basic Res Cardiol* 1995; 90: 29–31.

Schulz R, Rose J, Martin C, et al. Development of short-term myocardial hibernation: its limitation by the severity of ischemia and inotropic stimulation. *Circulation* 1993; 88: 684–695.

Schulz R, Rose J, Post H, Heusch G. Regional short-term hibernation in swine does not involve endogenous adenosine or K_{ATP} channels. *Am J Physiol* 1995; 268: H2294–H3201.

Shen Y-T, Vatner SF. Mechanism of impaired myocardial function during progressive coronary stenosis in conscious pigs. Hibernation versus stunning. *Circ Res* 1995; 76: 479–488.

Theroux P, Franklin D, Ross Jr J, Kemper WS. Regional myocardial function during acute coronary artery occlusion and its modification by pharmacological agents in the dog. *Circ Res* 1974; 35: 896–908.

Theroux P, Ross Jr J, Franklin D, et al. Regional myocardial function in the conscious dog during acute coronary occlusion and responses to morphine, propranolol, nitroglycerin, and lidocaine. *Circulation* 1976; 53: 302–314.

Vanoverschelde JLJ, Wijns W, Depré C, et al. Mechanisms of chronic region postischemic dysfunction in humans. New insights from the study of noninfarcted collateral-dependent myocardium. *Circulation* 1993; 87: 1513–1523.

Vatner SF. Correlation between acute reductions in myocardial blood flow and function in conscious dogs. *Circ Res* 1980; 47: 201–207.

CHAPTER 12

Myocardial Hibernation: An Adaptive Phenomenon?

Roberto Ferrari

Hibernation comes from the Latin word *hiberna*, meaning *winter*, and is a sort of dormancy occurring on a seasonal basis in many animals, including certain mammals. Under this condition, the metabolic rate falls to low levels so that the animal draws on its reserves very slowly.

In the context of coronary artery disease, the concept of myocardial hibernation was generated on clinical grounds in the early 1980s when Rahimtoola, in reviewing the results of coronary artery bypass surgery trials, identified patients with coronary artery disease and chronic LV dysfunction that improved on revascularization (Rahimtoola, 1981, 1985). Later, he defined myocardial hibernation as a state of persistently impaired myocardial and LV function at rest due to reduced coronary blood flow that can be partially or completely restored to normal, if the myocardial oxygen supply-demand relationship is favorably altered, either by improving blood flow and/or by reducing demand (Rahimtoola, 1989). Undoubtedly, the complexity of this condition is reflected by the complexity of its definition.

From the physiopathological point of view, perhaps the most important concept arising from this entity is that the ischemic chronic regional myocardial dysfunction could be viewed as a self-protective, adaptive process of down-regulation of contractile function and metabolism in response to chronic hypoperfusion. This new state of flow-function match could eventually remain stable for a prolonged period of time and be reversed on myocardial revascularization. While this hypothesis of functional and metabolic adaptation in response to chronic hypoperfusion remains mainly unproven (largely due to the absence of any experimental models of chronically hibernating myocardium), there is no doubt that on clinical grounds chronic dysfunctioning segments may regain function after myocardial revascularization. Before reviewing arguments in favor of or contrary to the view that myocardial hibernation may represent an adaptive process to chronic flow reduction, we shall precisely define, for the interest of the readers, the accepted as well as the unresolved features of this condition.

Myocardial Hibernation: Accepted and Unresolved Issues

Hibernating myocardium has so far been demonstrated to occur in the clinical syndromes of unstable angina, chronic stable angina, myocardial infarction with LV dysfunction and/or heart failure, and chronic hypoperfusion due to congenital anomalies of the coronary arteries (Ferrari et al., 1992; Rahimtoola, 1995). To sum up, we can say that

1. It is true that resting LV dysfunction resulting from coronary artery disease is not always irreversible. Quite a number of studies have confirmed that it improves on revascularization.

2. The exact frequency of occurrence of hibernating myocardium in coronary artery disease patients is not precisely known. One study showed it to be almost three times more common in unstable angina than in stable angina (75% vs. 28%) (Rahimtoola, 1995). It is known that incidence of hibernation in non-Q-wave infarction is 20% (Galli et al., 1994), and 11% of patients referred for cardiac transplantation have hibernating myocardium (Ferrari et al., 1994; Rahimtoola, 1995).

3. Hibernating myocardium has to be identified before revascularization. A number of methods are available to assess viability and contractile reserve in regions with hypokinetic or akinetic wall motion. These include cardiac imaging techniques that evaluate myocardial viability on the basis of myocardial perfusion and metabolic activity (Schelbert, 1991), cell membrane integrity (Dilsizian & Bonow, 1993), and infusion of low-dose, positive inotropic agents during echocardiography to evaluate contractile reserve (Bonow, 1995). The use of these techniques is essential to predict the likelihood of recovery and to estimate the operative risk, and it has provided much important physiopathological information.

4. PET studies have demonstrated that cardiac metabolism is maintained in hibernating myocardium, thus suggesting a normal or near-normal biochemical pathway. In addition, PET studies have originally demonstrated a reduction in myocardial blood flow in hibernating myocardium when compared to normals (Conversano et al., 1992). This latter point, anyway, does not appear to be a prerequisite for hibernation and has been recently reviewed (Vanoverschelde et al., 1993). In some cases basal regional perfusion in the hibernating segments can be nearly normal or only moderately reduced. This suggests that flow reduction might be not proportional to the severe depression in regional function, thus arguing against a perfect flow-function matching. In these cases coronary reserve is severely reduced, providing evidence that hibernation could be the result of multiple and repetitive bouts of myocardial stunning (Heyndrickx, 1995; Vanoverschelde et al., 1993). If this is the case, reperfusion is therapeutically performed to improve

coronary reserve, rather than actual flow. Arguments against this hypothesis, however, arise from the results of reperfusion often leading to immediate recovery of the hibernating myocardium, suggesting that readmission of flow is beneficial.

5. Estimation of cellular viability is crucial to the diagnosis of hibernation, but does not necessarily provide information on recovery of contraction on reperfusion. This latter event requires (1) integrity of cellular and subcellular membranes to provide adequate quantity of calcium to the myofilament, (2) availability of metabolic pathways to provide enough ATP to support contraction, and (3) persistence of adequate myofilaments and subendocardial layer to perform contraction. This last point, which is not evaluated by methodologies aimed at assessing viability (such as scintigraphic techniques or PET), obviously plays a fundamental role in the early recovery on reperfusion. If the akinetic area is lacking myofilaments or is extended to more than 20% of the subendocardium, one cannot expect an immediate recovery of contraction, despite the presence of viability (Ferrari, 1995; La Canna et al., 1994).

6. Dobutamine echocardiography has demonstrated that hibernating myocardium retains a certain amount of contractile reserve (La Canna et al., 1994). The contractile response is limited (which is implicit in the use of low-dose dobutamine instead of high-dose dobutamine) and quite often only temporary, reflecting the lack of normal coronary flow reserve. This technique will identify not only the segments with viability, but actually those with myofilaments able to contract. While this fact explains the higher specificity of this technique with respect to those assessing viability, it poses several problems about the results of biopsies so far taken from patients with hibernating myocardium diagnosed only on the basis of preserved viability.

7. Myocardial biopsies from chronic dysfunctioning segments performed at the time of surgery contain a variable amount of myocytes that display rather typical electron microscopic abnormalities. These are characterized by the loss of intracellular glycogen in the space left by the dissoluted sarcomeres and the presence of numerous, small, doughnutlike mitochondria in the areas adjacent to the glycogen-rich perinuclear zones (Borgers & Ausma, 1995; Elsässer & Schaper, 1995; Flameng et al., 1981). Despite these cardiomyocyte changes, alterations in the extracellular matrix and connective tissue remodeling are not uncommon, and might contribute to the abnormal wall motion of hibernating segments as well as to the rate of recovery. This observation in principle precludes the notion of immediate function normalization after reperfusion. These data, however, are strongly biased by the diagnostic inclusion criteria. Biopsies taken from patients with signs of viability and a preserved contractile reserve (positive echodo-

butamine) show a completely different picture, with almost normal myocytes (personal, unpublished data). These patients also show an immediate recovery of function (Ferrari, 1995; La Canna et al., 1994).

8. The rate of recovery of resting LV dysfunction after revascularization depends on the criteria selected for the diagnosis (viability vs. preserved contractile reserve, or both). It has been suggested that the hibernating myocardium recovering "immediately" or very rapidly, reflects a rather acute episode of ischemia. The myocardium that takes longer to recover (up to 1 year) might be considered more chronic (Rahimtoola, 1995).

9. An open question regarding myocardial hibernation is: How long can the ischemic myocardium maintain its metabolic integrity? It is possible that the metabolic status of hibernating myocardium deteriorates over time. If so, down-regulation of contraction during persistent hypoperfusion can be viewed as a temporary mechanism to prolong myocardial viability, but it is inevitably time limited. On the other hand, it is possible that the successfully adapted myocardium maintains such a state indefinitely, thereby causing long-term hibernation. This latter issue raises the problem whether hibernation could be considered an adaptive process to ischemia.

THE CONCEPT OF HIBERNATION AS AN ADAPTIVE PROCESS TO ISCHEMIA

When considering all of the previously mentioned points, hibernation appears as a hypokinetic, underperfused, or even normoperfused myocardium, with maintained aerobic metabolism, absence of ongoing signs of ischemia, no ST/T changes, no enzyme or lactate leakage, and ability to regain contraction on reperfusion, although with different speed and degree of recovery. Morphologically the hibernating myocyte does not exhibit typical signs of necrosis; it might show either classic signs of hibernation or a normal ultrastructure. Hibernating myocytes may remain hypokinetic for months or years. This latter finding challenges the long-held concept of ischemia as an imbalance between energy supply and demand, inevitably leading to necrosis.

Besides the clinical concept of hibernation, in the early 1980s several laboratories found that the reduction in regional contractile function may be proportional to the reduction in regional myocardial blood flow (Canty, 1988; Gallagher et al., 1983; Heusch, 1991; Vatner 1980). New terms were coined to explain such adaptive processes as *absolute ischemia* (Gallagher et al., 1983) and *perfusion-contraction matching* (Ross, 1991). The observed impairment of myocardial contractile function in hibernation, thus, is not regarded as a consequence of an energetic deficit, but instead as a regulatory event with a purpose of maintaining myocardial integrity and viability. The concept was taken further and it was even questioned whether the hibernating myocyte can be considered ischemic (Ferrari et al., 1994).

Obviously, this depends on the definition of myocardial ischemia, certainly a demanding task (Hearse, 1994).

Beyond definitions, hibernating myocytes are, in all probability, the end result of an ischemic insult, although not necessarily ischemic, as indicated by the lack of markers for ongoing ischemia (Fedele et al., 1988; Ferrari & Visioli, 1991; Pantely et al., 1990). At all events, we cannot consider hibernating myocytes as normal, simply because they do not contract. Once again, this is probably a sign of adaptation. Whenever a cell is under stress from external stimuli, the reaction is to self-protect, at the expense of its own function. Thus, down-regulation of contraction is probably the price to pay for maintenance of viability under circumstances of limited or altered perfusion.

Nevertheless, it is important to recognize that a perfusion-contraction matching was observed for a period of 5 hours of moderate ischemia in conscious, chronically instrumented dogs (Matsuzaki et al., 1983). Clinically, hibernation can be maintained over months or even years. In addition, if hibernation relies only on a perfect "matching," every coronary artery disease patient will exhibit hibernation, but we know this is not the case as the phenomenon is a rare event.

Thus, some other explanation must be proposed. Probably one such explanation has to do with the sequence of events occurring in patients with coronary artery disease and hibernating myocardium.

TIME SEQUENCE OF EVENTS FOLLOWING ACUTE ISCHEMIA AND HIBERNATION

On acute coronary artery occlusion, contractile function in the ischemic region rapidly ceases. Within a few cardiac cycles, systolic segment shortening and systolic wall thickening are reduced (hypokinesis) or abolished (akinesis). Within minutes, paradoxic systolic segment lengthening and systolic wall thinning (dyskinesis, bulging) occurs (Theroux et al., 1976). Electrophysiological changes in the surface ECG become evident only after the loss of systolic wall excursion, while changes in the local subendocardial ECG occur even later (Battler et al., 1980).

It is interesting to recall that patients with hibernating myocardium often have a history of an acute ischemic insult, either in the form of a transmural myocardial infarction or prolonged ischemic pain. Thereafter, the area of acute ischemia is likely to receive a residual collateral flow, as these patients show signs of chronic hypoperfusion, as demonstrated by PET or positive, late rest-redistribution thallium. It is therefore tempting to speculate that acute ischemia causes a rapid down-regulation of contraction, persisting even in the subsequent phase of hypoperfusion. Undoubtedly the loss of regional contractility in response to a loss of blood is an adaptive phenomenon, drastically reducing energy expenditure, thereby allowing a new, more favorable balance between energy supply and demand. Restoration of residual flow will provide a limited supply of oxygen and substrates that in some cases is enough to meet the metabolic and energetic need of the hypokinetic myocytes. Under

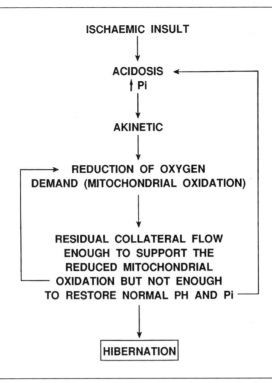

Figure 12-1. Schematic representation of the role of akinesia in the development of hibernation.

these circumstances myocytes can no longer be considered ischemic, since they receive enough oxygen to meet the rate of mitochondrial oxidation, which is in turn reduced by down-regulation of contraction.

Thus, hibernation could arise from this particular sequence of coronary flow restriction. The ultimate cause of contractile down-regulation during acute ischemia and/or hypoperfusion is not clear. We have undertaken a series of experiments to answer this question and it would appear that changes in interstitial pH might be involved (Ferrari et al., 1993, 1996).

Acute and global ischemia cause a rapid fall of pH, and an increase of P_i, which in turn brings about quiescence of the ischemic zone. Hypoperfusion following total ischemia does not restore pH to normal, which remains reduced, but probably allows a delivery of oxygen and substrate sufficient to maintain viability (Fig 12-1). This may contribute to keeping contraction down-regulated. Interestingly, it has been shown that metabolic acidosis, with a reduction in perfusate pH from 7.4 to 6.8–6.9, reduces hypoxic damage in the isolated heart by a mechanism related to a reduction in energy expenditure, while a further reduction in perfusate pH results in further damage (Nayler et al., 1979). This series of events, however, is unlikely to occur in the ischemic myocardium in vivo, where coronary flow is expected to fluctuate and myocytes are exposed to different, repetitive sequences of no, hypo-, and normal perfusion.

It is also possible that the acute ischemic insult (often reported by patients with hibernating myocardium and simulated in the laboratory by a brief episode of total, no-flow ischemia) preconditions and thereby protects the myocardium entering a hibernation phase (Ferrari et al., 1993; Schulz et al., 1995). The term *ischemic preconditioning* refers to a reduction in infarct size ensuing prolonged and severe myocardial ischemia by one or more preceding short episodes of ischemia and reperfusion (Murry et al., 1986, 1990). It is indeed possible that the two phenomena (ischemic preconditioning and hibernation), although different, are in some way linked. Coronary flow changes in patients with coronary artery disease are extremely complex, and acute short-term occlusion may be followed by full or partial reperfusion.

TIME SEQUENCE OF EVENTS ON REPERFUSION OF HIBERNATING MYOCARDIUM

At present it is unclear whether reperfusion of the hibernating myocardium causes an immediate or delayed recovery of function. Experimentally, acute hibernating myocardium may recover immediately or enter a stunning phase. Clinically, it is important to estimate the likely rate of recovery, as this constitutes a substantial part of the operative risk for each patient.

As pointed out earlier in this chapter, the estimation of the contractile reserve by echocardiography during low-dose dobutamine infusion permits accurate evaluation of such risk, as the test is highly dependent on the presence and functional status of the myofilaments in the hibernating area. On the contrary, techniques assessing viability do not explore the contractile apparatus of the hibernating myocytes, but rather the integrity of the membranes and metabolic pathways. It has been clearly demonstrated that hibernating myocytes of patients identified, for instance, by PET lack myofilaments and therefore cannot be expected to immediately recover contraction on reperfusion (Elsässer & Schaper, 1995; Flameng et al., 1981).

Thus, if the clinical question concerns not only the diagnosis of hibernation but also the likelihood of an early recovery, we believe that echocardiography during low-dose echodobutamine infusion should be utilized, ideally in conjuction with estimation of viability.

We have studied 55 patients in this manner and recovery of function estimated by intraoperative echocardiography fraction was immediate (Figs 12-2 and 12-3) (La Canna et al., 1994, 1996). The same evidence is available in the experimental setting (Mertes et al., 1995).

SUMMARY

Myocardial hibernation, as first defined by Rahimtoola (1981, 1985), is a state of chronic contractile dysfunction in patients with coronary artery disease that is fully reversible on reperfusion.

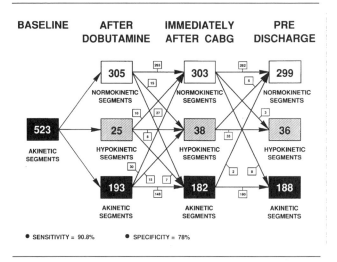

Figure 12-2. Changes in baseline akinetic segments detected after dobut-amine infusion (by transthoracic echocardiography), immediately after revascularization (CABG) (by intraoperative epicardial echocardiography), and 2 weeks later (PRE-DISCHARGE) (by transthoracic echocardiography).

% EJECTION FRACTION

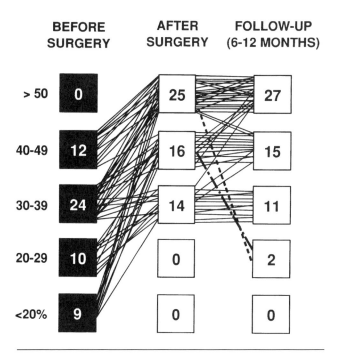

Figure 12-3. Changes in LV ejection fraction of patients with hibernating myocardium.

Clinical conditions consistent with the existence of myocardial hibernation include unstable and stable angina, myocardial infarction heart failure, and anomalous origin of coronary arteries. The mechanisms of hibernation are not known. Morphological alterations have been described in the hibernating area of patients, but this information is strongly affected by the diagnostic criteria utilized to screen patients. It has been postulated that hibernation is an adaptive phenomenon occurring during ischemia. In this context, down-regulation of contraction is not regarded as a consequence of energetic deficit, but as a regulatory event aimed at reducing energy expenditure, thereby maintaining integrity and viability. Thus, hibernation might bear a relationship to the phenomenon of low-flow perfusion-contraction matching, or repetitive stunning or preconditioning.

Clear-cut evidence for the mechanism of hibernation in the clinical setting seems likely to remain elusive because of the nature of the studies needed to document it. Current experimental evidence supports the view that hibernation, stunning, preconditioning, or their coexistence can be responsible for regional myocardial contractile dysfunction reversible on reperfusion. These are all adaptive and protective phenomena, independent of their terminology and strict definitions, that need not directly apply to the extremely complex situation arising from myocardial ischemia in humans.

ACKNOWLEDGMENTS

This work was supported by the National Research Council targeted project "Prevention and Control Disease Factors" no. 93.00656 PF 41/115 and "The New Ischemic Syndromes" European Commission project no. PL 950838. The authors thank Alessandro Colizzi and Roberta Bonetti for their editorial and secretarial assistance in preparing the manuscript.

REFERENCES

Battler A, Froelicher VF, Gallagher KP, et al. Dissociation between regional myocardial dysfunction and ECG changes during ischemia in the conscious dog. *Circulation* 1980; 62: 735–744.

Bonow RO. The hibernating myocardium: identification of viable myocardium in patients with coronary artery disease and chronic left ventricular dysfunction. *Basic Res Cardiol* 1995; 90: 49–51.

Borgers M, Ausma J. Structural aspects of the chronic hibernating myocardium in man. *Basic Res Cardiol* 1995; 90: 44–46.

Canty JM. Coronary pressure-function and steady-state pressure-flow relations during autoregulation in the unanesthetized dog. *Circ Res* 1988; 63: 821–836.

Conversano A, Herrero P, Geltman EM, et al. Differentiation of stunned from hibernating myocardium by positron emission tomography [abstract]. *Circulation* 1992; 86(Suppl I): I-108.

Dilsizian V, Bonow O. Current diagnostic techniques of assessing myocardial viability in patients with hibernating and stunned myocardium. *Circulation* 1993; 87: 1–20.

Elsässer A, Schaper J. Hibernating myocardium: adaptation or degeneration? *Basic Res Cardiol* 1995; 90: 47–48.

Fedele FA, Gewirtz H, Capone RJ, et al. Metabolic response to prolonged reduction of myocardial blood flow distal to a severe coronary artery stenosis. *Circulation* 1988; 78: 729–735.

Ferrari R. Commentary on hibernating myocardium and its clinical relevance. *Basic Res Cardiol* 1995; 90: 52–54.

Ferrari R, Cargnoni A, Bernocchi P, et al. Metabolic adaptation during a sequence of no-flow and low-flow ischemia: a possible trigger for hibernation. *Circulation* 1996; (in press).

Ferrari R, Cargnoni A, Curello S, et al. Metabolic adaptation of underperfused isolated rabbit heart: insight into molecular mechanisms underlying hibernation [abstract]. *Circulation* 1993; 88: 1004.

Ferrari R, La Canna G, Giubbini R, et al. Hibernating myocardium. In: Yacoub M, Papper J, eds. *Annual of cardiac surgery.* 1994: 28–32.

Ferrari R, La Canna G, Giubbini R, Visioli O. Stunned and hibernating myocardium: possibility of intervention. *J Cardiovasc Pharmacol* 1992; 20: 5–13.

Ferrari R, Visioli O. Stunning: damaging or protective to the myocardium? *Cardiovasc Drugs Ther* 1991; 5: 939–946.

Flameng W, Suy R, Schwarz F, et al. Ultrastructural correlates of left ventricular contraction abnormalities in patients with chronic ischemic heart disease: determinants of reversible segmental asynergy postrevascularization surgery. *Am Heart J* 1981; 102: 846–857.

Gallagher KP, Matsuzaki M, Osakada G, et al. Effect of exercise on the relationship between myocardial blood flow and systolic wall thickening in dogs with acute coronary stenosis. *Circ Res* 1983; 52: 716–729.

Galli M, Marcassa C, Bolli R, et al. Spontaneous delayed recovery of perfusion and contraction after the first 5 weeks after anterior infarction: evidence for the presence of hibernating myocardium in the infarcted area. *Circulation* 1994; 90: 1386–1397.

Hearse DJ. Myocardial ischemia: can we agree on a definition for the 21st century? *Cardiovasc Res* 1994; 28: 1737–1744.

Heusch G. The relationship between regional blood flow and contractile function in normal, ischemic, and reperfused myocardium. *Basic Res Cardiol* 1991; 86: 197–218.

Heyndrickx GR. Hibernating myocardium. *Basic Res Cardiol* 1995; 35–37.

La Canna G, Alfieri O, Giubbini R, et al. Echocardiography during infusion of dobutamine for identification of reversible dysfunction inpatients with chronic coronary artery disease. *J Am Coll Cardiol* 1994; 23: 617–622.

La Canna G, Giubbini R, Alfieri O, et al. Comparison of viability and contractile reserve for predicting early recovery of akinetic myocardium after surgical revascularization in patients with chronic coronary artery disease. *J Am Coll Cardiol* 1996; (in press).

Matsuzaki M, Gallagher KP, Kemper WS, et al. Sustained regional dysfunction produced by prolonged coronary stenosis: gradual recovery after reperfusion. *Circulation* 1983; 68: 170–182.

Mertes H, Seear DS, Johnson M, et al. Assessment of hibernating myocardium by dobutamine stimulation in a canine model. *J Am Coll Cardiol* 1995; 26(5): 1348–1355.

Murry CE, Jennings RB, Reimer KA. Preconditioning with ischemia: a delay of lethal cell injury in ischemic myocardium. *Circulation* 1986; 74: 1124–1136.

Murry CE, Richard VJ, Reimer KA, Jennings RB. Ischemic preconditioning slows energy metabolism and delays ultrastructural damage during a sustained ischemic episode. *Circ Res* 1990; 66: 913–931.

Nayler WG, Ferrari R, Poole-Wilson PA, Yepez CE. A protective effect of mild acidosis on hypoxic heart muscle. *J Moll Cell Cardiol* 1979; 11: 1053–1071.

Pantely GA, Malone SA, Rhen WS, et al. Regeneration of myocardial phosphocreatine in pigs despite continued moderate ischemia. *Circ Res* 1990; 67: 1481–1493.

Rahimtoola SH. Coronary bypass surgery for chronic angina. *Circulation* 1981; 65: 225–241.

Rahimtoola SH. A perspective on three large multicenter randomized clinical trials of coronary bypass surgery for chronic stable angina. *Circulation* 1985; 72: 123–135.

Rahimtoola SH. The hibernating myocardium. *Am Heart J* 1989; 117: 211–221.

Rahimtoola SH. Hibernating myocardium. A brief article. *Basic Res Cardiol* 1995; 90: 38–40.

Ross Jr J. Myocardial perfusion-contraction matching. Implications for coronary heart disease and hibernation. *Circulation* 1991; 83: 1076–1083.

Schelbert HR. Positron emission tomography for the assessment of myocardial viability. *Circulation* 1991; 84: 122–131.

Schulz R, Post H, Sakka S, et al. Intraischemic preconditioning. Increase tolerance to sustained low-flow ischemia by a brief episode of no-flow ischemia without intermittent reperfusion. *Circ Res* 1995; 76: 942–950.

Theroux P, Ross Jr J, Franklin D, et al. Regional myocardial function in the conscious dog during acute coronary occlusion and responses to morphine, propranolol, nitroglycerin, and lidocaine. *Circulation* 1976; 53: 202–314.

Vanoverschelde JLJ, Wijns W, Depré C, et al. Mechanisms of chronic regional postischemic dysfunction in humans. New insights from the study of noninfarcted collateral-dependent myocardium. *Circulation* 1993; 87: 1513–1523.

Vatner SF. Correlation between acute reductions in myocardial blood flow and function in conscious dogs. *Circ Res* 1980; 47: 201–207.

CHAPTER 13

Myocardial Hibernation: Current Clinical Perspectives

Shahbudin H. Rahimtoola

In the 1970s many workers (Anderson, 1972; Banka et al., 1976; Bodenheimer et al., 1978; Bonchek et al., 1974; Bourrassa et al., 1972; Chatterjee et al., 1973; Chesebro et al., 1978; Dyke et al., 1974; Helfant et al., 1974; Horn et al., 1974; Klausner et al., 1976; Massie et al., 1978; McAnulty et al., 1975; Popio et al., 1977; Rees et al., 1971; Stadius et al., 1980) focused their attention on proving the reversibility of resting LV dysfunction with coronary bypass surgery and on its detection preoperatively. In the 1980 Consensus Development Conference on Coronary Artery Bypass Surgery (1982), I failed to convince people about the presence of abnormal LV function at rest that was due to chronic, painless, persistent, severe myocardial ischemia at rest, which was reversible (Rahimtoola 1982a, 1982b). The reasons this concept was not accepted likely were (1) chronic, persistent, low-flow ischemia was not thought possible; (2) painless ischemia was not generally accepted, particularly in the United States; and (3) there were no experimental studies documenting its occurrence. At that time it was generally believed that persistent abnormal LV function at rest was due to irreversible myocardial necrosis and that prolonged "ischemia" with or without pain was not possible. Even though painless ischemia had been described in the 1970s, only in the 1980s did it become widely recognized that painless ischemia was quite common in patients with a variety of anginal syndromes (Deanfield et al., 1983; Maseri, 1983). From 1983 to 1985 I was unable to convince my colleagues at the national level that it was worth dedicating research funds to the study of the problem of chronic painless ischemia and the associated LV dysfunction. I realized that a short, less complex term was needed to describe this phenomenon (abnormal LV function at rest due to chronic, painless, resting, persistent myocardial "ischemia," which was reversible) before it would gain more widespread recognition and acceptance. Therefore, I used the term *hibernating myocardium* in 1984 (Rahimtoola, 1985a) in a National Heart, Lung, and Blood Institute (NHLBI) workshop (1984) on the treatment of coronary artery disease. It was better accepted than at the

1980 conference, probably because painless ischemia was being more widely recognized and attention was focused on the other more important statements about coronary bypass surgery. Bashour's editorial (1986) drew attention to hibernating myocardium and the concept of *electrical stunning* (transient Q-waves from profound myocardial ischemia). Braunwald and Rutherford's subsequent editorial (1986) propelled this topic to prominence. They emphasized the importance of recognizing the hibernating myocardium and that hibernating was an appropriate term for this clinical condition.

The hibernating myocardium must be distinguished from the stunned myocardium (Braunwald & Kloner, 1982) and also from transient LV dysfunction that is a result of stress-induced ischemia, although the hibernating myocardium may coexist with both conditions.

THE CONCEPT OF HIBERNATION

The clear clinical observation was that patients with LV systolic dysfunction could be shown to improve or even normalize LV systolic function with revascularization, that is, by increasing coronary blood flow. This is best illustrated by a single patient, a young patient with single-vessel disease (an occluded left anterior descending coronary artery) with minimal or no angina, akinetic anterior and apical walls, and no history or ECG evidence of previous myocardial in-

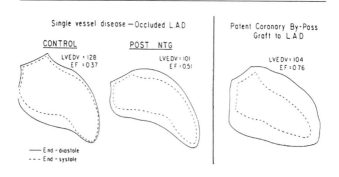

Figure 13-1. End diastolic (-) and end systolic (- -) silhouettes of the left ventricle from the right anterior oblique contrast ventriculogram. In the preoperative studies (A), the ejection fraction (EF) in the control state was 0.37 and there was a large akinetic area involving the anteroapical wall. After nitroglycerin (NTG), there was an improvement of wall motion of the akinetic zone, and EF improved to 0.51. The patient had no history of myocardial infarction. Coronary arteriography showed one-vessel disease with a totally occluded left anterior descending coronary artery (LAD). The distal LAD was filled by collaterals from the circumflex coronary artery and the posterior descending coronary artery. Eight months postoperatively (B) on routine study, the graft was fully patent and there was good filling of the LAD. The patient now shows normal LV wall-motion function and a normal EF of 0.76. LVEDV = left ventricular end diastolic volume. (From Rahimtoola [1982a], with permission.)

farction. Revascularization by coronary bypass surgery normalized LV function (Fig 13-1). These observations led to a simple but obvious concept that resting LV dysfunction could be reversed with increasing myocardial blood flow.

It was postulated (Rahimtoola, 1989) that persistently reduced coronary blood flow could lead to persistently reduced LV function such that blood flow and myocardial contraction were in equilibrium. As a result, ischemic symptoms/signs and/or myocardial infarction did not occur. However, it was recognized from the beginning that if blood flow was reduced further and/or myocardial O_2 needs were increased, then ischemic symptoms/signs and myocardial infarction could occur.

Seven studies in patients (six with PET using ^{13}N-ammonia and one using the inert gas technique) have documented reduced coronary blood flow in hibernating myocardium (Rahimtoola, 1996).

BENEFIT OF ACCEPTANCE OF THE CONCEPT

Acceptance of the concept of hibernating myocardium has had a considerable effect on cardiovascular medicine. These effects include (1) the occurrence of a great deal of basic and clinical research, (2) reassessment of the definition of ischemia, (3) development, and assessment of tests for the diagnosis of viable myocardium, and (4) better treatment of patients.

Definition

Hibernating myocardium can be described by the clinical situation, that is, it is *impaired LV function that is reversible by revascularization* (Rahimtoola, 1982a, 1982b, 1989, 1993, 1995a, 1995b).

Hearse has defined it as "exquisitely regulated tissue successfully adapting its activity to prevailing circumstances" (1994).

The question of whether hibernating myocardium is ischemia or not is to some extent a semantic one depending on the definition of ischemia. Surprisingly, even in the 1990s there is no uniform agreement of the definition of ischemia even by investigators in the field (Hearse, 1994). If one defines ischemia as a reduction in blood flow, then hibernating myocardium is ischemic myocardium. If one defines ischemia as a reduced blood flow that is associated with evidence of an effect of reduced blood flow (apart from reduced LV contraction), then hibernating myocardium is likely not ischemic myocardium.

Diagnosis

The clinical diagnosis of hibernating myocardium is based on (1) documenting LV dysfunction at rest and (2) documenting that this area of LV dysfunction at rest has viable myocardium.

Diagnosis of Hibernating Myocardium*

I. Documenting LV dysfunction at rest
   A. Two-dimensional echocardiography
   B. Radionuclide ventriculography
   C. Contrast ventriculography

II. Documenting area of LV dysfunction has viable myocardium
   A. Assessing regional function
      1. LV wall thickness
      2. Change in LV wall motion
         a. Nitroglycerin
         b. Postextrasystolic potentiation
         c. Exercise
         d. Catecholamine infusion (e.g., dobutamine)
   B. Assessing perfusion, membrane integrity, and metabolism
      1. Thallium-201/Tc-99m sestamibi scintigraphy
      2. PET

It is relatively easy to document LV dysfunction at rest by either two-dimensional echocardiography, or radionuclide or contrast ventriculography.

Demonstrating that the area of LV dysfunction has viable myocardium is easy in some patients and in others may be quite difficult. LV wall thickness at end diastole of less than 5 mm suggests that there is not likely to be a significant amount of viable myocardium in the area of LV dysfunction. Sublingual nitroglycerin (Banka et al., 1976; Chesebro et al., 1978; Helfant et al., 1974; Klausner et al., 1976; McAnulty et al., 1975) or postextrasystolic potentiation (Banka et al., 1976; Dyke et al., 1974; Horn et al., 1974; Klausner et al., 1976; Popio et al., 1977) can be used to show an improvement of the LV dysfunction either by two-dimensional echocardiography or contrast ventriculography. The sensitivity, specificity, and predictive accuracy of the nitroglycerin contrast ventriculogram is 67%, 73%, and 73%, respectively. The predictive accuracy of a positive test is 85%; that of a negative test is <50% (Rahimtoola, 1982a, 1982b; Stadius et al., 1980). A postextrasystolic ventriculogram is likely to have the same values for predictive accuracies (Banka et al., 1976; Klausner et al., 1976). Exercise ventriculography to demonstrate change in LV wall-motion function has been used only occasionally.

Clinically, the most frequently used test is dobutamine ventriculography using two-dimensional echocardiography (Aridi et al., 1995; Beleslin et al., 1994; Chen et al., 1995; Cigarro et al., 1993; La Canna et al., 1994; Smart et al., 1993). Dobutamine is infused in a dosage of 5 μg per kilogram per minute for 3 to 5 minutes, which is increased progressively if needed to doses of 10, 20, 30, and 40 μg per kilogram per minute (Aridi et al., 1995; Beleslin et al., 1994; Chen et al., 1995). The end points of the study are a positive echo test, heart rate of 85% of predicted maximum, hypertension (systolic blood pressure >220 mmHg, diastolic blood pressure >120 mmHg), hypotension (fall in systolic blood pressure ≥

---

* Outline copyrighted S.H. Rahimtoola, M.B., F.R.C.P., M.A.C.P.

TABLE 13-1. PREDICTIVE ACCURACY*

	No. of Studies	No. of Pts.	Predictive Positive	Accuracy Negative
DOB. Echo	15	402	83%	81%
Thallium spect	13	378	69%	90%
Rest-Redis-Reinj	9	295	69%	89%
Rest-Redis	4	83	69%	92%
PET	6	146	82%	83%

*From Bonow (1996), with permission.

10 mmHg over baseline), ventricular arrhythmia, sustained supraventricular arrhythmias, angina, ST-segment elevation or depression ≥ 1 to 2 mm on the ECG, or significant other symptoms. Ischemia or angina induced by dobutamine is treated with sublingual nitroglycerin or intravenous esmolol if it is necessary to do so. Viable myocardium is diagnosed if there is an improvement of LV wall-motion function with dobutamine (Aridi et al., 1995; Beleslin et al., 1994; Chen et al., 1995; Cigarro et al., 1993; La Canna et al., 1994; Smart et al., 1993). If the improvement is followed by deterioration "biphasic response" (Aridi et al., 1995; Chen et al., 1995), then the test is more specific for hibernating myocardium. If deterioration of LV function occurs early, then the test is compatible with the hypothesis that stress-induced ischemia was superimposed on hibernating myocardium. For dobutamine echocardiography, the predictive accuracy of a positive and negative test are 83% and 81%, respectively (Bonow, 1996) (Table 13-1).

The uptake and retention of thallium-201 and Tc-99m sestamibi by the myocardium is dependent on blood flow and on intact cell membrane activity and cell viability. Two tests can be performed: (1) stress-redistribution-reinjection (Dilsizian et al., 1990) and (2) rest-redistribution (Ragosta et al., 1993; Udelson et al., 1994). For stress-redistribution-reinjection, the predictive accuracies of a positive and negative test are 69% and 89%, respectively (Bonow, 1996). For rest-redistribution studies, both thallium-201 and Tc-99m sestamibi give similar results (Udelson et al., 1994). Currently, several centers are performing a combined thallium-201/Tc-99m sestamibi test. Thallium-201 is injected at rest followed by a stress-redistribution Tc-99m sestamibi test. This combination provides information about hibernating myocardium as well as stress-induced ischemia. This test is comparatively easy and quick to perform when both types of information are needed in a patient.

Positron emission tomography (PET) is another promising method for demonstrating viable myocardium using ammonia (NH_3) as the tracer for determining perfusion and F18-fluorodeoxyglucose to assess preservation of metabolic activity in areas of LV dysfunction (Tillisch et al., 1986). [11-C] acetate has also been used to assess metabolic activity (Gropler et al., 1992). Hibernating myocardium is diagnosed in areas of LV dysfunction that demonstrate enhanced F18-fluorodeoxyglucose uptake relative to perfusion, termed *metabolic/blood flow mismatch* (Tillisch et al., 1986). For PET studies, the predictive accuracy of a positive and negative test are 82% and 83%, respectively (Bonow, 1996).

It is clear that at the present time there is no perfect test for diagnosing hibernating myocardium. Thus, there is a need for *clinical judgment* in an individual patient. The most widely available and used test is dobutamine echocardiography. At most institutions, thallium and sestamibi are available but PET is not. Even in centers where PET is available for clinical studies, PET study is usually used in those with severe LV dysfunction, especially in those being considered for cardiac transplantation. The choice of a test depends on the clinical condition of the patient, on the tests available, and the expertise with a particular test in each institution. Thus, in an individual patient one could perform one test and if that is negative one could proceed to the next test if the index of suspicion of hibernating myocardium is high. On the other hand, if the index of suspicion is very low, one negative test may be adequate. Thus, the number of tests performed may range from one to four.

Clinical syndromes

Hibernating myocardium has been demonstrated to occur in patients with stable and unstable angina, AMI, and in patients with severe LV dysfunction in clinical heart failure.

Unstable and stable angina Angina is the result of myocardial ischemia, which results in LV dysfunction; LV wall motion may be hypokinetic, akinetic, or even dyskinetic.

A large number of clinical studies have documented that LV dysfunction at rest can improve with revascularization (Akins et al., 1980; Berger et al., 1979; Bonchek et al., 1974; Braunwald & Rutherford, 1986; Brundage et al., 1984; Carlson et al., 1989; Chatterjee et al., 1973; Cigarro et al., 1993; Cohen et al., 1988; Dilsizian et al., 1990; Elefteriades et al., 1993; Ferrari et al., 1992; Gibson et al., 1983; La Canna et al., 1994; Marwick et al., 1992; Mizuno et al., 1988; Ragosta et al., 1993; Rahimtoola, 1982a, 1982b, 1985a, 1985b, 1989; Rees et al., 1971; Takeishi et al., 1991; Tillisch et al., 1986; Topol et al., 1984; Van den Berg et al., 1990). These studies show that hibernating myocardium is common in these clinical syndromes. After coronary bypass surgery the best predictor of an improvement in resting LV ejection fraction is the number of viable, asynergic myocardial segments per patient, that is, the number of segments that were hibernating. There was no correlation with angina (Ragosta et al., 1993; Tillisch et al., 1986).

Earlier a group from the University of Virginia (Berger et al., 1979; Gibson et al., 1983), using quantitative thallium-201 imaging on exercise and redistribution, showed that 18 of 28 patients (64%) with persistent thallium defects of 25 to 50% showed improvement or normalization after revascularization, as did 3 of 14 patients (21%) with persistent thallium defects of >50%. More recently, the group from the National Institutes of Health (Bonow et al., 1991; Dilsizian et al., 1990) have shown that approximately 50% of LV wall segments that show a persistent thallium-201 defect on redistribution or delayed studies after exercise have hibernating myocardium that improves or returns to normal after revascularization. It appears that reinjection of thallium identifies viable myocardium in 31 to 49% of myocardial regions considered irreversible using conventional 3- to 4-hour redistribution images (Dilsizian et al., 1990; Ohtani et al., 1990; Rocco et al., 1990; Tamaki et al., 1990). More recently, La Canna and colleagues (1994) have studied 33 patients with dobutamine echocardiography. Of 314 myocardial segments that were akinetic preoperatively, 160 (51%) were normal and 19 (6%) were hypokinetic 3 months after coronary bypass surgery.

The frequency of hibernating myocardium in unstable and stable angina has been documented. Carlson and coworkers (1989) showed that it was present in 18 of 24 patients (75%) with unstable angina and in only 5 of 18 patients (28%) with stable angina. We have presented data to show that long-term (10-year) survival after coronary bypass surgery was significantly better in patients with unstable angina and preoperative LV dysfunction than in those with stable angina and preoperative LV dysfunction (Rahimtoola, 1989). In fact, up to 6 years after surgery, survival in patients with unstable angina was similar to that in patients with unstable or stable angina who had normal preoperative LV function (Rahimtoola, 1989). These data were compatible with the hypothesis that it is more usual for the preoperative abnormal left ventricle to improve or return to normal in patients with unstable angina than in those with stable angina.

Acute myocardial infarction　　Myocardial hibernation is known to occur in a region of LV wall at a distance from the area of infarction (Rahimtoola, 1989) and in the LV wall in the area of infarction (Kulick & Rahimtoola, 1991). More recently, Adams and coworkers (1995) have studied 41 patients an average of 8 days after a first AMI. Using PET they demonstrated mismatch (hibernation) in 78% of the patients; 31% of patients had a large area of mismatch.

Using PET, Tamaki and associates (1992) demonstrated increased F18-fluorodeoxyglucose uptake, indicating hibernating myocardium, in 48 of 84 patients (57%) after myocardial infarction. At follow-up, a cardiac event (cardiac death, nonfatal myocardial infarction, unstable angina, and late revascularization) occurred in 3% of patients with no increase in F18-fluorodeoxyglucose and in 33% of patients who had increased F18-fluorodeoxyglucose uptake. It is noteworthy that 16 of 17 patients who had a subsequent event had an increase in F18-fluorodeoxyglucose. Multivariate analysis showed that an increase in F18-fluorodeoxyglucose uptake was the most significant predictor of a subsequent cardiac event ($p = .0006$), followed by the number of diseased vessels ($p = .008$). This study demonstrates that hibernating myocardium occurs in many patients after myocardial infarction and is associated with a high incidence of subsequent cardiac events.

Montalescott and colleagues (1992) performed a randomized trial of PTCA versus no PTCA of the infarct-related artery 6 weeks after AMI in patients who had single-vessel disease with no clinical or exercise-induced evidence of myocardial ischemia. Patients who were randomized to PTCA had increased coronary blood flow, an improvement

TABLE 13-2. LEFT VENTRICULAR FUNCTION BEFORE AND AFTER CORONARY ARTERY BYPASS GRAFTING

Time	Left ventricular end diastolic dimension (mm)	Doppler mitral regurgitation	Radionuclide ejection fraction (%) Rest	Exercise
Initial	66	Severe	16	15
4 weeks postoperatively	68	Moderate	26	24
6 weeks postoperatively	52	Mild	33	34
1 year postoperatively*	50	—	52	—

* Personal communication with LW Stevenson, 1992.
(Reprinted with permission from Luu, 1990.)

in the thallium-201 pathologic/normal ratio after exercise and improved LV wall motion. LV ejection fraction did not change significantly (0.51 ± 0.03 to 0.52 ± 0.04) in the group randomized to no PTCA, whereas it increased from 0.48 ± 0.03 to 0.51 ± 0.04 ($p < .04$) in the PTCA group. These data clearly demonstrate the occurrence of hibernating myocardium in the infarcted area or in an area that was presumed to be infarcted.

Severe LV dysfunction and/or heart failure Akins and associates (1980) have reported on 2 patients with heart failure but without angina who were shown to have severe coronary artery disease and stress-induced ischemia. Coronary bypass surgery improved the abnormal resting LV function and clinical heart failure. Shanes and coworkers (1985) reported on a patient with presumed dilated cardiomyopathy. The patient had severe coronary artery disease with stress-induced ischemia and the LV dysfunction returned to normal after coronary bypass surgery.

Interesting data from patients referred for cardiac transplantation at the University of California, Los Angeles, have been presented. One patient, in whom revascularization instead of transplantation was carried out, had a gradual improvement in LV function over the 1-year postoperative period (Table 13-2) (Luu et al., 1990). Among 207 patients evaluated for heart transplantation from 1984 to 1990, 22 (11%) had revascularization instead of transplantation and their 40-month actuarial survival was 72%; most of the deaths were perioperative (Louie et al., 1991).

Lee and coworkers (1994) have shown that 50 patients with mismatch who were revascularized had a 4% mortality and a 4% incidence of angina/myocardial infarction, whereas in 21 patients who were not revascularized the incidence of mortality and of anginal/myocardial infarction was 14% and 62%, respectively. Using PET, Eitzman and colleagues (1992) studied 82 patients with an LV ejection fraction of 0.34 ± 0.13. Myocardial hibernation, indicated by a mismatch on PET, was present in 44 of 82 patients (54%). On follow-up, death or myocardial infarction had occurred in 2 of 38 (5%) patients who had no hibernation, in 1 of 26 patients (4%) who had hibernating myocardium and were revascularized, and in 9 of 18 patients (50%) who had hibernating myocardium but were not revascularized. DiCarli and coworkers (1994) have presented results in patients with severe LV dysfunction (ejection fraction, 0.25 ± 0.07) who had angina or were referred for cardiac transplantation. Hibernating myocardium, demonstrated by PET, was present in 43 of 93 patients (46%). Patients with hibernating myocardium who were revascularized had a much lower incidence of cardiac death than those who were not revascularized (4% vs. 33%; 2-year actuarial survival, 88 vs. 50%; $p = .03$). These studies demonstrate the presence of hibernating myocardium in many patients with or without heart failure; the incidence of death or infarction was high in patients not revascularized. As mentioned earlier, Ragosta and associates (1993) have shown that postoperative improvement in LV ejection fraction was predicted using multivariate analysis by the number of viable, asynergic myocardial segments per patient, that is, the number of myocardial segments that were hibernating. Angina was not correlated.

TREATMENT

Pouleur and colleagues (1992) have presented data that are compatible with the hypothesis that prolonged administration of nisoldipine may improve hibernating myocardium. Additional studies are needed.

The most definitive evidence of improvement of hibernating myocardium has been with revascularization either by percutaneous catheter techniques or coronary bypass surgery (Akins et al., 1980; Berger et al., 1979; Bonchek et al., 1974; Braunwald & Rutherford, 1986; Brundage et al., 1984; Carlson et al., 1989; Chatterjee et al., 1973; Cigarro et al., 1993; Cohen et al., 1988; Dilsizian et al., 1990; Elefteriades et al., 1993; Ferrari et al., 1992; Gibson et al., 1983; La Canna et al., 1994; Marwick et al., 1992; Mizuno et al., 1988; Ragosta et al., 1993; Rahimtoola, 1982a, 1982b, 1985a, 1985b, 1989; Rees et al., 1971; Takeishi et al., 1991; Tillisch et al., 1986; Topol et al., 1984; Van den Berg et al., 1990). The aim is to obtain complete myocardial revascularization or, alternatively, as complete a revascularization as possible. The decision to perform revascularization and by which technique is made after a consideration of several factors: (1) the suitability of the coronary arteries for revascularization, (2) the extent of hibernating myocardium, (3) the risks of revascularization, and (4) estimation of functional recovery after revascularization. Symptoms are of secondary consideration. The greater the severity of angina, the greater the need for revascularization. Heart failure symptoms also signify a very significant need for revascularization. Since all the factors to be considered in recommending revascularization cannot be accurately quantitated at the present time, there is a need for *clinical judgment* in the decision to recommend revascularization.

SOME COMPLEXITIES OF HIBERNATING MYOCARDIUM

Hibernating myocardium and heart failure in hibernation

LV dysfunction is an important consequence of coronary artery disease and results from acute myocardial ischemia, hibernating myocardium, or myocardial infarction. Stunning may be superimposed on any of these syndromes. It may eventually lead to heart failure (Fig 13-2). Occasionally, however, coronary artery disease may produce a mechanical defect (e.g., mitral regurgitation, ventricular septal defect) that results in clinical heart failure without significant LV dysfunction. Myocardial stunning, which is a "short-term" phenomenon (discussed later), may supervene on myocardial ischemia, hibernation, or infarction and exacerbates LV dysfunction. LV dysfunction from any cause results in or contributes to myocardial ischemia by increasing myocardial oxygen demand and reducing coronary blood flow, and, if it persists, structural changes commonly occur, leading to heart failure. Hibernating myocardium can be completely, or almost completely, restored to normal with therapy. Thus, LV dysfunction or heart failure caused or exacerbated by hibernating myocardium can be improved with appropriate therapy. On the other hand, if the hibernating myocardium is not appropriately treated in a timely manner, it may be associated with progressive cellular damage, recurrent myocardial ischemia, myocardial infarction, heart failure, and death.

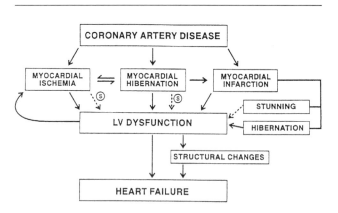

Figure 13-2. Sequelae of coronary artery disease. Coronary artery disease may result in myocardial ischemia, hibernation, or infarction, all of which are associated with LV dysfunction. Hibernation may also be associated with subsequent acute ischemia or infarction. Stunning may be superimposed on ischemia or hibernating myocardium on reperfusion. Both hibernating and stunned myocardium may be present in patients who have myocardial infarction. By definition, stunning usually improves spontaneously over a period of time. Left ventricular (LV) dysfunction, with or without associated structural changes, may produce clinical heart failure. Except for infarcted myocardial tissue, all other states are potentially reversible with appropriate and timely treatment. S = myocardial stunning (Rahimtoola, 1995a, with permission).

Recovery of myocardial hibernation

The rate of recovery of resting LV dysfunction after revascularization and the study of the morphologic changes in the dysfunctional myocardium have allowed the hibernating myocardium to be described as acute, subacute, or chronic (Rahimtoola, 1993, 1995a) (Fig 13-3).

Acute   When hibernating myocardium recovers "immediately" or very rapidly after revascularization (Cohen et al., 1988; La Canna et al., 1994; Topol et al., 1984) (Fig 13-4), it is presumptive evidence that the myocardium is normal or almost normal. This is confirmed by electron microscopic studies of transmural myocardial biopsy samples in patients undergoing coronary bypass surgery (Flameng et al., 1987) and by histological examination at autopsy (Cabin et al., 1987). Acute experimental studies of hibernation also confirm this (Arai et al., 1991, 1995; Pantely et al., 1990; Schulz et al., 1992, 1993).

Chronic   After revascularization, it may take hibernating myocardium up to 1 year to recover (Table 13-3). Electron microscopic studies of transmural myocardial biopsy samples taken at coronary bypass surgery have demonstrated marked abnormalities. The most striking features are loss of myofibrillar content and excessive accumulation of glycogen (Borgers et al., 1993; Flameng et al., 1981; Vanoverschelde et al., 1993). These can be expected to take time to recover after revascularization. Animal models of a longer duration of reduced coronary blood flow are being developed (Bolukoglu et al., 1992; Canty & Klocke, 1987; Fedele et al., 1988; Mills et al., 1994).

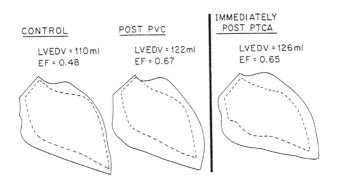

CONTROL

LVEDV = 110 ml
EF = 0.48

POST PVC

LVEDV = 122 ml
EF = 0.67

IMMEDIATELY
POST PTCA

LVEDV = 126 ml
EF = 0.65

Figure 13-3. *Example of hibernating myocardium. The patient had severe (95–99%) stenosis of the proximal left anterior descending coronary artery. At rest, the anterior LV wall is severely hypokinetic or akinetic and the LV ejection fraction (EF) is 0.48. In the postpremature ventricular contraction (post-PVC beat), the wall-motion function and ejection fraction are normal. Immediately after successful percutaneous transluminal coronary angioplasty (PTCA), LV wall motion and EF are normal. LVEDV = left ventricular end diastolic volume. (From Rahimtoola [1991], with permission.)*

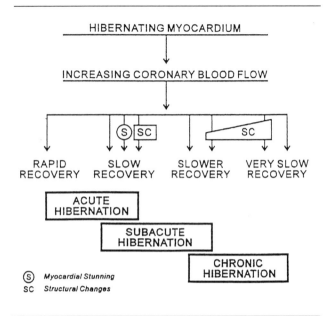

Figure 13-4. *Rates of recovery (rapid to very slow) of LV function after increasing coronary blood in hibernating myocardium. The role of stunned myocardium and of structural changes in the myocardium is shown. The possible range of acute, subacute, and chronic myocardial hibernation based on rate of recovery of LV function is illustrated. (From Rahimtoola [1995b], with permission.)*

Subacute Data presented by Matsuzaki and colleagues (1983) from an experimental study showed that after 5 hours of reduced perfusion, reduced contraction, and little or no myocardial infarction (hibernation), reperfusion was followed by a gradual recovery of LV function over a 7-day period. This most likely represents stunning following reperfusion of hibernating myocardium. In a patient with hibernating myocardium reported by Baker and colleagues (1991), recovery of LV function occurred over 10 to 60 weeks. Some patients revascularized with coronary bypass surgery (Marwick et al., 1992) and by PTCA (Nienaber et al., 1991) showed a similar slow recovery of LV function. Hibernation may have been subacute since it was likely to have been present for a long time prior to reperfusion. In addition, since ventricular function recovered over months after revascularization in these patients, there may have been changes in the myocardium, or early changes similar to those that may occur in chronic hibernation, that take time to return to normal. The delayed recovery in function might also represent stunning following hibernation (Kloner & Przyklenk, 1991). It is likely that both could occur, that is, in some patients reperfusion of hibernating myocardium is followed by stunning and in others myocardial abnormalities associated with subacute hibernation take time to recover after reperfusion.

The differences between short-term/acute and chronic hibernation are summarized in Table 13-3.

TABLE 13-3. HIBERNATING MYOCARDIUM

Experimental	Short term	Chronic
Clinical	Acute Subacute	Subacute Chronic
Myocardium	Normal Some structural changes	Near normal Some structural changes, Marked structural changes*
Adjacent myocardium	Infarcted Fibrotic Normal	Infarcted Fibrotic Normal
Prior to hibernation	Acute ischemic episode(s) Gradual reduction of blood flow Stunning?	Acute ischemic episode(s) Gradual reduction of blood flow Stunning?
Recovery from hibernation	Rapid/slow Stunning may occur LV Function: normal, or less normal	Rapid/slow/very slow Stunning? LV Function: normal or less abnormal

*Dedifferentiation or diffuse atrophy/wasting from reduced function.
Copyright S.H. Rahimtoola, M.B., F.R.C.P., M.A.C.P.

RELEVANCE TO CLINICIANS

Outcome of patients with coronary artery disease is importantly determined by the amount of LV myocardium that will be irreversibly damaged. This myocardium is composed of myocardium that is already irreversibly damaged and the amount of myocardium that is at risk, which is the myocardium that is hibernating and/or that is at risk from acute ischemic episodes (Table 13-4). In patients with LV dysfunction at rest, the combination(s) of irreversibly damaged myocardium and viable myocardium that may be present in many patients is shown in Table 13-5.

TABLE 13-4. LEFT VENTRICULAR MYOCARDIUM

Normal

Dysfunctional at rest

    Irreversibly damaged (infarcted)
    Stunned
    Hibernating

Ischemic with increased myocardial needs and/or reduced myocardial supply (of blood that contains O_2, substrates, etc.)

Copyright S.H. Rahimtoola, M.B., F.R.C.P., M.A.C.P.

TABLE 13-5. COMBINATIONS THAT MAY BE PRESENT IN PATIENTS

	LV dysfunction at rest				
Irreversible myocardial damage	+	+	+	0	0
Viable myocardium at risk					
Hibernating	0	+	0	+	+
Ischemic on "stress"	0	0	+	0	+

Copyright S.H. Rahimtoola, M.B., F.R.C.P., M.A.C.P.

TABLE 13-6. NEED TO ASSESS PRESENCE AND EXTENT OF HIBERNATING MYOCARDIUM

	Mild-moderate LV dysfunction at rest			
	LMCAD	3VD	LAD+1VD	1VD
Unstable angina	−	−	±	+
Stable angina, severe	−	−	±	+
mild	±	±	+	+
No angina	+	+	+	+
Heart failure	+	+	+	+

+ = yes; ± = varies; — = no;
LMCAD = left main coronary artery disease;
3VD = three-vessel disease;
1VD = one-vessel disease;
LAD = left anterior descending.
Copyright S.H. Rahimtoola, M.B., F.R.C.P., M.A.C.P.

TABLE 13-7. NEED TO ASSESS PRESENCE AND EXTENT OF HIBERNATING MYOCARDIUM

	Mild-moderate LV dysfunction at rest			
Objective evidence of stress-induced ischemia	LMCAD	3VD	LAD + 1VD	1VD
Moderate-severe	−	−	±	+
Mild	±	+	+	+
None	+	+	+	+

+ = yes; ± = varies; — = no;
LMCAD = left main coronary artery disease;
3VD = three-vessel disease;
1VD = one-vessel disease;
LAD = left anterior descending.
Copyright S.H. Rahimtoola, M.B., F.R.C.P., M.A.C.P.

One of the goals in clinical practice is to reduce the amount of irreversibly damaged myocardium. Therefore, in clinical practice when one sees a patient with LV dysfunction at rest one should ask the question whether there is hibernating (viable) myocardium in the area of LV dysfunction. The need to assess the presence and extent of hibernating myocardium in patients with mild to moderate LV dysfunction at rest depending on the extent of coronary artery disease, in those with various clinical syndromes, and in those with objective evidence of stress-induced ischemia is shown in Tables 13-6 and 13-7, respectively. In patients with severe LV dysfunction at rest, one usually needs to assess the presence and extent of coronary artery disease in almost all patients. At the present time, successful revascularization of the hibernating myocardium will reduce LV dysfunction and reduce the amount of myocardium at risk. It may prolong life, reduce and/or correct clinical heart failure, and improve the symptomatic state of the patient.

SUMMARY

The concept of hibernating myocardium that arose from clinical observations is now widely accepted and the original postulates have now been proven to be largely correct. It can be defined as *exquisitely regulated tissue successfully adapt-*

ing its activity to prevailing circumstances and can be described by the clinical situation as impaired LV function at rest that is reversible by revascularization.

The clinical diagnosis prior to revascularization is based on (1) documenting LV dysfunction at rest and (2) documenting that the area of LV dysfunction at rest has viable myocardium. The former is easy. The latter is more difficult; the two most commonly used tests are dobutamine echocardiography and radionuclide tests (PET, if available, is also very useful). None of these tests is perfect.

Hibernating myocardium has been documented in patients with unstable and stable angina, AMI, and severe LV dysfunction and/or heart failure.

Hibernating myocardium is definitively treated by successful revascularization. The decision to perform revascularization is made after considering (1) the suitability of the coronary arteries for revascularization, (2) the risks of revascularization, and (3) estimation of functional recovery after revascularization. After revascularization, hibernating myocardium may recover rapidly, more slowly, or very slowly.

In patients with LV dysfunction at rest, a variety of combinations of irreversibly damaged and viable myocardium may be present. The need to diagnose hibernating myocardium is different in different patients depending on the extent and severity of LV dysfunction at rest, the clinical syndrome, the extent and severity of coronary artery disease, and the extent and severity of stress-induced ischemia.

REFERENCES

Adams JN, Norton M, Trent R, et al. Hibernating myocardium after acute myocardial infarction treated with thrombolysis [abstract]. *Eur Heart J* 1995; 16: 36.

Akins CW, Pohost GM, DeSanctis RW, Block PC. Selection of angina-free patients with severe left ventricular dysfunction for myocardial revascularization. *Am J Cardiol* 1980; 46: 695–700.

Anderson RP. Effects of coronary bypass graft occlusion on left ventricular performance. *Circulation* 1972; 46: 507–513.

Arai AE, Grauer SE, Anselone CG, et al. Metabolic adaptation to a gradual reduction in myocardial blood flow. *Circulation* 1995; 92: 244–252.

Arai AE, Pantely GA, Anselone CG, et al. Active down-regulation of myocardial energy requirements during prolonged moderate ischemia in swine. *Circ Res* 1991; 69: 1458–1469.

Aridi I, Kleiman NS, Raizer AE, Zoghbi WA. Dobutamine echocardiography in myocardial hibernation. Optimal dose and accuracy in predicting recovery of ventricular function after coronary angioplasty. *Circulation* 1995; 91: 663–670.

Baker WB, Klein MS, Reardon MJ, et al. Reversible cardiac dysfunction (hibernation) from ischemia due to compression of the coronary arteries by a pseudoaneurysm. *N Engl J Med* 1991; 325: 1858–1861.

Banka VS, Bodenheimer MM, Shah R, Helfant RH. Intervention ventriculography: comparative value of nitroglycerin, post-extrasystolic potentiation and nitroglycerin plus post-extrasystolic potentiation. *Circulation* 1976; 53: 632–637.

Bashour TT. Of myocardial life, hibernation and death. *Am Heart J* 1986; 112: 427–428.

Beleslin BD, Ostojic M, Stepanovic J, et al. Stress echocardiography in the detection of myocardial ischemia. Head-to-head comparison of exercise, dobutamine, and dipyridamole tests. *Circulation* 1994; 90: 1168–1176.

Berger BC, Watson DD, Burwell LR, et al. Redistribution of thallium at rest in patients with stable and unstable angina and the effect of coronary artery bypass surgery. *Circulation* 1979; 60: 1114–1125.

Bodenheimer MM, Banka VS, Fooshee C, et al. Relationship between regional myocardial perfusion and the presence, severity and reversibility of asynergy in patients with coronary heart disease. *Circulation* 1978; 58: 789–795.

Bolukoglu H, Liedtke J, Nellis S, et al. An animal model of chronic coronary stenosis resulting in hibernating myocardium. *Am J Physiol* 1992; 263: H20–H29.

Bonchek LI, Rahimtoola SH, Chaitman BR, et al. Vein graft occlusion: immediate and late consequences and therapeutic implications. *Circulation* 1974; 50(Suppl II): 84–97.

Bonow RO. Identification of viable myocardium. *Circulation* 1996; 94: 2674–2680.

Bonow RO, Dilsizian V, Cuocolo A, Bacharach SL. Identification of viable myocardium in patients with coronary artery disease and left ventricular dysfunction: comparison of thallium scintigraphy with reinjection and PET imaging 18F-fluorodeoxyglucose. *Circulation* 1991; 83: 26–37.

Borgers M, Thone F, Wonters L, et al. Structural correlates of regional myocardial dysfunction in patients with critical coronary artery stenosis: chronic hibernation? *Cardiovasc Pathol* 1993; 2: 237–245.

Bourrassa M, Lesperance J, Campeau J, et al. Fate of left ventricular contraction following aortocoronary venous grafts: early and late post-operative modifications. *Circulation* 1972; 46: 724–730.

Braunwald E, Kloner RA. The stunned myocardium: prolonged, post-ischemic ventricular dysfunction. *Circulation* 1982; 66: 1146–1149.

Braunwald E, Rutherford JD. Reversible ischemic left ventricular dysfunction: evidence for the "hibernating myocardium." *J Am Coll Cardiol* 1986; 8: 1467–1470.

Brundage BH, Massie BM, Botvinick EH. Improved regional ventricular function after successful surgical revascularization. *J Am Coll Cardiol* 1984; 3: 902–908.

Cabin HS, Clubb S, Vita N, Zaret BL. Regional dysfunction by equilibrium radionuclide angiocardiography: a clinical-pathologic study evaluating the relation of degree of dysfunction to the presence and extent of myocardial infarction. *J Am Coll Cardiol* 1987; 10: 743–747.

Canty Jr JM, Klocke FJ. Reductions in regional myocardial function at rest in conscious dogs with chronically reduced regional coronary artery pressure. *Circ Res* 1987; 61 (Suppl II): 107–116.

Carlson EB, Cowley MJ, Wolfgang TC, Vetrovec GW. Acute changes in global and regional rest ventricular function after successful coronary angioplasty: comparative results in stable and unstable angina. *J Am Coll Cardiol* 1989; 13: 1262–1269.

Chatterjee K, Swan HJC, Parmley WW, et al. Influence of direct myocardial revascularization on left ventricular asynergy and function in patients with coronary heart disease. *Circulation* 1973; 47: 276–286.

Chen C, Li L, Chen LL, et al. Incremental doses of dobutamine induce a biphasic response in dysfunctional left ventricular regions subtending coronary stenoses. *Circulation* 1995; 92: 756–766.

Chesebro JH, Ritman EL, Frye RL, et al. Regional myocardial wall thickening response to nitroglycerin. A predictor of myocardial response to aortocoronary bypass surgery. *Circulation* 1978; 57: 952–957.

Cigarro CG, de Filippi CR, Brickner ME, et al. Dobutamine stress echocardiography identifies hibernating myocardium and predicts recovery of left ventricular function after coronary revascularization. *Circulation* 1993; 88: 430–436.

Cohen M, Chainey R, Hershman R, et al. Reversal of chronic ischemic myocardial dysfunction after transluminal coronary angioplasty. *J Am Coll Cardiol* 1988; 12: 1193–1198.

Consensus Development Conference on Coronary Artery Bypass Surgery. Medical and scientific aspects. NIH, December 3–5, 1980. Frye RL, Frommer PL, eds. *Circulation* 1982; (June Suppl).

Deanfield J, Maseri A, Selwyn AP, et al. Myocardial ischemia during daily life in patients with stable angina: its relation to symptoms and heart rate changes. *Lancet* 1983; 2: 753–758.

DiCarli M, Davidson M, Little R, et al. Value of metabolic imaging with positron emission tomography for evaluating prognosis in patients with coronary artery disease and left ventricular dysfunction. *Am J Cardiol* 1994; 73: 527–533.

Dilsizian V, Rocco TP, Freedman NMT, et al. Enhanced detection of ischemic but viable myocardium by the reinjection of thallium after stress redistribution imaging. *N Engl J Med* 1990; 323: 141–146.

Dyke SH, Cohn PF, Gorlin R, Sonnenblick EH. Detection of residual myocardial function in coronary artery disease using postextrasystolic potentiation. *Circulation* 1974; 50: 694–699.

Eitzman D, Al-Aonar Z, Kanter HL, et al. Clinical outcome of patients with advanced coronary artery disease after viability studies with positron emission tomography. *J Am Coll Cardiol* 1992; 20: 559–565.

Elefteriades JS, Tolis Jr G, Levi E, et al. Coronary artery bypass grafting in severe left ventricular dysfunction: excellent survival with improved ejection fraction and function state. *J Am Coll Cardiol* 1993; 22: 1411–1417.

Fedele FA, Gewirtz H, Capone RJ, et al. Metabolic response to prolonged reduction of myocardial blood flow distal to a severe coronary artery stenosis. *Circulation* 1988; 78: 729–735.

Ferrari R, La Canna G, Giubbini R, et al. Hibernating myocardium in patients with coronary artery disease: identification and clinical importance. *Cardiovasc Drugs Ther* 1992; 6: 287–293.

Flameng W, Suy R, Schwartz F, et al. Ultrastructural correlates of left ventricular contraction abnormalities in patients with chronic ischemic heart disease: determinants of reversible segmental asynergy postrevascularization surgery. *Am Heart J* 1981; 102: 846–857.

Flameng W, Vanhaecke J, Van Belle H, et al. Relation between coronary artery stenosis and myocardial purine metabolism, histology and regional function in humans. *J Am Coll Cardiol* 1987; 9: 1235–1242.

Gibson RS, Wats DD, Taylor CJ, et al. Prospective assessment of regional myocardial perfusion before and after coronary revascularization surgery by quantitative thallium-201 scintigraphy. *J Am Coll Cardiol* 1983; 1: 804–815.

Gropler RJ, Geltman EM, Sampathkumaran K, et al. Functional recovery after coronary revascularization for chronic coronary artery disease is dependent on maintenance of oxidative metabolism. *J Am Coll Cardiol* 1992; 20: 569–577.

Hearse JD. Myocardial ischemia: can we agree on a definition for the 21st century? *Cardiovasc Res* 1994; 28: 1737–1744.

Helfant RH, Pine R, Meister SG, et al. Nitroglycerin to unmask reversible asynergy. Correlation with post-coronary bypass ventriculography. *Circulation* 1974; 50: 108–113.

Horn HR, Teichholz LE, Cohen PF, et al. Augmentation of left ventricular contraction patency in coronary artery disease by an inotropic catecholamine: the epinephrine ventriculogram. *Circulation* 1974; 49: 1063–1071.

Klausner SC, Ratshin RA, Tybert JV, et al. The similarity of changes in segmental contraction patterns induced by post-extrasystolic potentiation and nitroglycerin. *Circulation* 1976; 54: 615–623.

Kloner RA, Przyklenk K. Hibernation and stunning of the myocardium. *N Engl J Med* 1991; 325: 1877–1879.

Kulick D, Rahimtoola SH. Assessment of the survivors of acute myocardial infarction: the case for coronary angiography. In: Gersh B, Rahimtoola SH, eds. *Acute myocardial infarction*. Amsterdam: Elsevier Science, 1991: 448–468.

La Canna G, Alfieri O, Giubbini R, et al. Echocardiography during infusion of dobutamine for identification of reversible dysfunction in patients with chronic coronary artery disease. *J Am Coll Cardiol* 1994; 23: 617–626.

Lee KS, Marwick TH, Cook SA, et al. Prognosis of patients with left ventricular dysfunction, with and without viable myocardium after myocardial infarction. Relative efficacy of medical therapy and vascularization. *Circulation* 1994; 90: 2687–2694.

Louie HW, Laks H, Milgalter E, et al. Ischemic cardiomyopathy: criteria for coronary revascularization and cardiac transplantation. *Circulation* 1991; 84(Suppl III): 290–295.

Luu M, Stevenson LW, Brunken RC, et al. Delayed recovery of revascularized myocardium after referral for cardiac transplantation. *Am Heart J* 1990; 119: 668–670.

Marwick TH, MacIntyre WJ, Lafont A, et al. Metabolic responses of hibernating and infarcted myocardium to revascularization: a follow-up study of regional perfusion, function, and metabolism. *Circulation* 1992; 85: 1347–1353.

Maseri A. The changing face of angina pectoris: practical implications. *Lancet* 1983; 1: 746–749.

Massie B, Botvinick EH, Brundage BH, et al. Relationship of regional myocardial perfusion to segmental wall motion. Physiological basis for understanding the presence and the reversibility of asynergy. *Circulation* 1978; 58: 1154–1163.

Matsuzaki M, Gallagher KP, White F, Ross Jr J. Sustained regional dysfunction produced by prolonged coronary stenosis: gradual recovery after reperfusion. *Circulation* 1983; 68: 170–182.

McAnulty JH, Hattenhauer MT, Rösch J, et al. Improvement in left ventricular wall motion following nitroglycerin. *Circulation* 1975; 51: 140–145.

Mills I, Fallon JT, Wrenn D, et al. Adaptive responses of coronary circulation and myocardium to chronic reduction in perfusion pressure and flow. *Am J Physiol* 1994; 266: H447–H457.

Mizuno K, Arakawa K, Shibuya T, et al. Improved regional and global diastolic performance in patients with coronary artery disease after percutaneous transluminal coronary angioplasty. *Am Heart J* 1988; 115: 302–306.

Montalescott G, Faraggi M, Drobinski G, et al. Myocardial viability in patients with Q wave myocardial infarction and no residual ischemia. *Circulation* 1992; 86: 47–55.

NHLBI workshop on surgery in the treatment of coronary artery disease, September 6 and 7, 1984, Bethesda, MD. Braunwald E, Hollingsworth C, Passamani E, eds. *Circulation* 1985; (Suppl V, December).

Nienaber CA, Brunken RC, Sherman CT. Metabolic and functional recovery of ischemic human myocardium after coronary angioplasty. *J Am Coll Cardiol* 1991; 18: 966–978.

Ohtani H, Tamaki N, Yonekura Y, et al. Value of thallium-201 reinjection after delayed aspect imaging for predicting reversible ischemia after coronary artery bypass grafting. *Am J Cardiol* 1990; 66: 394–399.

Pantely GA, Malone SA, Rhen WS, et al. Regeneration of myocardial phosphocreatinine in pigs despite continued moderate ischemia. *Circ Res* 1990; 67: 1481–1493.

Popio KA, Gorlin R, Bechtel D, Levine JA. Post-extrasystolic potentiation as a predictor of potential myocardial viability: preoperative analyses compared with studies after coronary bypass surgery. *Am J Cardiol* 1977; 39: 944–953.

Pouleur H, van Eyll C, Gurne O, Rosseau MF. Effects of prolonged nisoldipine administration on the "hibernating" myocardium. *J Cardiovasc Pharmacol* 1992; 22(Suppl 5): S73–S78.

Ragosta M, Beller GA, Watson DD, et al. Quantitative planar rest-redistribution thallium-201 imaging in detection of myocardial viability and prediction of improvement in left ventricular function after coronary bypass surgery in patients with severely depressed left ventricular function. *Circulation* 1993; 87: 1630–1641.

Rahimtoola SH. Coronary bypass surgery for chronic angina—1981: a perspective. *Circulation* 1982a; 65: 225–241.

Rahimtoola SH. Postoperative exercise response in the evaluation of the physiological status after coronary bypass surgery. *Circulation* 1982b; 65(Suppl II): 106–114.

Rahimtoola SH. A perspective on three large multicenter randomized clinical trials of coronary bypass surgery for chronic stable angina. *Circulation* 1985a; 72(Suppl V): 123–125.

Rahimtoola SH. Unstable angina: current status. *Mod Concepts Cardiovasc Dis* 1985b; 54: 19–23.

Rahimtoola SH. The hibernating myocardium. *Am Heart J* 1989; 117: 211–221.

Rahimtoola SH. The hibernating myocardium in ischaemic and congestive heart failure. *Eur Heart J* 1993; 14(Suppl A): A22–A26.

Rahimtoola SH. From coronary artery disease to heart failure: role of the hibernating myocardium. *Am J Cardiol* 1995a; 75: 16E–22E.

Rahimtoola SH. Hibernating myocardium: a brief article. *Basic Res Cardiol* 1995b; 90: 38–40.

Rahimtoola SH. Hibernating myocardium has reduced blood flow at rest that increases with low-dose dobutamine. *Circulation* 1996; 94: 3055–3061.

Rees G, Bristow JD, Kremkau EL, et al. Influence of aortocoronary bypass surgery on left ventricular performance. *N Engl J Med* 1971; 284: 1116–1120.

Rocco TP, Dilsizian V, McKusick KA, et al. Comparison of thallium redistribution with rest "reinjection" imaging for the detection of viable myocardium. *Am J Cardiol* 1990; 66: 158–163.

Schulz R, Guth BD, Pieper K, et al. Recruitment of an inotropic reserve in moderately ischemic myocardium at the expense of metabolic recovery. A model of short-term hibernation. *Circ Res* 1992; 70: 1282–1295.

Schulz R, Rose J, Martin C, et al. Development of short-term myocardial hibernation. Its limitation by the severity of ischemia and inotropic stimulation. *Circulation* 1993; 88: 684–695.

Shanes JG, Kondos GT, Levitsky S, et al. Coronary artery obstruction: a potentially reversible cause of dilated cardiomyopathy. *Am Heart J* 1985; 110: 173–178.

Smart SC, Sawada S, Ryan T, et al. Low-dose dobutamine echocardiography detects reversible dysfunction after thrombolytic therapy of acute myocardial infarction. *Circulation* 1993; 88: 405–411.

Stadius M, McAnulty JH, Culter J, et al. Specificity, sensitivity and accuracy of the nitroglycerin ventriculogram as a predictor of surgically reversible wall motion abnormalities [abstract]. *Am J Cardiol* 1980; 45: 399.

Takeishi Y, Tono-Oka I, Kuboba I, et al. Functional recovery of hibernating myocardium after coronary bypass surgery: does it coincide with improvement in perfusion? *Am Heart J* 1991; 122: 665–670.

Tamaki N, Kawamoto M, Takahashi N, et al. Prognostic value of an increase in fluorine-18 deoxyglucose uptake in patients with myocardial infarction: comparison with stress thallium imaging. *J Am Coll Cardiol* 1992; 22: 1621–1627.

Tamaki N, Ohtani H, Yonekura Y, et al. Significance of fill-in after thallium-201 reinjection following delayed imaging: comparison with regional wall motion and angiographic findings. *J Nucl Med* 1990; 31: 1617–1623.

Tillisch J, Brunken R, Marshall R, et al. Reversibility of cardiac wall motion abnormalities predicted by positron tomography. *N Engl J Med* 1986; 314: 884–888.

Topol EJ, Weiss JL, Guzman PA, et al. Immediate improvement of dysfunctional myocardial segments or after coronary revascularization: detection by intraoperative transesophageal echocardiography. *J Am Coll Cardiol* 1984; 4: 1123–1134.

Udelson JE, Coleman PS, Metherall J, et al. Predicting recovery of severe regional ventricular dysfunction. Comparison of resting scintigraphy with ^{201}T and ^{99m}Tc-sestamibi. *Circulation* 1994; 89: 2552–2561.

Van den Berg Jr EK, Popma JJ, Dehmer GJ, et al. Reversible segmental left ventricular dysfunction after coronary angioplasty. *Circulation* 1990; 81: 1210–1216.

Vanoverschelde J-LJ, Wijns W, Depre C, et al. Mechanisms of chronic regional post-ischemic dysfunction in humans: new insights from the study of noninfarcted collateral-dependent myocardium. *Circulation* 1993; 2: 237–245.